Electromyography in Clinical Practice
Electrodiagnostic Aspects of Neuromuscular Disease

Second Edition

Electromyography in Clinical Practice
Electrodiagnostic Aspects of Neuromuscular Disease

Second Edition

Michael J. Aminoff, M.D., F.R.C.P.

Professor, Department of Neurology
University of California, San Francisco, School of Medicine
Director, Clinical Neurophysiology Laboratories, and
Attending Physician, Department of Neurology
University of California Medical Center
San Francisco, California

Churchill Livingstone
New York, Edinburgh, London, Melbourne   1987

Library of Congress Cataloging in Publication Data

Aminoff, Michael J. (Michael Jeffrey)
  Electromyography in clinical practice.

  Includes bibliographies and index.
  1. Electromyography. 2. Neuromuscular diseases—
Diagnosis. I. Title. [DNLM: 1. Electromyography.
WE 141 A517e]
RC77.5.A44 1987   616.7′407547   87-18184
ISBN 0-443-08419-X

Second Edition © Churchill Livingstone Inc. 1987

First Edition © Addison-Wesley Publishing Company, Inc. 1978

Distributed in the United Kingdom by Churchill Livingstone,
Robert Stevenson House, 1-3 Baxter's Place, Leith Walk, Edinburgh
EH1 3AF, and by associated companies, branches, and representatives
throughout the world.

Accurate indications, adverse reactions, and dosage schedules for
drugs are provided in this book, but it is possible that they
may change. The reader is urged to review the package information
data of the manufacturers of the medications mentioned.

Acquisitions Editor: *Robert Hurley*
Copy Editor: *Margot Otway*
Production Supervisor: *Jocelyn Eckstein*

Printed in the United States of America

First published in 1987

Preface to Second Edition

Some 10 years have passed since I completed the manuscript of the first edition of this book, and these years have seen remarkable advances in the electrodiagnostic approaches used to study disorders of muscle and the peripheral nervous system. First, a more critical approach to the interpretation of the results of conventional studies has led clinicians to place greater reliance on electrophysiologic findings. Second, the development of new electrophysiologic techniques and the greater application of existing techniques to the study of neuromuscular disorders has broadened the scope of this form of investigation. In particular, the use of blink reflexes, H-reflexes, F-responses, and somatosensory evoked potentials has been helpful both for diagnostic and prognostic purposes and for providing new insights into the pathophysiologic basis of various disorders. Third, the increasing use of computers has made possible the use in clinical practice of techniques that were once of purely academic interest, and the development of techniques for studying conduction in different subpopulations of nerve fibers in individual nerve trunks now promises to become of major clinical significance. Fourth, the application of both new and more conventional techniques to the evaluation of patients with disorders of the central nervous system—an approach sometimes referred to as *central EMG*—has provided new means of analyzing these disorders.

These developments have made necessary this second edition, in which I have made numerous additions to the text and completely rewritten some sections. Inevitably, the book has become larger. However, I have kept very much in mind the primary purpose of the book as outlined in the preface to the first edition, namely, to provide a concise and practical account of the subject rather than a comprehensive account of all its aspects, which is now anyway available from larger, more encyclopedic texts. Techniques used solely for research have deliberately not been considered.

I am grateful to Dr. R.K. Olney for reading a number of the chapters and offering helpful suggestions and comments on the text, and to Ms. Susan Shaddick for her good-humored secretarial assistance. Furthermore, the encouragement and understanding of my wife, Jan, and our three children made it possible for me to find the time to bring this book to its conclusion. Finally, I am grateful to Churchill Livingstone for undertaking the publication of this second edition, and in particular to Mr. Robert Hurley and his staff for their help and advice during its production.

Michael J. Aminoff, M.D.

Preface to First Edition ⎯⎯⎯⎯⎯⎯⎯⎯⎯⎯⎯⎯⎯

Although the term *electromyography* refers strictly to methods used to record the electrical activity of muscle, it has come to have a wider meaning which encompasses also the electrodiagnostic techniques used to study the functional integrity of peripheral nerves and the neuromuscular junction. In recent years, the application of refined neurophysiologic techniques to the study of disorders of muscle and the peripheral nervous system has proved to be of considerable diagnostic value to the physician; this, in turn, has stimulated the further development and expansion of this branch of clinical neurophysiology into a separate specialty of its own. Perhaps because of its rapid advance, however, many clinicians are not fully aware of the scope and limitations of the investigative procedures in current use, and are uncertain about the interpretation and emphasis to be placed on the information obtained from them in relation to individual clinical problems. At the same time, an increasing number of those responsible for undertaking these procedures, or training in this field, have felt the need for a convenient summary of the physiologic basis of the specialty and the accumulated clinical experience of recent years, and for a resumé of those techniques which are most useful in practice.

Accordingly, the purpose of this book is to review the manner in which electromyography may be of value in the investigation of patients with neuromuscular disorders, and to provide a concise, practical guide to those procedures in current clinical use. The book contains an account of the fundamental physiologic principles on which this form of investigation depends, and describes the equipment and methods used in its practice. It also discusses the significance of observations made at electromyography and reviews the findings in various clinical disorders. It is not intended, however, to provide a comprehensive account of all aspects of electromyography, and those techniques developed and used solely for purposes of research are not considered.

The book is aimed at medical practicers concerned with the management of patients with neuromuscular disorders, and at clinical neurophysiologists. Sufficient clinical details are provided to enable those readers without formal neurologic training to grasp the nature of the diagnostic problems confronting the clinician, and the manner in which electromyography can contribute to their solution. Pertinent anatomic details are included in the text, but this book is written primarily for those who already have some knowledge of human anatomy.

The book was written partly in California, and partly in England while I was senior registrar at The National Hospitals for Nervous Diseases. I am grateful to a number of friends and colleagues in London and San Francisco who helped in its preparation, and particularly to Dr. P.C. Gautier-Smith, Dr. M.J.G. Harrison, and Dr. R.A. Jaffe for their advice, to Dr. J.B. Pickett for providing some of the material used for illustrations, and to Miss Beryl Laatz for her invaluable secretarial assistance. Finally, I wish to thank my wife, Jan, for her encouragement and help, and the staff of the Addison-Wesley Publishing Company for their patient cooperation and advice during the production of this book.

Michael J. Aminoff, M.D.

Contents

Electrodiagnostic Methods for the Study of Nerve and Muscle

Electrophysiologic methods for studying the function of nerve and muscle were first introduced in the nineteenth century, but only within the last 30 to 40 years have they come to be used widely in a clinical context. Their widespread clinical application came about because of improvements in apparatus design that reduced the practical difficulties of using electrophysiologic methods and permitted the introduction of more refined techniques, thereby expanding considerably the scope of this form of investigation.

The accumulated experience of recent years has shown that electrophysiologic methods have a definite place in the investigation and diagnosis of certain categories of clinical disorder, as is discussed in general terms in the latter part of this chapter. In addition, these methods have enabled the physiologic characteristics of muscle and the peripheral nervous system to be studied in health and disease, and have provided insight into the pathophysiologic basis of many neurologic symptoms. Such studies have also led to both a re-examination of traditional concepts which, until recently, were accepted without question and, in some instances, to the more precise definition of neuromuscular disorders.

The application of electrophysiologic techniques to the study of neuromuscular disorders has also contributed to a general resurgence of interest in these conditions. In recent years, considerable new information has been accumulated regarding the ultrastructural, histochemical, biochemical, pharmacologic, and physiologic aspects of these disorders, and attempts have been made to integrate these data with observations made by clinical neurophysiologists. A multidisciplinary approach of this sort offers the greatest hope for ultimately finding a solution to fundamental problems concerning the development, prevention, and treatment of neuromuscular disorders.

CLINICAL APPLICATIONS

The electrophysiologic examination of patients with suspected neuromuscular disorders is no more than an extension of the clinical examination. As such, it should be performed by a physician who is experienced in the clinical evaluation of neuro-muscular disorders, familiar with the ana-tomic intricacies of the peripheral nervous system, and appreciative of the scope and limitations of the methods in use. Because the procedure is more than a laboratory test, it does not provide a simple, unquali-fied answer to the clinical problem that has prompted referral, but instead yields infor-mation that must then be integrated with that already available.

Patients are referred to the laboratory for electrophysiologic evaluation for a variety of reasons. Some patients who are referred have clinical problems or questions that cannot fully be assessed or answered by the electrophysiologic techniques in current use. In many instances, referral is merely a means of obtaining a second clinical opin-ion when there is uncertainty about the di-agnosis or management of a disorder. In other cases, a referral is made to obtain information that may help to establish the diagnosis or provide a guide to prognosis, to serve as a baseline or a means of com-parison in following the course of a disor-der, or to provide supportive evidence in a medicolegal context. It is important for the clinical neurophysiologist to determine the reason for each patient's referral if a sat-isfactory service is to be provided. An ad-equate electrophysiologic examination can-not even be planned unless the clinical history and physical findings are known. Unlike a simple laboratory test, the pro-cedure for electrophysiologic examination does not follow a rigid, predetermined pro-tocol, but is modified according to the clin-ical context in which it is requested, as well as by the initial findings that are obtained.

Electromyography

Electromyography, in the strict sense of the word, refers to methods of studying the electrical activity of muscle. It had little di-rect relevance to clinical neurology until the introduction of the concentric needle elec-trode in 1929.[1] By inserting this electrode directly into a muscle, electrical activity within circumscribed regions of that muscle and, in particular, the electrical events ac-companying the activation of muscle fibers and single motor units, could be recorded. The pattern of electrical activity in normal muscle thus came to be characterized, and this permitted departures from normal ac-tivity to be recognized and correlated with the presence of disorders of the motor unit. Electromyography is discussed in detail in later chapters, but it is appropriate to con-sider here its clinical usefulness.

The term *motor unit*, first used in 1925 by Liddell and Sherrington,[2] describes a single lower motor neuron and the muscle fibers that it innervates. The term therefore encompasses the cell body of the lower motor neuron in the spinal cord; its axon, which emerges from the cord to become a constituent fiber of a nerve root and, ulti-mately, of a peripheral nerve; its terminal arborizations and the neuromuscular junc-tions with which they are associated, and all of the muscle fibers that are innervated by it. The concept of the motor unit is a phys-iologic one because the activity of a muscle cell cannot properly be considered without reference to the nerve cell governing it.

The function of the normal motor unit can be disturbed at several sites. A lesion af-fecting either the cell body of a lower motor neuron or its axon may prevent the acti-vation of the muscle fibers of that unit. Al-ternatively, the function of a motor unit may be disturbed because of some disorder af-fecting its constituent muscle fibers. Each of these conditions may give rise to char-acteristic changes in the electrical activity recorded from the affected muscle. Elec-tromyography is often helpful, therefore, in detecting disorders of motor units and in determining the site of the underlying le-sion. Furthermore, if electrical evidence of a neurogenic lesion is present, the pattern of affected muscles and other electrophysiologic findings may indicate whether it is at the level of the root, plexus, or peripheral nerve.

As emphasized by Lambert,[3] such information may sometimes be obtained by electromyography when it cannot be obtained by clinical examination, either because the disease is only mildly advanced, because the presence of emotional overlay or of other symptoms and signs (such as pain or deformity) makes clinical evaluation difficult, or because clinical signs, such as weakness in individual muscles, are obscured by the compensatory action of unaffected, synergistic muscles. It must again be stressed, however, that electromyography is not a substitute for detailed clinical examination, but is complementary to it. Indeed, an adequate electromyographic study cannot be performed unless the clinical background of the patient and the diagnostic problems facing the clinician are known. The patient's history and physical signs govern which muscles are examined first, whereas the related diagnostic problem determines which other muscles are subsequently examined.

In some patients with weakness that is predominantly upper motor neuron in type but of uncertain etiology, the presence of a coexisting lower motor neuron deficit affects the diagnostic possibilities. Similarly, in patients with clinical evidence of a focal lower motor neuron deficit, the presence of more widespread denervation (even though subclinical) may profoundly influence the diagnostic considerations. In such circumstances, then, the findings obtained by the needle examination may be of special significance.

Electromyographic findings do not, in themselves, provide a clinical diagnosis, for there are no potentials that are pathognomonic of specific diseases.[3] The pattern of activity detected by electromyography does, however, provide a guide to the site and, in some instances, to the nature of the lesion. In arriving at a final diagnosis, the information so obtained should be considered in relation to the other available clinical and laboratory data. Conclusions based solely upon electromyographic findings must never be relied upon to the extent that clinical judgment is neglected.

Information derived from electromyography may also provide a guide to prognosis. For example, in patients with Bell's palsy, electromyographic evidence of denervation of the facial muscles indicates a less favorable prognosis than when denervation has not occurred. Similarly, when used to determine whether denervation is partial or complete, electromyographic sampling may reveal surviving motor units in a muscle that appears clinically to be totally inactive,[4] which would be of prognostic significance. Indeed, the findings and results of nerve stimulation may govern whether a peripheral nerve is explored after injury.

Electrical Stimulation of Peripheral Nerve

THE MUSCLE RESPONSE EVOKED BY NERVE STIMULATION

In addition to recording the electrical activity of muscle at rest or under voluntary control, the response of a muscle to supramaximal electrical stimulation of its motor nerve can be studied with surface electrodes. The size of the electrical response evoked in this way normally varies widely in different individuals and in different muscles, and depends on many factors, including the precise recording arrangements. Within these limitations, however, size of the electrical response correlates with the number of muscle fibers that can be activated by excitation of the nerve. Thus, an abnormally small response indicates loss or disease of motor units, although a response of amplitude within the normal range does not exclude such pathology. Accordingly, this procedure may provide evidence of motor unit pathology—an evoked response that is abnormally small—in patients with symptoms that might otherwise be attributed to nonorganic causes or to disease of upper motor neurons.[5] In such circumstances, needle electromyography is necessary to determine whether the underlying pathology is in the muscle itself or in its nerve supply.

Examination of the electrical response of a muscle to supramaximal stimulation of its motor nerve is also useful in defining the site of a focal lesion of the nerve, in determining whether axonal degeneration has occurred, in studying the completeness of the lesion after a peripheral nerve injury, and in detecting anomalous patterns of muscle innervation in the extremities.[3] Furthermore, when repetitive stimuli are used, changes in the size of the evoked response may enable disorders of transmission at the neuromuscular junction to be detected and classified. Such disorders include myasthenia gravis, Lambert-Eaton syndrome, and botulism.

NERVE CONDUCTION STUDIES

By recording the electrical response of a muscle to stimulation of its motor nerve at two points along its course, conduction velocity in the fastest conducting motor fibers along the intervening segment of the nerve can be calculated. This is of considerable value in distinguishing between disorders of the peripheral nerves and those affecting primarily either muscle or the cell bodies of the lower motor neurons. Similarly, the conduction velocity and amplitude of the action potential in sensory nerves can be measured by stimulating sensory fibers at one point and recording from them at another. Such a procedure is helpful in determining whether sensory symptoms are attributable to a disturbance of peripheral

nerve function or to a lesion proximal to the dorsal root ganglia.

Nerve conduction studies thus provide a means of demonstrating the presence and extent of a peripheral neuropathy, and are particularly helpful when clinical examination is difficult, such as when evaluating young children. These studies are useful in a number of different contexts. First, they may be used to determine whether patients with a mononeuropathy have an underlying, subclinical polyneuropathy. Second, in patients who do have a mononeuropathy, the site of the focal lesion may be identified. Third, nerve conduction studies, in combination with needle electromyography, are an important means of determining the severity of a focal nerve lesion, and thus may guide management. Fourth, they provide a means of distinguishing between a polyneuropathy and mononeuritis multiplex when the two are clinically indistinguishable. Fifth, in patients with an established polyneuropathy, they may be used to determine the extent to which the disability relates to the superadded compressive focal neuropathies that are likely to occur in this context and that are potentially reversible. Sixth, nerve conduction studies provide a means of following the course of peripheral nerve disorders and of determining a patient's prognosis. The findings, especially when considered in conjunction with the results of needle examination, may indicate the extent of axonal loss and the presence or absence of reinnervation. Finally, nerve conduction studies may provide a clue to the underlying pathology. In recent years, studies on human neuropathies and on experimental neuropathies in animals have revealed that the predominant pathologic change may be either axonal degeneration or segmental demyelination, depending on the etiology of the disorder. A distinction between these two pathologic processes may not be possible on clinical grounds. However, conduction velocity is usually markedly reduced in primary demyelinative neuropathies, whereas it is either unaffected or only mildly reduced in axonal neuropathies. Other electrophysiologic distinguishing features include the occurrence of dispersed muscle and nerve action potentials, areas of focal conduction block, and markedly prolonged terminal latencies in demyelinative neuropathies. By contrast, in axonal disorders, the muscle response to stimulation of motor nerves and the action potentials recorded from sensory fibers may be unrecordable or markedly reduced in amplitude, and needle examination of affected muscles reveals evidence of denervation. On the basis of the electrophysiologic changes, therefore, it is frequently possible to predict the underlying pathology, thereby reducing the number of possible etiologies to be considered, without resorting to biopsy.

The measurement of conduction velocity has been used in genetic and epidemiologic studies as a means of detecting hereditary disorders of the peripheral nerves prior to the development of clinical signs,[6] and as a means of detecting heterogeneity in clinically similar cases. For example, it has been shown that patients with peroneal muscular atrophy may have either a markedly reduced or a relatively normal conduction velocity in motor nerves. This distinction is probably genetically determined since values for conduction velocity are consistent within families.[7-9]

The development of techniques for evaluating nerve conduction has thus added a new dimension to the study of disorders of the peripheral nervous system. Practical details of the techniques concerned, as well as their application to specific clinical problems, are discussed in detail in later chapters.

H REFLEX

The H reflex is a monosynaptic reflex that is easily recorded from the soleus muscle in adults in response to low-intensity stimulation of the tibial nerve. As discussed in later chapters, the response may be delayed or lost in a number of peripheral neuropathies, even though the results of conventional motor and sensory conduction studies are normal.[10] The response may also be abnormal in patients with S1 radiculopathies. Although H reflexes have been used for some years to study motor neuron excitability in different contexts, this use has no immediate clinical application and will be considered only briefly.

F RESPONSE

The F response may be useful in the evaluation of patients with peripheral neuropathies, radiculopathies, or plexopathies. It is sometimes abnormal even when conventional nerve conduction studies are normal, and it is especially useful in assessing the function of those proximal portions of the peripheral nervous system, such as the roots or plexuses, that are not easily evaluated by conventional techniques because of their inaccessibility. Unlike the H reflex, F responses can be recorded without difficulty from most skeletal muscles by stimulation of their motor nerves. These responses occur as a result of the discharge of a few anterior horn cells by antidromic impulses reaching the cell bodies along their axons from the site of nerve stimulation.

BLINK REFLEX

The blink reflex, which is well known to clinical neurologists, can also be elicited by an electrical stimulus to a branch of the trigeminal nerve, and the response of the orbicularis oculi muscles on each side may be recorded on an oscilloscope. This technique has been used, especially by Kimura,[11] to monitor function of the trigeminal and facial nerves when an isolated lesion of these nerves is suspected, or in patients with polyneuropathies. It has also been used to provide evidence of pontine dysfunction when this is not clinically evident, as in patients with suspected multiple sclerosis. The blink reflex has been studied in a variety of other contexts, but the findings have then been notable more for their academic interest than for any immediate clinical relevance.

SOMATOSENSORY EVOKED POTENTIALS

Electrical stimulation of an accessible sensory or mixed peripheral nerve elicits potentials that can be recorded from selected locations over the scalp and spine, as well as peripherally. These somatosensory evoked potentials have been used to identify and localize lesions involving the somatosensory pathways, especially those segments that traverse the central nervous system. Their major application has been in the detection of subclinical lesions in patients with suspected multiple sclerosis. Their utility in the evaluation of spinal injuries, in predicting the outcome of post-traumatic coma, and in monitoring patients undergoing spinal surgery is less clear.[12] These potentials have also been used to evaluate lesions of the peripheral nervous system, especially when inaccessible proximal portions of peripheral nerves or a limb plexus are involved.

Electrical Stimulation of Muscle

There is a difference in the excitability response of innervated and denervated muscle to electrical stimulation. This difference forms the basis of a simple test for determining whether or not a particular muscle is denervated and, if the test is repeated at intervals, whether the extent of denervation is increasing or reinnervation is occurring. The most satisfactory form of

this test involves determining the relationship between the intensity and the duration of current necessary to produce a minimal contraction of the muscle, with the duration being shortened incrementally. Strength-duration curves were first applied in a clinical context by Adrian.[13] Their use has declined with the development of needle electromyography and methods for measuring nerve conduction velocity, and in many laboratories they are no longer undertaken. Although they provide no clue to the site of the underlying lesion, they can nevertheless be used to follow the course of a disorder and to determine whether or not it is progressing.

OTHER APPLICATIONS

The preceding discussion emphasizes the clinical value of electrophysiologic methods for studying the neuromuscular system. These methods have also been used in a wider context to examine the activity of individual muscles in the maintenance of posture and during normal movement. Such studies have provided information of considerable academic interest and have advanced knowledge of normal physiologic mechanisms. They are not, however, of immediate clinical relevance, and so are beyond the scope of this book. The application of similar methods to the analysis of various movement disorders and their underlying pathophysiology is of unquestionable clinical utility, and electrophysiologic techniques are also being widely used to study the functional integrity of the autonomic nervous system. These applications are, therefore, reviewed briefly in Chapter 15.

REFERENCES

1. Adrian ED, Bronk DW: The discharge of impulses in motor conduction nerve fibres. Part II. The frequency of discharge in reflex

and voluntary contractions. J Physiol 67:119, 1929

2. Liddell EGT, Sherrington CS: Recruitment and some other features of reflex inhibition. Proc R Soc Lond [Biol] 97:488, 1925

3. Lambert EH: Electromyography and electrical stimulation of peripheral nerves and muscle. p. 311. In Mayo Clinic and Mayo Foundation: Clinical Examinations in Neurology. W. B. Saunders, Philadelphia, 1969

4. Gilliatt RW, Taylor JC: Electrical changes following section of the facial nerve. Proc R Soc Med 52:1080, 1959

5. Hodes R, Larrabee MG, German W: The human electromyogram in response to nerve stimulation and the conduction velocity of motor axons. Studies on normal and on injured peripheral nerves. Arch Neurol Psychiatry 60:340, 1948

6. Lambert EH: Neurophysiological techniques useful in the study of neuromuscular disorders. p. 247. In Neuromuscular Disorders (The Motor Unit and Its Disorders). Vol. 38. Research Publications, Association for Research in Nervous and Mental Disease, Williams & Wilkins, Baltimore, 1960

7. Dyck PJ, Lambert EH: Lower motor and primary sensory neuron diseases with peroneal muscular atrophy. 1. Neurologic, genetic, and electrophysiologic findings in hereditary polyneuropathies. Arch Neurol 18:603, 1968

8. Dyck PJ, Lambert EH: Lower motor and primary sensory neuron diseases with peroneal muscular atrophy. 2. Neurologic, genetic, and electrophysiologic findings in various neuronal degenerations. Arch Neurol 18:619, 1968

9. Thomas PK, Calne DB: Motor nerve conduction velocity in peroneal muscular atrophy: Evidence for genetic heterogeneity. J Neurol Neurosurg Psychiatry 37:68, 1974

10. Shahani BT: Late responses and the "silent period." p. 333. In Aminoff MJ (ed): Electrodiagnosis in Clinical Neurology. Churchill Livingstone, New York, 1986

11. Kimura J: The blink reflex as a clinical test. p. 347. In Aminoff MJ (ed): Electrodiagnosis in Clinical Neurology. Churchill Livingstone, New York, 1986

12. Aminoff MJ: The clinical role of somatosensory evoked potential studies: A critical appraisal. Muscle Nerve 7:345, 1984

13. Adrian ED: The electrical reactions of muscles before and after nerve injury. Brain 39:1, 1916

2

Aspects of Nerve and Muscle Physiology

Modern electrodiagnostic techniques involve recording the electrical activity of striated muscle and peripheral nerves. It is of some importance, therefore, to appreciate the physiologic basis of such activity, which is discussed in this chapter. The physiology of muscle and the peripheral nervous system is also considered in relation to certain other factors that have direct relevance for those undertaking electrodiagnostic procedures in clinical practice. However, in view of the particular importance of the functional organization of the motor unit to the interpretation of the electromyogram, this is discussed separately in the next chapter. Throughout this chapter and the next, deliberate emphasis is placed not only on current physiologic concepts, but also on the experimental observations that have led to their development.

THE ELECTRICAL ACTIVITY OF NERVE AND MUSCLE

The nature and ionic basis of the electrical activity of striated muscle fibers are qualitatively similar to that of nerve cells. The following account, therefore, refers to both types of cell.

The Resting Membrane Potential

The inside of a muscle or nerve cell is electrically negative with respect to its exterior. This potential difference across the cell membrane is called the resting membrane potential, and is on the order of -90 mV for striated muscle cells and -70 mV for lower motor neurons, the sign indicating the polarity of the inside of the cell relative to its exterior. The resting membrane potential primarily reflects differences in ionic concentration that exist across the cell membrane and the selective permeability of the cell membrane.

The cell membrane separates two aqueous solutions—intracellular and interstitial fluids—each of which contains ions, particles that carry an electrical charge. The intracellular and interstitial fluids are in osmotic equilibrium with each other, and in each the total number of anions and cations is equal, so that both are electrically neutral. However, the distribution of ions between these two solutions is unequal. The intracellular concentration of potassium is relatively high, and the concentration of sodium and chloride is relatively low compared with the concentration of these ions outside the cell. These inequalities in ionic concentration are created and maintained by a transport mechanism requiring the expenditure of energy by the cell, and are related also to the varying degree of permeability that the cell membrane has for different ionic species.

In discussing the manner in which these differences in ionic concentration lead to a potential difference across the cell membrane, the effect of the active transport mechanism will initially be neglected for the sake of simplicity. There are, however, two important passive forces—forces not requiring the expenditure of energy—that affect the movement of ions, and these are relevant to any discussion of membrane potentials. First, particles unequally distributed in a solution will tend to move by diffusion from areas of high concentration to areas of low concentration, moving down their concentration gradients until these are abolished. Second, the movement of ions will be influenced by voltage gradients, with positive ions being attracted down the electrical gradient toward the cathode, and negative ions moving similarly toward the anode.

It was originally proposed by Bernstein that only one species of ion—potassium—could diffuse across the resting cell membrane.[1] If this were the case, potassium ions would tend to move out of the cell and down their concentration gradient, thereby producing an excess of anions within the cell and of cations outside of it. These excess ions of opposite polarity would attract each other across the cell membrane, collecting in the vicinity of the membrane. This would then set up an electrical gradient across the membrane, opposing further outward movement of potassium ions. Eventually, this gradient would become large enough to cause an influx of potassium ions in a number just sufficient to counteract their efflux down the concentration gradient. The electrical potential difference needed to counteract completely the tendency of potas-

sium ions to diffuse out of the cell along their concentration gradient—that is, to maintain in a steady state the unequal distribution of potassium ions on either side of the membrane—is called the equilibrium potential for potassium. Its magnitude at 37°C can be calculated from the Nernst equation, a convenient form of which is

$$E_k = 61 \log \frac{[K]_O}{[K]_I}$$

where E_k is the equilibrium potential for potassium, expressed in millivolts, and $[K]_O$ and $[K]_I$ are the potassium concentrations outside and inside the cell, respectively. It should be noted that the Nernst equation can actually be applied to any permeant ionic species unequally distributed across the cell membrane.

Bernstein's theory provided an explanation for the existence and polarity of the resting membrane potential, and for the changes in potential that appeared to occur when a nerve or muscle cell is excited. However, experimental studies subsequently provided data that could not easily be reconciled with his theory. The magnitude of the resting membrane potential was found to differ from that predicted by the Nernst equation for the unequal potassium distribution. Furthermore, it was discovered that the cell membrane is permeable to other ions, including sodium and chloride, and that excitation of the cell led not to abolition of the resting membrane potential, as was originally supposed, but to its reversal.

The demonstration, with radioisotopes, that the cell membrane is permeable to sodium, and that this ion is in a continuous state of flux across it, was of particular significance in the development of present concepts concerning the origin of the resting membrane potential. Passive electrochemical factors alone could not account for the efflux of sodium ions from the cell because this efflux must occur against both the concentration and the electrical gradients for this ionic species. Accordingly, it was necessary to postulate some mechanism by which the cell, through the expenditure of energy, could actively expel sodium ions at the same rate as they passively entered it. Considerable evidence has now accumulated to suggest that such a mechanism does indeed exist.

Hodgkin and Keynes, in their study of the giant axons of cuttlefish, found that the efflux of sodium ions is usually roughly proportional to their inflow, and that metabolic inhibitors could block this efflux.[2] They also found that metabolic inhibitors could reduce the influx of potassium ions, that the efflux of sodium ions is immediately reduced to about one third if potassium is removed from the external medium, and that both sodium efflux and potassium influx are temperature-dependent. These findings not only support the concept of an active (energy-dependent) sodium transport process in the cell, but suggest that there is, at least in part, an active uptake of potassium ions that is coupled with the expulsion of sodium ions. The remainder of the potassium flux is passive and relates to the potassium concentration gradient and the membrane potential. The active transport mechanism responsible for this process is generally referred to as the sodium pump, or the sodium-potassium exchange pump. The precise manner in which it operates is not entirely clear, but certain aspects of it that relate to the resting membrane potential must briefly be considered.

It was initially assumed by many that the expulsion of sodium ions was tightly coupled with the influx of potassium on a one-to-one basis—that is, that sodium expulsion was an electrically neutral process, with a positively charged ion entering the cell for every ion expelled. If this were the case, the active transport process would have no immediate or direct effect on the membrane potential. The pump, and the selective permeability of the membrane to different ionic species, would merely produce a chemical gradient across the membrane; this would then lead to passive ionic fluxes, thereby generating a potential difference across the membrane. However, evidence suggests that the expulsion of sodium ions often exceeds the influx of potassium, with the coupling ratio in nerve cells usually approximating 3:2. This means that the number of positive ions expelled usually exceeds that transported into the cell, and this, in itself, will lead to a potential difference across the membrane. The subject has been reviewed by Thomas, who believes that the sodium pump often—perhaps always—makes a direct contribution in this way to the resting membrane potential.[3] Nevertheless, experimental observations suggest that normally this difference is no more than a few millivolts, the greater part of the potential difference across the membrane being generated by passive ionic movements.

When the membrane potential of a cell has the same value as the equilibrium potential (Nernst potential) for a particular species of ion, influx of that species of ion will be equal to its efflux, unless active transport mechanisms are operating. Conversely, ionic movements will occur passively when these two potentials have different values. Thus, if the cell membrane potential is changed so that it reaches the same level as the equilibrium potential for a species of ion to which the membrane is permeable, net movement of this ion by passive processes will cease.

In the resting cell, the movement of ions across the cell membrane is in a steady state, so that the influx of any ionic species is equal to its efflux. Since the membrane is permeable, to a variable extent, to a number of ionic species with different equilibrium potentials, these factors have to be taken into account in any quantitative description of the resting membrane potential. The membrane potential necessary to counteract fully any passive movement of potassium, sodium, and chloride ions along their concentration gradients is given approximately by the Goldman-Hodgkin-Katz equation. This equation relates the resting membrane potential to the concentration gradients of the diffusible ions and to the specific permeability of the membrane to each of them, but neglects any direct contribution to it by the sodium pump. At a temperature of 37°C, the equation takes the form of

$$E_M = 61 \log \frac{P_k[K]_O + P_{Na}[Na]_O + P_{Cl}[Cl]_I}{P_k[K]_I + P_{Na}[Na]_I + P_{Cl}[Cl]_O}$$

where E_M is the resting membrane potential expressed in millivolts, P is the specific permeability of the membrane to the ionic species indicated, and the subscripts I and O refer to the concentration of the ionic species inside and outside the cell, respectively.

Apart from these three species of ions, the only other important ions that need to be considered are the impermeant organic anions within the cell. These have an important role in maintaining the osmotic equilibrium of the cell. They also help to maintain the electroneutrality of the intracellular medium and may, therefore, influence the distribution of permeant ions across the cell membrane.

In summary, there is an unequal distribution of ions across the cell membrane as a result of active transport processes and the different permeability of the membrane to different ionic species. This unequal distribution leads to the passive movement of ions down their concentration gradients, and thus to a potential difference across the membrane. In addition, there is evidence that the sodium pump itself generates an ionic current across the cell membrane, thereby making a small, direct contribution to the resting membrane potential.

It should be noted that the cell membrane has the electrical characteristics of a capacitor, and these are believed to contribute to its overall biophysical properties. For present purposes, however, sufficient insight into the basis of the resting membrane potential and the generation and propagation of an action potential can be gained without considering this complex aspect and its associated mathematical analysis.

The Action Potential

Nerve and muscle cells are excitable; that is, they are able to produce an action potential after the application of a suitable stimulus. The action potential is a transient reversal of the membrane potential caused by a temporary alteration in membrane permeability. This change in potential is actively propagated along the fiber without decrement. If a stimulus below the threshold required to produce an action potential is applied, it reduces but does not reverse the membrane potential. This change in membrane potential is not actively propagated along the fiber, but decreases as it spreads from the point of stimulation. As the intensity of a subthreshold electrical stimulus is increased, the potential difference across the membrane is reduced until it reaches a critical level. At this threshold level, it may either trigger an abrupt self-generating mechanism so that an action potential is produced, or it may return to the baseline again, as shown in Figure 2.1. A stimulus that reduces the membrane potential beyond this threshold value normally leads to the automatic generation of an action potential.

The ionic basis of these events is complex. The ability to generate an action potential depends on the presence of sodium in the external medium, and the action potential itself is characterized by a brief reversal of the resting membrane potential, rather than by simple depolarization to zero. This suggests that a change in the membrane permeability to sodium, with a consequent influx of sodium ions into the

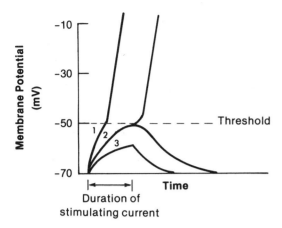

Fig. 2.1 Variation in the membrane potential caused by stimuli of different intensities. The responses recorded close to the stimulating electrode are superimposed on the same time scale. *1*, response to a suprathreshold stimulus showing generation of an action potential; *2*, responses to a stimulus of threshold intensity showing generation of an action potential in one case, and a slow decrement to the baseline without generation of an action potential in another; *3*, response to a subthreshold stimulus showing the gradual return of the membrane potential to its resting level without the generation of an action potential.

cell, is implicated in the process. The nature of the self-generating mechanism involved in the development of the action potential is demonstrated by the work of Hodgkin and Huxley,[4] who found that membrane permeability to sodium is voltage-dependent—that is, it is increased when the membrane potential is reduced. This means that if the membrane potential is reduced by a stimulus, sodium ions will enter the cell at an increased rate, thereby further reducing the membrane potential.

The changes that occur in ionic permeability during activity have been examined by several methods. The manner in which changes in the concentration of ions in the external environment of the cell alter the action potential has been studied, and radioisotopes have been used to follow ionic

flux during activity. The most precise method, however, is the voltage clamp technique whereby electrodes are placed on either side of the cell membrane and an external source supplies the amount of current necessary to keep the membrane potential at any selected level, with total current flow being measured in relation to time.[5] This technique permits the membrane potential to be changed without the explosive development of an action potential as a result of any self-generating interaction between membrane potential and sodium permeability.

With moderate depolarization of the membrane, Hodgkin and Huxley found that the ionic current is essentially biphasic, there being an initial inward flow of current, followed by a longer outward flow.[4] The initial phase of the ionic current is related to an influx of sodium ions into the cell. Thus, the membrane potential at which the initial current flow is just abolished was found to have a linear relationship with the logarithm of the external sodium concentration when this is varied, in accordance with the Nernst equation. The later and more prolonged outward flow of current results from an efflux of potassium, which has been shown by radioactive tracer studies to occur with membrane depolarization.[6]

Sudden depolarization of the cell membrane thus causes a rapid increase in its permeability, first to sodium and then to potassium, so that these ions can move down their concentration gradients. As can be seen from Figure 2.2, the former event results in reversal of the membrane potential, the latter in its returning to the resting level—that is, in repolarization of the membrane. The increase in sodium permeability declines rapidly, and repolarization occurs because of this, and because of the increase in potassium permeability. Because of the different time courses of the permeability changes to these two ionic species, however, potassium permeability is still higher than normal when repolarization is complete. As a consequence, the membrane hy-

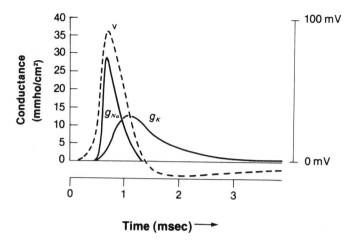

Fig. 2.2 Changes in sodium (g_{Na}) and potassium (g_K) conductance during an action potential (v). Ionic conductance is a measure of the permeability of the cell membrane to that species of ion and is measured in mmho. (Modified from Hodgkin AL, Huxley AF: A quantitative description of membrane current and its application to conduction and excitation in nerve. J Physiol 117:500, 1952.)

perpolarizes; that is, the inside of the cell becomes more negative than it is at rest, the potential difference across it being driven toward the equilibrium potential of potassium. This is followed by a gradual return of potassium permeability and membrane potential to their resting levels.

Immediately after a cell has produced an action potential, it is impossible to produce another one. This absolute refractory period occurs because of the decline in sodium permeability and the increase in potassium permeability that follow the generation of an action potential. A short while later, as repolarization occurs, the cell becomes able to respond to stimuli of greater intensity than normal by producing another action potential. During this relative refractory period, the threshold returns gradually to normal levels.

Propagation of Action Potentials in Muscle and in Unmyelinated Nerve Fibers

As indicated above, in the active region of the fiber, there is a transient influx of sodium ions; consequently, the inside of the fiber becomes positively charged with respect to its exterior. In the immediately adjacent, inactive region, however, the inside of the fiber remains negatively charged and, accordingly, current flows in a local circuit between these two regions, as illustrated in Figure 2.3. This leads to depolarization of the membrane ahead of the action potential. The depolarization causes a local increase in sodium permeability that produces a further depolarization, and eventually an action potential is generated ahead of the previous one. In other words, generation of an action potential in one region of the fiber depolarizes the immediately adjacent regions. This local depolarization is above the threshold for generating a further action potential, so that the process is self-propagating.

The importance of this local flow of current between resting and active regions to the propagation of an action potential can be demonstrated experimentally. The external environment of a nerve fiber can be altered so that its electrical resistance is increased without a change in its chemical or ionic constitution. In such circumstances, the speed of propagation of an action potential is reduced.[7]

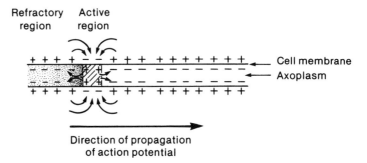

Fig. 2.3 Local current circuits between the active region and the adjacent inactive region of an unmyelinated nerve fiber during propagation of an action potential.

Propagation of Action Potential in Myelinated Nerve Fibers

Conduction in myelinated nerve fibers occurs in a slightly different manner than that described above. The myelin acts as an insulator, and effective contact of the cell membrane with the external medium occurs only at the nodes of Ranvier, which interrupt the myelin sheath at intervals of about 1 to 2 mm. The ionic permeability changes described above, and hence the ability to generate an action potential, are, therefore, restricted to these sites. During activity, current flows in a local circuit between one node and the next, with the flow directed toward the inactive node—and so in the direction of propagation—in the axoplasm, and toward the active node in the interstitial fluid, as shown in Figure 2.4. Thus, when one node is active, that is, generating an action potential, the neighboring node becomes depolarized and generates a further action potential. In this way, the action potential is relayed from node to node, the process being called *saltatory conduction* (from the Latin *saltare:* to dance).

Since the local current circuits produce an action potential only at the nodes of Ranvier, the nearest of which is some distance ahead of the active region, conduction velocity is faster in myelinated than in unmyelinated fibers. Because it limits ionic exchange to the nodal regions, the presence of myelin also reduces energy expenditure

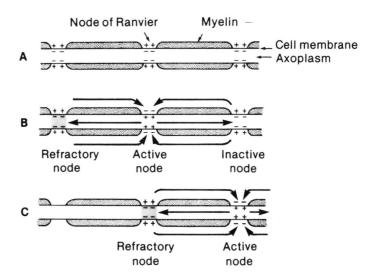

Fig. 2.4 Local current circuits during the propagation of an action potential in a myelinated nerve fiber. The direction of propagation is from left to right, and the arrows indicate the direction of current flow between active and inactive nodes. (**A**) Nerve fiber at rest. (**B**) Impulse at node in center. (**C**) Impulse at node on right.

by the cell during propagation of an action potential.

A considerable amount of experimental evidence supports the concept that conduction occurs in this saltatory manner in myelinated fibers. Thus, the intensity of current necessary to stimulate a myelinated fiber is lower at the nodes than in the internodal regions. Similarly, agents, such as narcotics, that block conduction are more effective when applied at the nodes than when they are applied between them. Furthermore, the amplitude of the action potential increases abruptly at each node, the membrane current during activity has a large inward component only in the nodal regions, and conduction is reversibly blocked by increasing the external resistance between two adjacent nodes.[8]

OTHER ASPECTS OF NERVE PHYSIOLOGY

Nerve Fiber Conduction Velocity

The rate at which a nerve fiber propagates an action potential correlates with several of its morphologic features. The conduction velocity is directly related to the diameter of the axon. This is because the diameter is inversely related to the internal electrical resistance of the fiber, and conduction velocity increases as the electrical resistance is reduced. Myelinated fibers conduct faster than unmyelinated ones because the local current circuits are confined to regions some distance ahead of the active region. For the same reason, fibers with a large internodal length conduct faster than those with a smaller spacing between nodes. Finally, a direct relationship has been shown to exist between conduction velocity and the thickness of the myelin sheath surrounding the axon. There is, however, a lack of unanimity concerning the precise

relationship that exists between each of these morphologic features and conduction velocity.

The Compound Action Potential of a Peripheral Nerve

The compound action potential recorded from a multifiber peripheral nerve represents the sum of the electrical events that occur in those of its fibers that are excited by the stimulus. If a peripheral nerve is excited by successive electrical stimuli that gradually increase in intensity from a very weak level while recordings are made from the nerve a short distance away, a small nerve action potential will eventually be seen as the stimulus intensity reaches threshold level. As the intensity of stimulation is increased further, the size of this compound action potential will increase to a maximal value. This incremental change occurs because the various fibers that constitute the nerve differ in their excitability. In general, the threshold of excitability of a myelinated nerve fiber is inversely proportional to the internodal spacing in that fiber, and thus to the size of the fiber. A stimulus of an intensity just above the nerve threshold activates only the most excitable fibers. As the intensity of the stimulus is increased from this level, more and more fibers, which differ by small amounts in their excitability, are activated, and the compound action potential therefore increases in size. Eventually, all of these fibers are activated so that the compound action potential reaches a maximum, and further increase of the stimulus intensity produces no further increment.

The appearance of the compound action potential is influenced also by differences in conduction velocity among the fibers constituting the nerve. If the stimulus to the nerve is increased in intensity beyond that evoking a response of maximal size, smaller potentials will be found to follow the main one, as illustrated in Figure 2.5. These smaller potentials occur as a result of the activation of fibers that have a still higher threshold for excitation. These potentials are not incorporated into the main one because they arise from fibers that have a much slower conduction velocity than those giving rise to the large initial spike; thus, they arrive at the recording electrodes after the larger potential. This explanation of these later potentials may be supported experimentally. Thus, if the compound action potential is recorded at increasing distances from the site of stimulation, thereby increasing the conduction distance, the separation between these peaks will also increase.

It is clear that the electrical activity recorded from a peripheral nerve in response to a maximal or supramaximal stimulus represents the compound action potential of its constituent fibers, and its form relates to their conduction velocities. If sub-maximal stimuli are used, the dimensions of the compound action potential also relate to the excitability of the fibers.

Classification of Nerve Fibers

Peripheral nerves contain a variety of fibers that differ in their origin and ultimate destination, as well as in their morphologic and neurophysiologic characteristics. Through analysis of the various peaks of the compound action potential of peripheral nerves, fibers were initially divided into several groups according to their conduction velocities, as shown in Table 2.1. However, this system of classification has proved to be unsatisfactory for various technical reasons, as well as because a given group might contain several functionally different types of fiber.

Recently, therefore, afferent fibers have been classified on the basis of size and function, as shown in Table 2.2. A similar classification of efferent fibers is also possible,

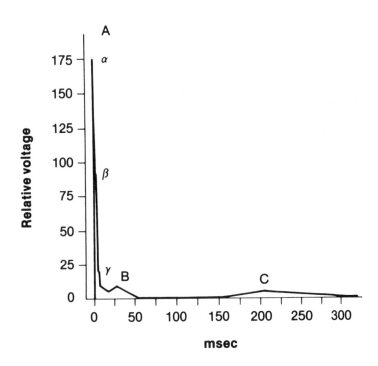

Fig. 2.5 Compound action potential of a peripheral nerve showing the relative sizes and time relationships of its components. (Ganong WF: Review of Medical Physiology. 7th ed. Copyright 1975 by Lange Medical Publications, Los Altos, CA. Modified from Erlanger J, Gasser HS: Electrical Signs of Nervous Activity. University of Pennsylvania Press, Philadelphia, 1937.)

Table 2.1. Electrophysiologic Classification of Nerve Fibers On the Basis of Conduction Velocity

Group	Fiber Diameter (μm)	Conduction Velocity (m/sec)	Anatomic Features
A	1–22	5–120	Myelinated somatic afferent and efferent
B	<3	3–15	Myelinated efferent preganglionic autonomic
sC	0.3–1.3	0.7–2.3	Unmyelinated efferent postganglionic sympathetic
drC	0.4–1.2	0.6–2.0	Unmyelinated somatic afferent

Note: The A fibers have been subdivided into various groups on the basis of their conduction velocities; they are traditionally labeled with the first four letters of the Greek alphabet.

since the largest (12 to 20 μm) innervate extrafusal muscle fibers, whereas the others (2 to 8 μm) innervate the intrafusal muscle fibers of the spindles.

OTHER ASPECTS OF MUSCLE PHYSIOLOGY

A detailed account of the physiology of neuromuscular transmission may be found in Chapter 14, which describes the various transmission defects that may occur. In essence, however, arrival of an impulse at the neuromuscular junction leads to release of acetylcholine from the nerve terminal. This causes a change in permeability of the post-synaptic membrane in the end-plate region of the muscle fiber, leading to its depolarization. This depolarization causes local current circuits that depolarize the adjacent membrane, whence an action potential is generated and propagated along the muscle

fiber. The muscle fiber action potential is a precursor to fiber contraction; as a consequence of its rapid propagation, tension is developed almost simultaneously along the length of the fiber. The structural basis of this contraction, and the manner in which it is initiated by the action potential, must now be considered.

The Structural Basis of Muscle Fiber Contraction

The individual cell or fiber of a voluntary muscle contains longitudinally oriented myofibrils that are composed of overlapping myofilaments, the latter being made up of long protein molecules. The muscle fiber has a cross-striated appearance as a result of regularly alternating light (I) and dark (A) bands which occur in phase in each myofibril. The I band is bisected by a dark Z line, whereas the A band is bisected by a light

Table 2.2. Classification of Afferent Nerve Fibers

Group	Fiber Diameter (μm)	Conduction Velocity (m/sec)	Source of Fiber	Electrophysiologic Equivalent
Ia	12–22	70–120	Spindle annulospiral endings	A
Ib	12–22	70–120	Golgi tendon receptors	A
II	5–12	30–70	Flower-spray spindle endings Touch and pressure receptors	A and ?B
III	2–5	12–30	Pain and temperature receptors Unidentified muscle receptors	A
IV	0.5–1	0.5–2	Pain and temperature receptors Unidentified muscle receptors	C

H zone which, in turn, is divided by a dark M line. The lightness of the I band is related to the presence of thin filaments of actin, associated with troponin and tropomyosin. These thin filaments extend through the I band from the Z line, and are present in the A band at the beginning of the H zone. The A band contains parallel, thick filaments of myosin, and it is dark where these overlap with the terminal portions of the thin filaments extending into the A band from the I band. The precise relationship of these interdigitating filaments to the various bands visible by light and electron microscopy is shown in Figure 2.6. The thin actin filaments are arranged in groups of six around a single, thick myosin filament, and in the A bands the thin and thick filaments are linked by transverse cross-bridges. These cross-bridges project out from the myosin filaments and are the sites at which actin and myosin interact during contraction.

During contraction of the muscle fiber, the length and diameter of each set of filaments remain unchanged, but the degree to which the filaments interdigitate increases, with the thin filaments being drawn into the A bands. Thus, the A bands remain constant in length during contraction, whereas the I bands shorten.[9,10] This concept of the structural basis of muscular contraction has been confirmed by experimental studies in which the tension produced by single muscle fibers has been shown to relate to the degree of interdigitation of the filaments within them.[11]

The Activation of Contraction

Two independent systems of tubules, formed by smooth membranes, lie in the sarcoplasm between the myofibrils. Their arrangement is shown in Figure 2.7. One of them, the sarcoplasmic reticulum, runs parallel to and tortuously between the myofibrils, and does not open onto the exterior of the cell. The other is known as the transverse tubular (or T) system. It consists of

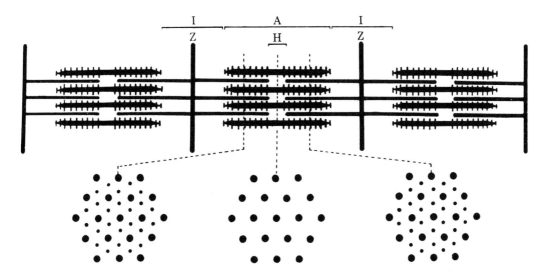

Fig. 2.6 Diagrammatic representation of part of a skeletal muscle fiber showing the arrangement of its constituent filaments and their relationship to the bands visible by light and electron microscopy. The myosin filaments are thick, with transverse cross-bridges projecting from them, whereas the actin filaments are thin. For convenience, the structure has been drawn with considerable longitudinal foreshortening. (Huxley HE: The structural basis of muscular contraction. Proc R Soc Lond [Biol] 178:131, 1971.)

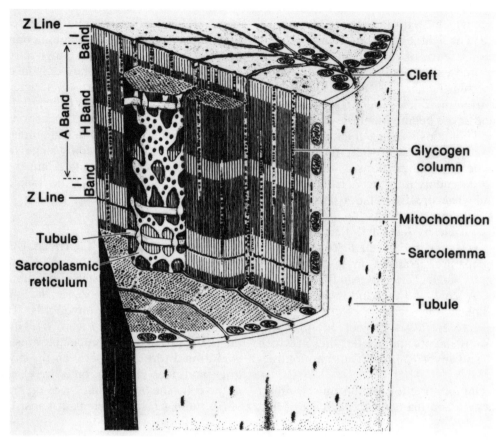

Fig. 2.7 Structure of a skeletal muscle fiber. The relationship of the sarcoplasmic reticulum to the system of transverse tubules is shown. (Hoyle G: How is muscle turned on and off? Sci Am 222:84, 1970. Copyright © 1970 by Scientific American, Inc. All rights reserved.)

invaginations of the cell membrane that form a ring around every myofibril either at its Z band or at the A and I band junctions, depending upon the animal species and speed of muscle contraction. These rings interconnect with each other and permit the interstitial fluid to penetrate close to the individual myofibrils within the cell. Each of these rings is situated between, and comes into intimate contact with, dilated terminal portions of the sarcoplasmic reticulum, thereby forming a structural complex called a triad. Individual triads thus constitute the junction between the sarcoplasmic reticulum and the T system.

The manner in which depolarization of the muscle fiber leads to activation of the contractile process is not fully understood, but the nature of the underlying process is becoming more apparent. In 1949, Hill pointed out that contraction begins too soon after the action potential to be accounted for by diffusion to the contractile elements of any hypothetical substance that might be liberated at the cell surface by depolarization of the cell membrane.[12] On the basis of their electron microscopic studies of the form and distribution of the sarcoplasmic reticulum, Porter and Palade first suggested in 1957 that the intracellular membrane system might function to conduct excitation inward from the cell surface.[13] In the following year, Huxley and Taylor reported that the application of a weak current to discrete regions of the cell membrane of an isolated muscle fiber led to contraction only when the membrane was depolarized at certain positions in relation to the striatal pattern.[14] These regions corresponded to the position of origin of the T system. Finally, Howell found that when the T system was selectively ruptured, fibers were unable to contract in response to chemical or electrical depolarization of the cell membrane.[15] These findings all suggest that when an action potential is propagated along the muscle fiber, depolarization spreads down the system of T tubules into the substance of the fiber. However, it is uncertain whether this occurs by active propagation or as a result of passive processes.

Depolarization of the membrane of the T tubule leads to the release of calcium ions from the sarcoplasmic reticulum. The mechanism by which this occurs is becoming clarified. In rested muscle, calcium ions are concentrated in those components of the sarcoplasmic reticulum that make up the tubular triads discussed earlier, and which are, therefore, closely related to the T system.[16–18] It has recently been shown that inositol 1,4,5-triphosphate mobilizes calcium ions from intracellular stores referable to endoplasmic reticulum in a variety of cell types, including purified sarcoplasmic reticulum fractions of rabbit fast-twitch skeletal muscle.[19] The released calcium ions then pass to the myofilaments and activate the contractile mechanism.

Contraction is a manifestation of the physicochemical interaction between the thick myosin and thin actin filaments. This occurs in conjunction with the energy-yielding hydrolysis of adenosine triphosphate (ATP) by an enzyme site on the myosin molecule. In the thin filaments, tropomyosin is bound to the actin; troponin, in turn, is bound to the tropomyosin. The troponin-tropomyosin complex inhibits the enzyme responsible for the hydrolysis of ATP. The inhibitory action of this complex is regulated by the presence of free calcium ions.

When these are released from the sarcoplasmic reticulum, they bind to the troponin, permitting the contractile process to proceed. During relaxation, calcium ions are taken up into the sarcoplasmic reticulum and returned to its terminal portions in the triads. The mechanisms involved in calcium ion transport by sarcoplasmic reticulum have recently been reviewed in detail elsewhere.[20]

Contractile Properties of Muscle

When a mammalian muscle is stimulated by a single shock applied to its motor nerve, it responds with a single contraction or twitch. The interval between the start of contraction and the development of peak tension varies widely in different muscles, as does the total duration of the twitch. Muscles have, therefore, been divided into those with a fast-twitch response and those with a slow one. In the limbs, for example, the time taken to develop peak tension after the start of contraction may be approximately 25 msec for a fast-twitch muscle and 100 msec for a slow one.

The mechanical response of the muscle to a single shock lasts longer than its electrical response. Repetitive stimuli can, therefore, be given at a rate that ensures their arrival after the refractory period from the preceding stimulus, but while the mechanical response is still occurring. In such circumstances, the tension developed by the muscle is greater than its response to a single shock because there is a summation of contractions. At rates of stimulation above a certain level, the individual mechanical responses fuse into a continuous tetanic contraction, during which the tension developed may be three or four times greater than that of the twitch response. Muscles differ in the frequency of stimulation required to develop their maximal tension and in their susceptibility to fatigue when repeated stimuli are applied at a rapid rate. These differences closely relate to the speed of the twitch response of the individual muscles. Thus, the stimulation rate needed to produce a tetanic contraction is higher for fast-twitch than for slow-twitch muscles.

In some laboratory animals, such as the cat, it is possible to correlate the contractile properties of certain muscles with their color, with fast-twitch muscles tending to be paler than slow-twitch ones. However, such a distinction cannot be made in humans. The basis for and implications of these differences in the contractile properties of muscle are considered further in the next chapter, where the functional organization of the motor unit is discussed.

With muscle strength training—i.e., frequent muscle activity produced against resistance—the size (cross-sectional area) of muscle fibers increases, especially in fast-twitch muscle fibers, without any change in the total number of muscle fibers in a given muscle. In animal experiments, increased activity has sometimes been associated with an increase in fiber number, but this is a result of longitudinal division (splitting) of existing fibers.[21] It is likely, then, that an exercise-induced increase in muscle volume is caused predominantly by an increase in the size of individual muscle fibers.

REFERENCES

1. Bernstein J: Untersuchungen zur Thermodynamik der bioelektrischen Strome. Pflugers Arch 92:521, 1902
2. Hodgkin AL, Keynes RD: Active transport of cations in giant axons from *Sepia* and *Loligo*. J Physiol 128:28, 1955
3. Thomas RC: Electrogenic sodium pump in nerve and muscle cells. Physiol Rev 52:563, 1972
4. Hodgkin AL, Huxley AF: Currents carried by sodium and potassium ions through the membrane of the giant axons of *Loligo*. J Physiol 116:449, 1952
5. Hodgkin AL, Huxley AF, Katz B: Measurement of current-voltage relations in the membrane of the giant axon of *Loligo*. J Physiol 116:424, 1952
6. Hodgkin AL, Huxley AF: Movement of radioactive potassium and membrane current in a giant axon. J Physiol 121:403, 1953
7. Hodgkin AL: The relation between conduction velocity and the electrical resistance outside a nerve fibre. J Physiol 94:560, 1939
8. Huxley AF, Stampfli R: Evidence for saltatory conduction in peripheral myelinated nerve fibres. J Physiol 108:315, 1949
9. Huxley H, Hanson J: Changes in the cross-striations of muscle during contraction and stretch and their structural interpretation. Nature 173:973, 1954
10. Huxley AF, Niedergerke R: Structural changes in muscle during contraction. Interference microscopy of living muscle fibres. Nature 173:971, 1954
11. Gordon AM, Huxley AF, Julian FJ: The variation in isometric tension with sarcomere length in vertebrate muscle fibres. J Physiol 184:170, 1966
12. Hill AV: The abrupt transition from rest to activity in muscle. Proc R Soc Lond [Biol] 136:399, 1949
13. Porter KR, Palade GE: Studies on the endoplasmic reticulum. III: Its form and distribution in striated muscle cells. J Biophys Biochem Cytol 3:269, 1957
14. Huxley AF, Taylor RE: Local activation of striated muscle fibres. J Physiol 144:426, 1958
15. Howell JN: A lesion of the transverse tubules of skeletal muscle. J Physiol 201:515, 1969
16. Hasselbach W: ATP-driven active transport of calcium in the membranes of the sarcoplasmic reticulum. Proc R Soc Lond [Biol] 160:501, 1964
17. Constantin LL, Franzini-Armstrong C, Podolsky RJ: Localization of calcium-accumulating structures in striated muscle fibers. Science 147:158, 1965
18. Winegrad S: Autoradiographic studies of intracellular calcium in frog skeletal muscle. J Gen Physiol 48:455, 1965

19. Volpe P, Salviati G, Di Virgilio F, Pozzan T: Inositol 1,4,5-triphosphate induces calcium release from sarcoplasmic reticulum of skeletal muscle. Nature 316:347, 1985

20. Martonosi AN, Beeler TJ: Mechanism of Ca^{2+} transport by sarcoplasmic reticulum. p. 417. In Peachey LD, Adrian RH, Geiger SR (eds): Handbook of Physiology. Section 10: Skeletal Muscle. American Physiological Society, Bethesda, Maryland, 1983

21. Gonyea W, Ericson GC, Bonde-Petersen F: Skeletal muscle fiber splitting induced by weight-lifting exercise in cats. Acta Physiol Scand 99:105, 1977

3

Properties and Functional Organization of Motor Units

A motor unit consists of one lower motor neuron and all the muscle fibers that it innervates. Little direct information concerning the structural or functional characteristics of individual motor units was available until recently, when these subjects were approached with new experimental techniques. To some extent, the information given in this chapter is an oversimplification, but frequent references to original sources are made in the text for the benefit of readers who require more detailed information.

THE MUSCLE COMPONENT OF MOTOR UNITS

Average Size

The average number of muscle fibers in the motor units of an individual muscle is indicated approximately by the innervation ratio of that muscle. This is the ratio of the total number of extrafusal muscle fibers to the total number of motor axons supplying them. Many early estimates failed to take into account the presence within a nerve of sensory axons, and of small motor axons

innervating the muscle spindles. If a correction is made for this, the innervation ratio in humans ranges from 25 or less in the external rectus, tensor tympani, and platysma muscles to 1,600 to 1,700 in the medial head of the gastrocnemius muscle. Such variation probably relates to the function of different muscles. It has frequently been noted that the facial or external ocular muscles, which are required to perform finely graded movements, have a lower innervation ratio than do the proximal limb muscles which subserve coarser activity. It has also been emphasized that the innervation ratio probably relates to the inertial load on the muscle. Thus, even slight movements of the mass of a limb will necessitate the simultaneous action of many muscle fibers, and the innervation ratio of muscles subserving such movements is usually high.

Distribution

It was originally believed, based on histologic[1] and electrophysiologic[2] grounds, that the constituent muscle fibers of individual motor units were arranged in scattered groups in normal muscle, with each group containing about 10 to 30 fibers. However, subsequent electrophysiologic studies provided data that did not agree with this premise, suggesting instead that the muscle fibers of individual units were scattered diffusely in the muscle, without any grouping.[3,4] Support for the latter view was subsequently provided by Ekstedt,[5] who reported that the electrical activity that Buchthal and co-workers[2] presumed to arise from a group of muscle fibers could, in fact, arise from single fibers. In recent years, more compelling data have accumulated, permitting resolution of this controversy.

Single motor nerve fibers can be dissected out from the anterior spinal roots in laboratory animals. Repeated electrical stimulation of one of these nerve fibers leads to a marked reduction in the glycogen content of the muscle fibers that it innervates,[6] and the distribution of these glycogen-depleted fibers can be studied histochemically. By such means, the distribution of the muscle fibers in a single motor unit was studied directly, and the fibers were found to be scattered diffusely over a wide cross-sectional area of the muscle, intermingling with fibers of other motor units and showing no evidence of any arrangement into groups.[7-9]

Histochemistry

Histochemical studies have revealed prominent differences in the staining characteristics of muscle fibers, leading to the recognition of two basic types.[10,11] In general, type 1 fibers are rich in mitochondrial oxidative enzymes but poor in myofibrillar ATPase, whereas for type 2 fibers the reverse is true. Intermediate forms and a certain number of subtypes have also been recognized, depending on the muscle and animal species under investigation. Some authors have, therefore, preferred classifications based on three or more principal types of fiber, but these will not be used in this account.

On the basis of indirect evidence, it has been assumed for some time that the muscle fibers of an individual motor unit are all of the same histochemical type. This concept is supported by experimental studies in cats and rats, utilizing the glycogen depletion method to visualize directly the fibers of a single motor unit.[7-9,12,13]

Contractile Properties and Their Histochemical Correlations

In some animals, the color of certain muscles correlates with the contractile properties of those muscles. Histochemical studies have revealed that some of these muscles are composed completely or predominantly of one or the other of the histochemical types of fiber described above. These studies have, therefore, led to the belief that the contractile properties of slow-twitch muscles are derived from type 1 fibers, whereas type 2 fibers are responsible for the properties of the fast-twitch muscles. This premise implies that motor units vary in the characteristics of their mechanical response to a stimulus since, as indicated above, the fibers of a given motor unit are all of the same histochemical type.

Physiologic studies in animals[14-17] and in humans[18,19] have demonstrated that this is, in fact, the case, with some units giving a fast-twitch response to a single stimulus, and others responding with a slow twitch. It follows, then, that motor units must differ also in the frequency of stimulation required to produce a fused tetanic contraction. This fact has been confirmed experimentally, and slow-twitch units have been found to require lower rates than fast-twitch ones. A number of other differences have also been found, as detailed in Table 3.1. For example, the slow-twitch units usually generate smaller twitch and tetanic tensions.[15-17,20]

Furthermore, they are extremely resistant to fatigue during repetitive stimulation. In contrast, fast-twitch units may be characterized as either moderately resistant or very sensitive to fatigue.[12]

The distinctive contractile properties of individual motor units indicate that their constituent fibers are physiologically, as well as histochemically, homogeneous. If this were not the case, and if, for example, very slow units contained some fast-twitch fibers, they would not develop their maximal tetanic tension at low frequencies of stimulation.[16]

Direct confirmation of the relationship between the contractile properties of individual motor units and the histochemical staining properties of their muscle fibers has been provided by several researchers.[7,12,13] They used the glycogen depletion method to identify the fibers constituting a unit after the mechanical properties of the unit had been characterized. The contractile speed of motor units appears to relate to the intensity with which they stain for myofibrillar ATPase; their resistance to fatigue relates to their affinity for stains of oxidative enzymes. Histochemical methods have also been used to demonstrate the presence of glycogen and of enzymes, such as phosphorylase, which are connected with glycogen metabolism. In general, a reciprocal relationship exists between the content of phosphorylase and of oxidative enzymes in muscles.[10] This suggests that type 1 fibers depend primarily on aerobic pathways for their energy requirements, whereas type 2 fibers depend, to a variable extent, on anaerobic glycolysis. The sensitivity of type 2 fibers to fatigue has tentatively been related to the depletion of their glycogen content by repetitive stimulation.[6,12]

The histochemical and contractile properties of motor units suggest that those containing type 1 fibers are capable of tonic activity, whereas those with type 2 fibers are better suited for phasic activity. However, to date, the properties of individual units have been studied in only a few species of animals and in a very limited number of muscles. It is, therefore, premature to assume that the correlations described above are applicable generally.

NEURAL INFLUENCE ON THE PROPERTIES OF MUSCLE

The nerves to fast-twitch and slow-twitch muscles can be sectioned and cross-united so that the fast-twitch muscle becomes innervated by the nerve that originally supplied the slow-twitch one, and vice versa. In such circumstances, the characteristic mechanical responses of the two muscles become reversed,[21–23] and there is a partial reversal of the histochemical profile of their constituent muscle fibers.[23–26] These findings, and the changes that are induced in muscle by denervation, indicate that the nervous system has an important role in influencing the metabolic activity of muscle and thus, its structural and functional properties. The nature of this neural influence and the site at which it is exerted are uncertain, but the results of cross-innervation experiments suggest that both the contractile material and the noncontractile components of muscle are affected. This provides an explanation for the histochemical and physiologic homogeneity of muscle fibers that belong to the same motor unit, but it implies that specific differences exist between the nerve cells of fast- and slow-twitch motor units. Some of these differences have been recognized and are discussed in the following section.

The neural influence on muscle appears to correlate, at least in part, with the amount and pattern of neuronal activity. Fast-twitch fibers can be converted to slow-twitch fibers by long-term, low-frequency electrical stimulation.[27] This transformation is not a result of hypertrophy or proliferation of slow-twitch fibers with concomitant atrophy of fast-twitch fibers, for there are no signs of extensive degeneration or regeneration in the stimulated muscles, nor of collateral sprouting.[27] Conversely, Lomo et al., using intermittent, 100-Hz, direct muscle stimulation, converted the denervated slow-twitch soleus muscle of the rat to a muscle with several properties characteristic of fast-twitch muscles.[28]

NEURONAL COMPONENTS OF MOTOR UNITS

An individual motor neuron summates the various excitatory and inhibitory inputs that it receives, and responds by firing if it is depolarized beyond a certain level. There is mounting evidence to suggest that the motor neurons of different units within the same muscle receive synaptic inputs that differ both quantitatively and qualitatively. However, a detailed account of this aspect is not required in this text, and attention will, therefore, be confined to some of the differences that exist in the intrinsic properties of motor neurons. These differences can tentatively be correlated with the contractile and functional properties of individual motor units, as shown in Table 3.1, but they are not sufficient to permit the separation of motor neurons into two qualitatively distinct groups.

Motor Neuron Size

Slow-twitch muscle tends to be supplied by nerve fibers with a lower conduction velocity than those supplying fast-twitch muscle,[14,29] and a similar relationship has recently been shown to apply to individual motor units.[16,17,20] Borg and co-workers studied the axonal conduction velocity and voluntary discharge properties of 120 motor units in the extensor digitorum brevis of human volunteers.[30] They found that motor units that could voluntarily be driven continuously at frequencies less than 10 per second (and that were thought to represent type 1 motor units) had axonal conduction velocities of between 35 and 45 m/sec, whereas those units which, on voluntary drive, responded only in high-frequency bursts (and were thought to represent type 2 units) had conduction velocities of between 40 and 54 m/sec.

Since the conduction velocity of an axon bears a direct relationship to its diameter, this suggests that the axons of slow-twitch units—and thus the size of their parent motor neurons—are generally smaller than those of fast-twitch units. This difference in motor neuron size has an important bearing on the functional properties of different motor units. Moreover, there is a direct relationship between the tension generated by a motor unit and the size of its motor neuron, as inferred from axonal conduction velocity,[16,17] and this relationship is significant in terms of the gradation of muscular contraction. It must be pointed out, however, that this relationship between axonal conduction velocity and the contractile properties of motor units is not always found.[31]

Motor Neuron Excitability

The resistance of the cell membrane to an electric current passing through it is called its *input resistance,* and this can now be measured directly. It follows from Ohm's law, which is defined in Chapter 4, that a current of fixed size will alter the membrane potential to a greater extent in a cell with a high input resistance than in one with a low input resistance. The input resistance of motor neurons has an inverse relationship to their size, whether the latter is measured directly[32] or is inferred from measurements of axonal conduction velocity.[20,33] This means that the relative excitability of a motor neuron is a function of its size—the smaller the cell, the lower is the intensity

Table 3.1. Comparison of the Properties of Type 1 and Type 2 Motor Units

Properties	Type 1 Motor Unit	Type 2 Motor Unit
Properties of Muscle Component		
Reactivity with histochemical stains for:		
Mitochondrial oxidative enzymes	High	Low to moderately high
Myofibrillar ATPase	Low	High
Phosphorylase	Low	High
Energy-yielding metabolic pathways	Oxidative	Anaerobic glycolysis ± oxidative
Contractile properties		
Twitch response	Slow	Fast
Stimulation rate for fused tetanic contraction	Low	High
Twitch and tetanus tensions	Small	Large
Resistance to fatigue during repetitive stimulation	High	Low to moderate
Properties of Motor Neuron Component		
Size	Small	Large
Intensity of stimulation required for activation	Low	High
Power of accommodation	Low	High to low
Duration of after-hyperpolarization	Long	Short

of stimulation that it requires to reach the threshold for firing, and thus the more excitable it is. Experimental studies have confirmed this relationship, with small motor neurons being recruited at a lower intensity of reflex[34] or intracellular electrical stimulation[33] than large ones.

Burke measured the input resistances of different motor neurons and the contractile properties of the motor units to which they belonged.[20] He found that the input resistance of neurons in slow-twitch units is generally higher than that in fast-twitch ones, although this distinction was not absolute. The motor neurons of slow-twitch units are thus more easily excited, presumably because of their smaller size.

The Accommodative Properties of Motor Neurons

The level of depolarization that is necessary to generate an action potential depends upon the rate at which the stimulus changes the membrane potential. A prolonged subthreshold depolarization may, for example, reduce the excitability of the cell. This occurs because the ability of the cell membrane to increase its permeability to sodium ions is impaired by the subthreshold depolarization; a concurrent increase in potassium permeability may also be involved. In general, the slower the rate at which a stimulus depolarizes the membrane, the greater is the level of depolarization that must occur in order to generate an action potential. The cell membrane thus accommodates to a persisting stimulus by becoming less excitable; presumably, this is one mechanism that limits the duration of the motor neuron response to a steady synaptic input.

The work of Burke and Nelson has shown that, in general, the tendency to accommodate to a slowly increasing stimulus is less in neurons belonging to slow-twitch motor units than in those belonging to fast-twitch ones, although about 50 percent of the latter show no accommodative response.[35] This suggests that the motor neurons of slow-twitch units can respond by tonic firing to a steady synaptic input, whereas the motor neurons of many fast-twitch units can only respond by firing in bursts. Indeed, such a difference in firing pattern has been found by Mishelevich to occur in response to a steady depolarizing current applied intracellularly.[36] The histochemical profile and contractile responses of many fast-twitch units imply that they are best suited for phasic activity; thus, the ability of their motor neurons to accommodate to a steady input would be one means of limiting the duration of their activity.

In humans, the voluntary discharge properties of motor units in the extensor digitorum brevis muscle have been related to contraction times of the individual units, as determined by selective electrical nerve stimulation or by averaging the increase in force related to its electromyographic potential in tonic voluntary contraction.[37] It was found that units with a contraction time of between 60 and 90 msec could be driven continuously, and had minimum firing rates of about 10 per second and maximum rates of about 30 per second. Units with contraction times of between 40 and 55 msec could not be driven continuously, and had a minimum rate of about 20 per second and maximum rates greater than 40 per second. Units with contraction times and firing properties intermediate to these were also found. These findings are, therefore, in general accord with the results of experimental studies in animals.

The Duration of After-Hyperpolarization of Motor Neurons

It will be recalled from Chapter 2 that, after the generation of an action potential, the cell membrane hyperpolarizes as a result of the relatively long-lasting increase in its permeability to potassium that occurs. This after-hyperpolarization has a shorter duration in motor neurons innervating a fast-twitch muscle than in those supplying a short-twitch one.[14,29] In the belief that the duration of after-hyperpolarization limits the rate of firing of motor neurons when they are "subjected to continuous synaptic bombardment," Eccles and associates suggested that duration of after-hyperpolarization is matched to the twitch characteristics of the muscle innervated.[14] Kernell subsequently confirmed that, under conditions of maintained activation, motor neurons discharge at different minimal and maximal frequencies depending on the duration of their after-hyperpolarization.[38] Moreover, in a study of the electrical and mechanical properties of individual motor units, Burke found that the motor neurons of fast-twitch units do, indeed, have a shorter after-hyperpolarization than do those of slow-twitch ones.[20]

It thus seems likely that the duration of after-hyperpolarization is such that individual motor neurons discharge at frequencies appropriate to the contractile responses of the muscle fibers they innervate, thereby ensuring optimal functional efficiency. Slow-twitch muscle fibers respond with a fused tetanus to the relatively low discharge frequency of the motor neurons governing them. Similarly, the higher discharge frequency of the neurons that innervate fast-twitch fibers is matched by the rapid stimulation required by these fibers to develop maximal tension. As mentioned earlier, the matching of these properties is but one example of the neural influence on muscle.

Motor Neuron Histochemistry

The neurophysiologic differences that exist between neurons belonging to fast-twitch motor units and those of slow-twitch motor units prompted Campa and Engel to study the histochemical reactions of these cells.[39] However, no distinguishing features were found.

MOTOR UNIT ACTIVITY DURING GRADATION OF MUSCLE CONTRACTION

The tension generated by the contraction of a muscle is the sum of the tensions developed by its constituent motor units. This tension can, therefore, be increased by two mechanisms. The rate of firing of active motor units may be increased (frequency or rate coding), or the number of active motor units may be increased (recruitment).

The firing rate of motor units influences the tension generated because, as the rate exceeds a certain level, the contractile responses of the units summate, thereby increasing the tension generated until a maximal tetanic contraction occurs. Electromyographic studies have confirmed that the firing rate of individual motor units normally increases as the force of muscular contraction is increased.[40,41] There is, however, a limit to the normal firing rate of a particular motor unit, and this may well relate to the frequency of stimulation that it requires to produce a maximal tetanic contraction. The precise mechanisms limiting the normal firing rate may include the duration of after-hyperpolarization of the motor neurons, as discussed earlier, but impaired peripheral feedback from the muscle may alter the limitation of firing rate. For example, Marsden and associates found that, when the ulnar nerve was blocked at the elbow by lidocaine so that the adductor pollicis muscle was denervated except for a few aberrant motor axons passing from the median to the ulnar nerve in the forearm, these few motor units could fire at rates of up to 150 Hz.[42] The limiting frequency can apparently be raised in conditions associated with weakness, with units firing at a faster rate in such circumstances.[43] Miller and Sherratt found that the firing rates of surviving motor units in the partially denervated first dorsal interosseous muscle rose to much higher levels than in normal muscle in order to generate a given amount of absolute force, but that mean firing rates were not significantly different from normal at corresponding levels of maximal voluntary contractions.[44]

Since the firing rate of individual motor units is limited, an increasing force of contraction is associated also with the recruitment of additional units. This depends on the differences that exist in the thresholds for excitation of the various motor units comprising the muscle, as discussed in the following section. The relative contribution of each of these mechanisms to the gradation of muscular contraction is not entirely clear, and different researchers have preferentially emphasized one or the other mechanism. As the tension in the muscle is increased, however, recruitment of motor units becomes less important than the rate of firing as the main regulator of force during tonic contractions. Depending upon the muscle involved, there is some variation in the highest tension at which new motor units are recruited. In some muscles (e.g., the adductor pollicis muscle), few, if any, motor units are recruited after the contraction has produced a tension that is 50 percent or more of maximal, whereas in other muscles (e.g., the brachial biceps or short extensor muscles of the toes), the recruitment of new motor units continues until almost 90 percent of maximal tension has been generated.[41,45,46]

In the anterior tibial and extensor digitorum brevis muscles, motor units with the lowest threshold and longest contraction times start firing at 5 to 10 Hz, and units with the highest threshold and shortest contraction times start firing at 15 to 20 Hz or at even faster rates during voluntary effort that slowly increases.[37,47] There is some controversy in the literature concerning maximal voluntary firing rates. Some authors have reported frequencies no higher than about 20 per second, whereas others have found frequency rates in excess of 50 or 60 per second. The issue is confounded because a variety of different muscles and of different motor unit types have been studied, different time periods have been used to calculate firing rates (so that static and dynamic phases are confused), and studies have been undertaken during different levels of fatigue,[48] with "maximum frequency" being measured in a number of different ways.

THE RECRUITMENT ORDER OF MOTOR UNITS

As indicated earlier, motor neuron excitability is inversely related to cell size. This implies that motor units are activated in a fixed order during graded muscular contractions, and that this order is the same regardless of the source of excitation leading to contraction. Experimental studies in animals confirm that this is the case during graded motor activity elicited by reflex or by supraspinal electrical stimulation.[49,50] Similarly, in normal human subjects, identical motor units are recruited in the same order by both voluntary and reflex activity in most instances.[51]

Earlier, it was stated that there is a direct relationship between motor neuron size and the amount of tension that a motor unit can

generate. This suggests that the units recruited first are those that generate the smallest tension, a fact which has been confirmed in human subjects.[52]

The order in which motor units are recruited may be modified to some extent, presumably because synaptic input is not distributed homogeneously to the motor neuron pool under study. Consequently, some cells are stimulated more intensely than others. This fact is exemplified by the work of Grimby and Hannerz, who found that, during voluntary contractions, the recruitment order of motor units with closely related thresholds for excitation was altered by proprioceptive afferent activity.[53]

Similarly, cutaneous stimulation may change the recruitment threshold of motor units in humans. Thus, stimulation of the digital nerves of the index finger may have both excitatory and inhibitory effects on the probability of firing of motor units of the first dorsal interosseous muscle during steady contractions. Fast-twitch, high-threshold units show an increased probability of firing, whereas low-threshold, slow-twitch units are more likely to exhibit a reduced probability of firing.[54] The overall effect of continuous electrical stimulation of the index finger is that recruitment of high-threshold units is increased and recruitment of low-threshold units is reduced.[55]

Desmedt and Godaux found that when a muscle acted as a synergist in one movement, as opposed to a prime mover in another, the order of motor unit recruitment consistently reversed in about 8 percent of motor unit pairs.[56] They also found that movements in a particular direction activate the motor neuron pool in a consistent order, independent of the speed of movement.

However, different modes of voluntary contraction have been shown to influence the firing rate and recruitment order of motor units. Grimby and Hannerz found that, in the short toe extensor muscle of human volunteers, certain motor units could be driven continuously and fired at regular rates, and that their firing rate increased slowly as contraction strength increased, with a maximal firing rate of less than 30 Hz during sustained contraction but greater than 60 Hz in twitch contraction.[45] Other units could not be driven continuously, did not fire repeatedly at rates of less than 20 Hz, showed a rapid increase in firing rate when the strength of contraction increased, and could fire at rates in excess of 100 Hz. Units with discharge properties intermediate to these were also found. Only continuously firing motor units were active in prolonged contractions of constant strength, whereas both continuously and intermittently firing units were active in rapid accelerations. Selective activation of intermittently firing units occurred in twitch concentrations if the muscle was relaxed before the twitch, if great effort was used to elicit the twitch, and if minimal duration of the twitch was intended.

Some researchers have demonstrated that human subjects have a small measure of voluntary control over the recruitment order of units with excitation thresholds that are close to each other.[51,57] They were unable, however, to confirm the finding of Basmajian that human subjects can exercise a considerable degree of voluntary control over the activity of individual motor units by singling them out and controlling their isolated contraction.[58] In patients with spasticity or upper motor neuron lesions, motor units may fire at a reduced rate, but whether this relates to a change in membrane properties of the motor neurons (e.g., increased duration of after-hyperpolarization), to a bias in the sampling of motor units toward slow-twitch units, or to other factors is unclear.[59] Some authors have also found disturbances in the recruitment order of motor units in the presence of fatigue[60] but this has not been confirmed by the experience of others.[59] Other studies have shown that the physiologic properties of motor units may be altered in patients with upper

motor neuron lesions. In patients with long-term spastic hemiplegia, for instance, some units develop increased fatigability and prolonged contraction times, reflecting the dynamic properties of muscle.[61]

REFERENCES

1. Wohlfart G: Muscular atrophy in disease of the lower motor neuron. Contribution to the anatomy of the motor units. Arch Neurol Psychiatry 61:599, 1949
2. Buchthal F, Guld C, Rosenfalck P: Volume conduction of the spike of the motor unit potential investigated with a new type of multielectrode. Acta Physiol Scand 38:331, 1957
3. Krnjevic K, Miledi R: Motor units in the rat diaphragm. J Physiol 140:427, 1958
4. Norris FH, Irwin RL: Motor unit area in a rat muscle. Am J Physiol 200:944, 1961
5. Ekstedt J: Human single muscle fiber action potentials. Acta Physiol Scand 61:suppl. 226, 1, 1964
6. Kugelberg E, Edstrom L: Differential histochemical effects of muscle contractions on phosphorylase and glycogen in various types of fibers: Relation to fatigue. J Neurol Neurosurg Psychiatry 31:415, 1968
7. Edstrom L, Kugelberg E: Histochemical composition, distribution of fibres and fatigability of single motor units. Anterior tibial muscle of the rat. J Neurol Neurosurg Psychiatry 31:424, 1968
8. Doyle AM, Mayer RF: Studies of the motor unit in the cat. A preliminary report. Bull Sch Med Univ Maryland 54:11, 1969
9. Brandstater ME, Lambert EH: Motor unit anatomy. Type and spatial arrangement of muscle fibers. p. 14. In Desmedt JE (ed): New Developments in Electromyography and Clinical Neurophysiology. Vol. 1. S. Karger AG, Basel, 1973
10. Dubowitz V, Pearse AGE: A comparative histochemical study of oxidative enzyme and phosphorylase activity in skeletal muscle. Histochemie 2:105, 1960
11. Engel WK: The essentiality of histo- and cytochemical studies of skeletal muscle in the investigation of neuromuscular disease. Neurology 12:778, 1962

12. Burke RE, Levine DN, Zajac FE, Tsairis P, Engel WK: Mammalian motor units: Physiological-histochemical correlation in three types in cat gastrocnemius. Science 174:709, 1971

13. Kugelberg E: Properties of rat hind-limb motor units. p. 2. In Desmedt JE (ed): New Developments in Electromyography and Clinical Neurophysiology. Vol. 1. S. Karger AG, Basel, 1973

14. Eccles JC, Eccles RM, Lundberg A: The action potentials of the alpha motoneurones supplying fast and slow muscles. J Physiol 142:275, 1958

15. Andersen P, Sears TA: The mechanical properties and innervation of fast and slow motor units in the intercostal muscles of the cat. J Physiol 173:114, 1964

16. Wuerker RB, McPhedran AM, Henneman E: Properties of motor units in a heterogeneous pale muscle (m. gastrocnemius) of the cat. J Neurophysiol 28:85, 1965

17. Appelberg B, Emonet-Denand F: Motor units of the first superficial lumbrical muscle of the cat. J Neurophysiol 30:154, 1967

18. Buchthal F, Schmalbruch H: Contraction times and fibre types in intact human muscle. Acta Physiol Scand 79:435, 1970

19. Sica REP, McComas AJ: Fast and slow twitch units in a human muscle. J Neurol Neurosurg Psychiatry 34:113, 1971

20. Burke RE: Motor unit types of cat triceps surae muscle. J Physiol 193:141, 1967

21. Buller AJ, Eccles JC, Eccles RM: Interactions between motoneurones and muscles in respect of the characteristic speeds of their responses. J Physiol 150:417, 1960

22. Close R: Effects of cross-union of motor nerves to fast and slow skeletal muscle. Nature 206:831, 1965

23. Romanul FCA, van der Meulen JP: Slow and fast muscles after cross innervation. Enzymatic and physiological changes. Arch Neurol 17:387, 1967

24. Dubowitz V: Pathology of experimentally re-innervated skeletal muscle. J Neurol Neurosurg Psychiatry 30:99, 1967

25. Yellin H: Neural regulation of enzymes in muscle fibers of red and white muscle. Exp Neurol 19:92, 1967

26. Robbins N, Karpati G, Engel WK: Histochemical and contractile properties in the cross-innervated guinea pig soleus muscle. Arch Neurol 20:318, 1969

27. Salmons S, Henriksson J: The adaptive response of skeletal muscle to increased use. Muscle Nerve 4:94, 1981

28. Lomo T, Westergaard RH, Dahl HA: Contractile properties of muscle: Control by pattern of muscle activity in the rat. Proc R Soc Lond [Biol] 187:99, 1974

29. Kuno M: Excitability following antidromic activation in spinal motoneurones supplying red muscles. J Physiol 149:374, 1959

30. Borg J, Grimby L, Hannerz J: Axonal conduction velocity and voluntary discharge properties of individual short toe extensor motor units in man. J Physiol 277:143, 1978

31. Eccles RM, Phillips CG, Chien-Ping W: Motor innervation, motor unit organization and afferent innervation of m. extensor digitorum communis of the baboon's forearm. J Physiol 198:179, 1968

32. Barrett JN, Crill WE: Specific membrane resistivity of dye-injected cat motoneurons. Brain Res 28:556, 1971

33. Kernell D: Input resistance, electrical excitability, and size of ventral horn cells in cat spinal cord. Science 152:1637, 1966

34. Granit R, Phillips CG, Skoglund S, Steg G: Differentiation of tonic from phasic alpha ventral horn cells by stretch, pinna, and crossed extensor reflexes. J Neurophysiol 20:470, 1957

35. Burke RE, Nelson PG: Accommodation to current ramps in motoneurons of fast and slow twitch motor units. Int J Neurosci 1:347, 1971

36. Mishelevich DJ: Repetitive firing to current in cat motoneurons as a function of motor unit twitch type. Exp Neurol 25:401, 1969

37. Grimby L, Hannerz J, Hedman B: Contraction time and voluntary discharge properties of individual short toe extensor motor units in man. J Physiol 289:191, 1979

38. Kernell D: The limits of firing frequency in cat lumbosacral motoneurones possessing different time course of after-hyperpolarization. Acta Physiol Scand 68:87, 1965

39. Campa JF, Engel WK: Histochemical and functional correlations in anterior horn neurons of the cat spinal cord. Science 171:198, 1971

40. Adrian ED, Bronk DW: The discharge of

impulses in motor nerve fibres. Part II. The frequency of discharge in reflex and voluntary contractions. J Physiol 167:119, 1929

41. Milner-Brown HS, Stein RB, Yemm R: Changes in firing rate of human motor units during linearly changing voluntary contractions. J Physiol 230:371, 1973

42. Marsden CD, Meadows JC, Merton PA: Isolated single motor units in human muscle and their rate of discharge during maximal voluntary effort. J Physiol 217:12P, 1971

43. Simpson JA: Control of muscle in health and disease. p. 171. In Andrew BL (ed): Control and Innervation of Skeletal Muscle. Churchill Livingstone, Edinburgh, 1966

44. Miller RG, Sherratt M: Firing rates of human motor units in partially denervated muscle. Neurology 28:1241, 1978

45. Grimby L, Hannerz J: Firing rate and recruitment order of toe extensor motor units in different modes of voluntary contraction. J Physiol 264:865, 1977

46. Kukulka CG, Clamann HP: Comparison of the recruitment and discharge properties of motor units in human brachial biceps and adductor pollicis during isometric contractions. Brain Res 219:45, 1981

47. Hannerz J: Discharge properties of motor units in relation to recruitment order in voluntary contraction. Acta Physiol Scand 91:374, 1974

48. Edstrom L, Grimby L: Effect of exercise on the motor unit. Muscle Nerve 9:104, 1986

49. Henneman E, Somjen G, Carpenter DO: Excitability and inhibitability of motoneurons of different sizes. J Neurophysiol 28:599, 1965

50. Somjen G, Carpenter DO, Henneman E: Responses of motoneurons of different sizes to graded stimulation of supraspinal centers of the brain. J Neurophysiol 28:958, 1965

51. Ashworth B, Grimby L, Kugelberg E: Comparison of voluntary and reflex activation of motor units. Functional organization of motor neurones. J Neurol Neurosurg Psychiatry 30:91, 1967

52. Milner-Brown HS, Stein RB, Yemm R: The orderly recruitment of human motor units during voluntary isometric contractions. J Physiol 230:359, 1973

53. Grimby L, Hannerz J: Recruitment order of motor units on voluntary contraction: Changes induced by proprioceptive afferent activity. J Neurol Neurosurg Psychiatry 31:565, 1968

54. Garnett R, Stephens JA: The reflex responses of single motor units in human first dorsal interosseous muscle following cutaneous afferent stimulation. J Physiol 303:351, 1980

55. Garnett R, Stephens JA: Changes in the recruitment threshold of motor units produced by cutaneous stimulation in man. J Physiol 311:463, 1981

56. Desmedt JE, Godaux E: Spinal motoneuron recruitment in man: Rank deordering with direction but not with speed of voluntary movement. Science 214:933, 1981

57. Henneman E, Shahani BT, Young RR: Voluntary control of human motor units. Neurology 25:368, 1975

58. Basmajian JV: Control and training of individual motor units. Science 141:440, 1963

59. Rosenfalck A, Andreassen S: Impaired regulation of force and firing pattern of single motor units in patients with spasticity. J Neurol Neurosurg Psychiatry 43:907, 1980

60. Grimby L, Hannerz J, Ranlund T: Disturbances in the voluntary recruitment order of anterior tibial motor units in spastic paraparesis upon fatigue. J Neurol Neurosurg Psychiatry 37:40, 1974

61. Young JL, Mayer RF: Physiological alterations of motor units in hemiplegia. J Neurol Sci 54:401, 1982

4

Electromyographic Apparatus

The development of commercially manufactured electromyographic systems has obviated the need for clinical neurophysiologists to have a detailed knowledge of the theoretical basis and mode of operation of electronic apparatus. Nevertheless, it is useful to have some knowledge of the underlying principles involved so that equipment may be handled with confidence and facility and used in a manner consonant with its limitations. A brief account of the apparatus used in clinical electromyography is, therefore, given in this chapter, but technical terms and mathematical analyses have been largely avoided in the interest of simplicity. Indeed, the account provided should be regarded as no more than an introduction to the subject. A brief list of general references is provided for those who require more detailed technical information. In addition, the attention of readers is drawn to the report by the Special Committee on EMG Instrumentation[1] which deals with various technical aspects and will be of particular value to those concerned with the design and purchase of equipment.

BASIC ELECTRICAL THEORY

Electric current is produced when a potential difference exists between two points on a conductor. A *conductor* is a substance that has only a slight opposition or resistance to the flow of current. The amount of current in a circuit depends on the potential difference that exists across it, as well as on the resistance of the circuit, such that $I = E/R$, where I is the current measured in amps, E is the potential difference expressed in volts, and R is the resistance in ohms (Ohm's law).

A conductor can induce a voltage in itself when the current varies, and this property is called its *inductance*. When an alternating current (AC) flows in a conductor with inductance, the amount of current is reduced because the additional voltage generated by the inductance opposes the applied voltage. This hindrance to the flow of an alternating current is called *inductive reactance,* and its magnitude relates directly to the frequency of the current.

A *capacitative circuit* is one that can store electricity, and alternating current will flow in such a circuit when an alternating voltage is applied. For a given voltage of fixed frequency, a small capacitor allows less current to flow than a large one. In other words, the smaller the capacitor, the more it opposes the flow of alternating current. This opposition to current flow, which is called *capacitative reactance*, is inversely proportional not only to the capacitance but also to the frequency of the alternating current.

The total opposition of a circuit to the flow of current is called its *impedance*. With direct current (DC) circuits, opposition by reactance does not occur, and impedance is purely resistive. In AC circuits, however, the flow is opposed by the inductive and capacitative reactance as well as by the resistance of the circuit, and this combined opposition represents the impedance. Since both inductive and capacitative reactance depend on frequency, the impedance in an AC circuit will vary with frequency.

THE ELECTROMYOGRAPHIC SYSTEM

The basic arrangement of a typical electromyographic system is shown diagrammatically in Figure 4.1. Bioelectric potentials from the tissue under study are picked up by a recording electrode and fed to an amplifier which is connected to a cathode ray oscilloscope, a loudspeaker system, and a magnetic tape recorder. The amplified signals can thus be monitored visually and acoustically, and stored for further analysis at a later date. In addition, some sort of photographic device is usually available so that a permanent record can be made of the oscilloscope display when necessary. In order that stimulation techniques can be employed, an electrical stimulator is incorporated into the system; this is connected to the oscilloscope so that it can trigger the sweep of the latter. These various components are discussed below in further detail.

RECORDING ELECTRODES

The flow of current in living tissues occurs as a result of the movement of ions, whereas in a wire it occurs as a result of the movement of electrons. Accordingly, in order to measure the electrical events that occur in tissues, ionic activity must be converted into electron movement. This conversion occurs at the junction of the electrode with the tissue from which the electrical activity is to be recorded.

An electrode is usually made of a metal, which is a good conductor of electricity. When it is placed in or on the tissue, a metal-electrolyte interface is formed. The electrolytes are contained in the fluids that come into contact with an electrode inserted directly into the tissue, or in the jelly or paste that is used with surface electrodes. At this interface, two opposing reactions occur: the electrode gives off ions into solution, and metallic ions in the solution combine with the electrons in the metal. In other words, there is an exchange of ions between the metal electrode and the electrolyte. Eventually, this leads to the development of a charge gradient, a layer of charge of one sign forming adjacent to the electrode, and another of opposite sign forming in the solution.

The presence of this electrical double layer has two important consequences. In the first place, it acts as a voltage source. The voltage generated may be several hundred millivolts, but the nature of the recording system is such that large standing potentials are neglected. However, when two electrodes are used to record the potential changes occurring in the tissue, a potential difference develops between them because there is a slight difference in the voltage that each generates at the metal-electrolyte interface. This potential difference is variable, and constitutes a source of artifact. Mechanical disturbances will alter the potential difference between the electrodes by changing the voltage gener-

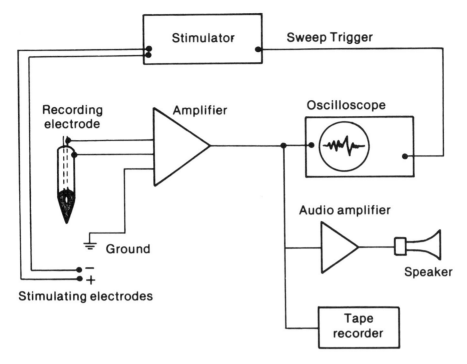

Fig. 4.1 The components of an electromyographic system.

ated by one or both of them, and the resulting voltage fluctuation may be sufficient to interfere with the bioelectrical events being recorded. This is one cause of movement artifact.

Second, each electrode exhibits some impedance to the flow of current. This has both resistive and reactive components, varies with frequency, and relates inversely to the electrode area. Its significance is discussed further in the section in this chapter dealing with amplifiers.

Electrodes are made of chemically inert conductors, and are constructed so that they are easily cleaned and mechanically robust. Two principal types of electrodes are used in clinical practice, depending on the nature of the information that is desired. The first is fixed to the skin overlying the muscle or nerve from which activity is to be recorded and is, therefore, called a surface electrode. The second type is called a needle electrode because it is inserted into, or close to, the tissue under study.

Surface Electrodes

Surface electrodes are used in studies of nerve conduction velocity and neuromuscular transmission, and whenever it is necessary for other reasons to determine the size of the electrical response of a muscle to stimulation of its motor nerve. The potential that is recorded represents the sum of the individual potentials produced by all of the nerve or muscle fibers that are activated. Surface electrodes are consequently not suitable for recording details of the electrical events accompanying the activation of individual motor units.

When surface electrodes are used, the impedance between them and the skin must be reduced. This is accomplished by washing the skin with acetone to remove surface grease; abrading it with pumice, sandpaper, or a fine needle to remove the superficial, scaly layer; and applying a conductive electrode paste to moisten the skin and to ensure good electrical contact. Care is taken not to use too much electrode paste and to prevent smearing of the paste beyond the confines of the electrodes in order to limit the spread of any applied electrical stimuli and to reduce attenuation of the response by shunting. The electrodes are fixed firmly to the skin with adhesive tape or an elastic strap. They usually consist of metal discs, varying in diameter from 0.5 to 2.5 cm, which are attached individually to the patient. Alternatively, they may consist of a pair of metal plates or "buttons" that are assembled in a plastic frame so that the distance between them is constant. However, specially designed electrodes can be used for recording from the digits of the hands or feet. These consist of either a spring-loaded metal clip or an adjustable noose made of coiled metal wire that is placed over the digit and then drawn tight.

In practice, the potential difference between two suitably placed electrodes is recorded by connecting each to one side of the differential amplifier. A third electrode is used to connect the patient with ground.

Needle Electrodes

Needle electrodes are inserted into, or close to, the tissue from which electrical activity is to be recorded. When used to sample a muscle, they permit the muscle to be explored systematically. Needle electrodes will record activity from a much smaller area than surface electrodes, and therefore permit the activity of single motor units to be studied. The outer shaft of the electrode is usually made of stainless steel, because of this material's mechanical strength. Several types of needle electrodes used in clinical practice are illustrated in

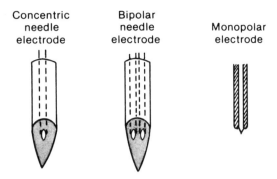

Fig. 4.2 Needle electrodes used in clinical practice.

Figure 4.2. They are manufactured commercially in a variety of sizes, but their recording area is usually less than 1 mm^2.

If needle electrodes are to be used on more than one patient, scrupulous care must be taken to clean and sterilize them between examinations. Sterilization can usually be achieved by autoclaving or by a gas procedure, but may alter the electrical characteristics of the electrodes.[1] The procedure selected will depend, in part, on the construction of the electrodes. Some materials or components cannot be autoclaved, and the instructions of the manufacturer concerning sterilization procedures should be followed. There is, however, some concern about the optimal way to sterilize electrodes that have been used in patients with suspected Creutzfeldt-Jakob disease, a transmissible disorder which may be caused by a slow virus infection or a novel proteinaceous agent. The easiest solution is to use disposable needle electrodes in such patients; otherwise, steam autoclaving at 132°C for at least 1 hour or immersion in 1 N sodium hydroxide at room temperature for 1 hour is recommended.[2] The needle electrodes used on patients with acquired immunodeficiency syndrome (AIDS) are probably best discarded, and care must be taken to avoid accidental puncture of laboratory personnel.

Before electrodes are sterilized, they

should be cleaned of all foreign debris and inspected with care. Concentric needle electrodes with blunted, bent, or broken points should be resharpened. Monopolar needle electrodes with bent, broken, or excessively exposed tips, or those with a break in the insulating material along the shaft, must be discarded. The electrical continuity of all electrodes should also be ensured before they are resterilized.

The biophysical characteristics of needle electrodes influence the parameters of the bioelectric potentials that are recorded with them. This makes it important to compare the findings in patients to those obtained in normal subjects using the same type of recording electrode. Further, when reporting the findings, the type of electrode used should be clearly indicated, and further details, such as the size of the recording surface, should be provided as necessary.

CONCENTRIC NEEDLE ELECTRODE

The concentric needle electrode consists of a hollow steel needle through which runs a silver, steel, or platinum wire which is fully insulated except at its tip. The potential difference between the outer shaft and the tip of its contained wire is measured by connecting each to one side of the differential amplifier. The patient is grounded by a separate surface electrode connected to the amplifier.

This type of electrode is mechanically robust, and its tip can be resharpened as necessary. It is much favored by clinical electromyographers, but it has certain disadvantages. In particular, because the electrode cannula acts as a shield, the electrode has directional recording characteristics, and simple rotation of the electrode may alter the configuration of individual potentials remarkably.

Of interest is a recent study by Dorfman and co-workers on the electrical properties of commercial concentric needle electrodes.[3] These authors found consistent differences in the properties of electrodes from different manufacturers due to differences in design, materials, and construction. The external diameter of the electrodes ranged between 0.41 and 0.46 mm, and core surface varied between 0.008 and 0.100 mm^2. Electrodes with smaller core lead-off surfaces generally had higher impedances and higher levels of broad-band noise and line noise.

Buchthal and co-workers described a technique of passing current through these electrodes to reduce their impedance.[4] The mechanism involved is unclear. It has been suggested that ionic movement or formation and release of gas bubbles, or both, may dislodge foreign matter adhering to the metal recording surface, or that ionic flow causes pitting of the core lead-off surface, with a resultant increase in its area. Dorfman and associates attribute the effect to some type of transient surface electrochemical phenomenon.[3]

BIPOLAR NEEDLE ELECTRODE

The bipolar needle electrode is a hollow needle containing two pieces of platinum wire, each of which is insulated except at its tip. The outer shaft is grounded, and the two inner wires are each connected to one side of the differential amplifier so that the potential difference between them is measured. However, the restricted recording range of this electrode makes it unsatisfactory for routine clinical purposes even though this type of electrode is least susceptible to electrical artifact. Potentials are shorter and of lower voltage than those recorded with the concentric needle electrode.

MONOPOLAR NEEDLE ELECTRODE

The monopolar needle electrode is a solid, stainless steel needle that is fully insulated except at its tip, and the potential

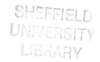

recorded with it is fed to one side of a differential amplifier. The potential recorded from a distant surface electrode, or from a second needle electrode inserted subcutaneously, is fed to the other side of the amplifier, and the patient is grounded separately.

The recording area from this electrode is circular and, in contrast to the concentric needle electrode, is not directional. Consequently, potentials recorded from the muscle tend to be larger and have more phases than those recorded with a concentric needle electrode because more muscle fibers of a motor unit are within the pick-up zone. Moreover, in further contrast to the concentric needle electrode, potentials recorded from muscle with this type of electrode have a longer duration because there is no cancellation effect due to potentials also being recorded from the cannula of the electrode. However, the Teflon insulating material has poor mechanical properties and, as it deteriorates at the distal end of the electrode, the size of the recording zone increases. This influences the parameters of the potentials that are recorded. Damage to the Teflon along the shaft of the needle may also occur.

OTHER TYPES OF ELECTRODES

A number of other types of electrodes, such as the multilead electrode and the electrode for single fiber electromyography, have been described and are considered separately in Chapter 8, where their specialized use is discussed.

AMPLIFIER AND PREAMPLIFIER

Recording electrodes pick up various interference signals, as well as the desired bioelectric activity. The bioelectric activity, however, is generally enhanced by a preamplifier that is placed relatively close to the electrodes in order to reduce the likelihood that the activity of interest will be contaminated by additional interference signals.

The bioelectric potentials must be amplified further before they can be displayed or recorded satisfactorily. By using a differential amplifier, it is possible to achieve this while simultaneously rejecting any interference signals. This instrument amplifies differences that exist in the signals from its two inputs, but rejects signals that are common to both inputs, such as those caused by interference. The ability of an amplifier to reject such common mode signals is indicated by its common mode rejection ratio (CMRR). The higher this ratio is, the greater is the ability of the amplifier to reject common mode potentials. A CMRR of 10,000, for example, means that the amplifier will amplify potential differences between its two inputs 10,000 times more than it amplifies the same potential when this is common to both inputs.

As indicated earlier, the impedance of some electrodes is quite large. This is particularly true of needle electrodes, which have a small surface area. The electrode impedance is in series with the voltage source in the tissue from which activity is being recorded, and with the input impedance of the amplifier. When two (or more) resistors are connected in series across a voltage source, the total resistance is equal to the sum of the individual resistances. It follows, from Ohm's law, that the fraction of the source voltage that can be recorded across one of the two resistors is directly proportional to the fraction that this resistor contributes to the total resistance. If the two resistors are of equal value, half of the applied voltage will be recorded across each, whereas if one is much larger than the other, the voltage measured across it will be proportionately larger. The voltage recorded across each resistor, therefore, represents the amount by which the voltage available for the remaining resistor is reduced. Since impedance can be substituted for resistance in Ohm's law, the impedances of the electrode and amplifier input can similarly be considered to act as a voltage divider. Accordingly, the input impedance of the amplifier should be large with respect to that of the electrodes in order to prevent loss of the bioelectric signal.

If the impedance of the two recording electrodes is not equal, the effective CMRR of the amplifier is reduced. In the concentric needle electrode, for example, the impedance of the inner wire electrode is greater than that of the outer shaft because of its smaller area. This means that there is an unequal loss of voltage of a common interference signal at the electrodes, and a proportion of this signal will, therefore, appear as a differential signal to the amplifier. Its effective CMRR thus depends on the type of electrodes used, and will be higher with surface electrodes than with concentric needle electrodes. The CMRR also depends on the size of the electrode impedance with respect to the input impedance of the amplifier; the lower the electrode impedance, the less the voltage loss at the electrodes, and thus the higher the CMRR will be.

Another important characteristic of the amplifier is the ratio of its output voltage to its input voltage—that is, its gain—over the range of frequencies of the signal with which it is presented. It must be able to amplify these signals uniformly, without distortion. The frequency range over which a particular amplifier is able to accomplish this is indicated by its stated frequency response. Amplification is uniform over the greater part of this range, but the gain diminishes at the upper and lower frequency limits. The point at which the gain is reduced to 0.707 of its original value is defined as the *cut-off frequency*. The *frequency response* is the range of frequencies between the low and high cut-off points. Gains are often expressed logarithmically, as this permits the overall gain of a series of amplifiers

to be determined by addition rather than multiplication. The units of gain are called decibels (dB), and using this notation, the gain of an amplifier may be expressed by the formula

$$\text{Gain (dB)} = 20 \log \frac{\text{Output voltage}}{\text{Input voltage}}$$

The gain of an amplifier at the low- and high-frequency cut-off points is reduced by 3 dB; for clinical purposes, the cut-off or -3 dB points of the amplifier in an electromyographic system should be 2 Hz and 10,000 Hz. In addition, the gain itself should be adjustable in selected steps so that a 1-cm vertical deflection on the screen of a standard cathode ray oscilloscope represents a potential difference of between 5 μV and 25 mV in magnitude.

If the frequency response of the amplifier is 2 to 10,000 Hz, it follows that the frequency response of the recording equipment with which it is connected should at least cover this range. Depending upon the type of investigation being conducted, it is sometimes necessary to alter the frequency response of the amplifier by the use of filters. These filters eliminate or attenuate noise and interference signals with a different frequency from that of the bioelectric signals being observed. A high-frequency filter allows low frequencies to pass, but attenuates signals with high frequencies; the reverse is true of low-frequency filters. The manner in which filters are used may be illustrated by a simple example. When surface electrodes are used to record bioelectric potentials, baseline drift—attributable to electrode or movement artifact—is sometimes troublesome, but may be reduced by adjusting the low-frequency filter of the system so that the amplifier cannot respond to such slow (that is, low-frequency) changes in potential. Conversely, if the frequency response of the amplifier is extended to below 2 Hz by adjusting the low-frequency filters, low-frequency potentials resulting from electrode or movement artifact will cause excessive baseline drift. Similarly, high-frequency noise becomes an increasing problem as the frequency response is extended beyond 10,000 Hz. Even when it is limited to 10,000 Hz, noise may still be conspicuous at the high sensitivity level required to record sensory action potentials. In the latter context, then, the high-frequency limit can be reduced to 3,000 Hz.

The filters used in an electromyographic system usually consist of a variable resistance-capacitance circuit. The principles governing their mode of operation have been alluded to earlier in this chapter. The capacitative reactance of a circuit is one component of its impedance to the flow of an electric current, and is inversely proportional to the frequency of the current. Accordingly, if a capacitor is placed in series with the line carrying the bioelectric signal, low-frequency signals will be impeded to a greater extent than those of high frequency. This forms the basis of a low-frequency filter. In contrast, if a capacitor is placed in a circuit that provides a bypass across the line transmitting the signal, high-frequency activity, which is impeded by the capacitor to a lesser extent than low-frequency activity, is filtered out, and a high-frequency filter results. These simple filter circuits are illustrated in Figure 4.3. Filters can also be constructed with inductors rather than capacitors, but for technical and economic reasons, capacitors are generally preferred.

The cut-off frequency of a filter circuit, or the frequency at which there is a 3-dB loss in gain of the signal through it, is directly related to the product of the resistance and capacitance of the circuit. It can thus be altered by varying one or another of these parameters, which is accomplished by changing the filter settings of an electromyographic system.

CATHODE RAY OSCILLOSCOPE

The cathode ray oscilloscope allows instantaneous changes in potential to be recorded. Electrons are emitted from a "gun," focused into a narrow beam and aimed at a fluorescent screen that emits light when hit by the electrons. The beams of electrons can be deflected in horizontal and vertical planes by applying a potential difference between suitably placed plates. The potential difference needed to move the

A

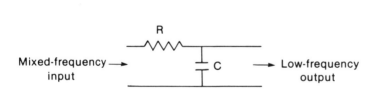

Mixed-frequency input → [R, C] → Low-frequency output

Fig. 4.3 Simple filter circuits. (**A**) High-frequency filter. (**B**) Low-frequency filter showing capacitor (C) and resistance (R).

B

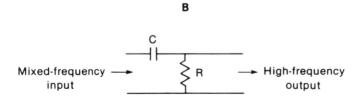

Mixed-frequency input → [C, R] → High-frequency output

beam from left to right is maintained across a pair of horizontal deflection plates. The voltage applied to these plates is increased at a constant rate so that the beam moves to the right at a constant speed, thereby providing a measure of time. When it reaches the extreme right-hand border of the screen, the voltage between the deflection plates is reset to its starting value so that the beam returns to the left side of the screen. The process is then repeated. The amplified bioelectric potential difference between the recording electrodes is fed to a second pair of plates that deflects the electron beam vertically so that, in this plane, it follows the potential changes in the tissue under study.

The cathode ray oscilloscope thus permits the voltage changes recorded in tissue to be displayed on a linear time scale. The time taken for the beam to move from left to right, known as the *sweep time*, is adjustable in selected steps in most electromyographic systems. Some systems also have a second time-marker trace that is also influenced by the voltage maintained across the pair of horizontal deflection plates. This permits accurate time measurements to be made when necessary, regardless of any nonlinearity in the horizontal deflections of the beam. Nonlinearity will cause the beam to move from left to right at an inconstant or variable rate, so that the time calibration will differ at various points along the lengths of the trace. This will affect both traces equally, however, so that if the time relations of a potential on the first trace are measured by reference to the second time-marker trace, errors due to nonlinearity of the display will be avoided.

When the spontaneous or voluntary action of a muscle is being examined by needle electromyography, the time base is allowed to run freely, sweeping repetitively from left to right. When stimulation techniques are being used, however, the stimulus is made to trigger a single sweep of the time base. The stimulus itself produces a change of potential that is picked up by the recording electrode, and this stimulus artifact will appear on the trace as a vertical deflection. Provided that it is small and does not interfere with the response to be recorded, this artifact is useful since it provides an indication of the precise time at which the stimulus was applied.

In some electromyographic systems, potentials occurring at random can be used to trigger a sweep of the time base if they are larger than other potentials. In other systems, more selective "triggers" are available so that, for example, potentials with an amplitude that is between preselected upper and lower levels or those with an amplitude that exceeds a preselected size and that are greater or less than a certain duration will generate a sweep of the time base.

A special type of oscilloscope—the "storage" oscilloscope—is sometimes used when nerve conduction studies are being performed. This instrument permits the trace to be retained on the screen, thereby allowing the latency and amplitude of the response to be measured without making a permanent photographic record. The trace can rapidly be erased electronically when it is no longer needed. Some storage oscilloscopes permit a number of sweeps to be displayed without superimposition; after each sweep, the beam moves back to the left side of the screen, as well as to a part of the screen that has not yet been used. For example, each new sweep may begin immediately beneath the preceding sweep, thereby facilitating study of randomly occurring potentials of interest.

AUDIO MONITOR

In addition to being displayed on the oscilloscope for visual analysis, bioelectric potentials are fed from the amplifier to an audio amplifier and then to a loudspeaker, enabling the examiner to listen to the electrical activity recorded from the tissue under study. This audio capability is especially valuable when a muscle is being examined by needle electromyography, because it is often possible to differentiate types of activity by their sound.

PHOTOGRAPHIC AND TAPE RECORDERS

A permanent record of the oscilloscope trace can be made photographically, facilitating analysis of the activity displayed. A conventional or Polaroid camera, or an ultraviolet photographic or metalized paper recorder, is used for this purpose. Records should include appropriate time and amplitude calibration signals.

In many electromyographic systems, a magnetic tape recorder is connected to the output of the differential amplifier. This permits the activity recorded from muscle and nerve to be stored and reviewed as needed.

NOISE

Noise appears on the oscilloscope as random fluctuations of the baseline, producing a humming or hissing sound over the loudspeaker. As it may obscure bioelectric signals of low amplitude, it is one factor that limits the recording of such signals. Noise may arise from movement of the electrodes or input leads. It is also generated within the amplifier for a variety of reasons; the extent to which this occurs depends upon the design of the amplifier. Noise can be diminished somewhat by using filters to limit the frequency response of the amplifier provided this does not distort the bioelectric potentials that are being studied (p. 43).

Noise generated within the amplifier can be measured if the input terminals are shorted (switched to the internal calibrator circuit) and the filters are adjusted for maximal bandwidth. With the amplifier set at maximum gain and the display sensitivity also set at a maximal level, the noise of the amplifier will appear as random, baseline fluctuations, causing a thickening of the oscilloscope trace. Peak-to-peak measurements of the noise are then made, but these are subject to observer bias and depend on various factors such as beam intensity. Noise can also be measured with a meter and expressed as microvolts root mean square, but this value can be misleading because the peak-to-peak value seen on the trace is generally much larger.

Methods of Improving the Signal-to-Noise Ratio

Under ordinary circumstances, the bioelectric signal is only recorded satisfactorily if it is of greater amplitude than the background noise—that is, if the signal-to-noise ratio is greater than 1. Although this ratio is sometimes particularly low, such as when sensory action potentials are being recorded, it can be improved by the use of an electronic signal averager. The signal averager produces a single trace that represents the average of a large number of sweeps of the oscilloscope. In practice, it is adjusted to analyze that part of the sweep that is believed to contain the bioelectric signal under study. This part of the sweep is divided by the averager into a number of smaller "points" or time intervals. The voltages of the signal and noise are measured in each point for a predetermined number of sweeps, and the values are then added and displayed as a single trace on the oscilloscope. Such a procedure enhances a signal that recurs at a constant time on the sweep while diminishing any random fluctuations of the baseline, which tend to average out. Averagers are generally equipped with sweep counters so that the progress of the test can be monitored, and can often be set so that stimulation is discontinued after a preselected number of stimuli have been delivered. Many commercially available averagers also have automatic artifact-rejection capability, so that any sweep with a potential that exceeds a predetermined level can be discounted.

When the signal-to-noise ratio is low, resolution of the signal can also be improved by photographically superimposing a number of faint traces from the oscilloscope so that the recurring bioelectric signal is enhanced with respect to the background noise. This approach yields much less satisfactory results, however, than does the use of an averager.

Finally, when the internal noise from the amplifier is particularly great in relation to that generated by the electrodes, the signal-to-noise ratio can be improved by the use of an input step-up transformer.

INTERFERENCE

The bioelectric signal may be obscured by unwanted signals picked up by the recording apparatus, as well as by noise. Such interference may be biologic in origin, but its most common source is the AC power line. The manner in which this power line generates an interference signal requires brief comment.

When two conductors are separated by a nonconductor, they act as a capacitor and are thus able to store electrical charges. When alternating current is applied to such a circuit, the capacitor alternately charges and discharges. Either the patient or the input leads of the electromyographic system act as one side of a capacitor, and a wire connected with the main power line acts as the other. Capacitative coupling between the main power line and the patient allows current to flow through the latter, producing an interference signal with the same frequency as the power in the main line (that is, 60 Hz in North America or 50 Hz in Great Britain). Since the signal is common to both electrodes, it is diminished by the use of an amplifier with a high CMRR and a high input impedance compared with the electrode impedance.

Capacitative coupling between one or both input leads and the main power line poses a greater problem. The induced current flows through the impedances of the electrodes to ground and, because these impedances are not uniform, the interference signal generated differs at each electrode. In such circumstances, it is usually necessary to place a grounded metal shield around the source of the interference or the input leads, thereby providing an alternative pathway for the electrostatically induced current.

Care must be taken to ensure that the patient and the recording system are grounded at only one point. If two separate grounding wires are connected to the patient, a so-called "ground loop" is created. The magnetic field from adjacent power lines can induce an electromotive force in this loop, such as occurs in a transformer. This causes an alternating current to flow through the patient, thereby generating an interference signal.

One final point must be made. Radios, televisions, paging systems, fluorescent lights, and some electrical appliances may also generate interference signals. It may not be possible to avoid interference from these sources without moving the electromyographic apparatus or using it in a screened room.

STIMULATOR AND STIMULATING ELECTRODES

In many electrodiagnostic procedures, it is necessary to stimulate nerve or muscle electrically. For this purpose, a generator is used to pass a rectangular pulse of current for a brief period. The duration of this stimulus is usually adjustable, ranging from 0.05 to 1 msec. The current is generally passed through two surface electrodes that are placed in such a way that the current flow between them passes through the nerve or muscle to be stimulated. The resistance of dry skin to the flow of an electric current is reduced by lightly covering the electrodes with electrode jelly. There are two types of stimulators, or pulse generators, in common use. The first type has a constant current source. The total current it generates between the two stimulating electrodes is independent of the external load resistance, that is, the resistance of and between the electrodes. In contrast, the second type generates a constant voltage. In either case, the stimulator provided in commercially manufactured electromyographic systems permits the intensity, duration, and frequency (repetition rate) of the stimulus to be controlled in preselected steps within a specified range.

Any part of the stimulating current that flows near the recording electrodes will lead to a potential difference between them, which will be recorded on the cathode ray oscilloscope as a stimulus artifact. It is, therefore, important to reduce the spread of stimulating current to a minimum. This is achieved by making the impedance very high between the stimulator and ground by isolating the stimulator from the ground. This is usually accomplished through the use of an isolation transformer in which current in a coil connected with the electromyographic system induces a current in a second coil which is spaced apart from, and has no electrical connection with, the first one, and which is connected to the stimulating electrodes. Although the stimulus artifact is not abolished by these means, it is markedly reduced in amplitude and duration and does not usually interfere with the response recorded on the oscilloscope. In-

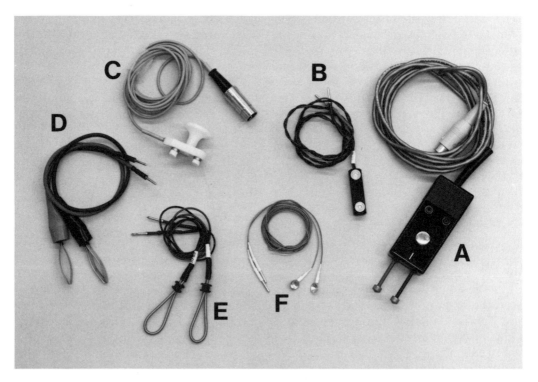

Fig. 4.4 Stimulating electrodes. (**A**) Metal prongs set in a plastic handle (often available with controls set in the handle). (**B**) Metal discs set in a plastic block. (**C**) Felt-covered ''buttons'' set in a plastic block. (**D**) Spring-loaded metal clips. (**E**) Adjustable noose of coiled metal wire. (**F**) Disc electrodes.

deed, it is useful to retain a small stimulus artifact to indicate the precise time at which the stimulus was applied, thereby permitting accurate measurement of the interval between the stimulus and response. Accordingly, the stimulator should be able to trigger the horizontal sweep of the oscilloscope before the stimulus is delivered, so that the stimulus artifact appears in full on the trace.

Stimulating electrodes are usually of the surface type (Fig. 4.4). However, if a deeply situated structure, such as the sciatic nerve, must be stimulated, needle electrodes may be used. Surface electrodes commonly consist of two protruding metal (silver or steel) or felt "buttons" that are fixed in a small plastic block. In order to stimulate digital nerve fibers, individual, ring-shaped electrodes can be wrapped around the fingers; alternatively (and more conveniently), spring-loaded metal clip electrodes, or adjustable electrodes consisting of a noose of coiled metal wire (p. 40), can be used. A particularly convenient, commercially available stimulator consists of two metal prongs set in a plastic handle that also contains the controls for adjusting the stimulus. Metal surface electrodes are lightly covered with electrode jelly before use, whereas the felt type are moistened with saline. Current is passed between the two electrodes by the pulse generator, causing excitation to occur at the cathode.

SAFETY CONSIDERATIONS

The following section indicates some of the possible hazards associated with the use of an electromyographic system, but is not intended to provide a comprehensive account of this topic. Specific regulations concerning the safety of electrical apparatus exist in many countries, and the reader should be familiar with those that are locally applicable. In addition, whenever new apparatus is installed for use on patients, it should first be thoroughly checked for safety, in the environment in which it is to be used, by a suitably qualified person.

Currents may "leak" from an electromyographic system, largely as a result of the capacitative coupling that occurs between two conductors separated by a nonconductor. These leakage currents may lead to the death of a patient, usually by causing ventricular fibrillation. Electromyographic systems are generally designed, therefore, so that their outer cases are grounded, allowing leakage currents to flow to ground via their power cords rather than by flowing through the patient. As an added precaution, however, it is wise to ensure that the patient is not in electrical contact with grounded metal objects or with other devices operated by the main power line. Moreover, the patient undergoing electromyographic examination should be lying on a bed or table that is constructed from a poor conductor of electricity (such as wood), isolated from the ground, or grounded but isolated from the patient. The patient should be grounded at one point via the apparatus, and ground, stimulating, and recording electrodes should be located on the same limb in order to minimize the path of any leakage through the body.

It is not widely appreciated that a potential difference may exist between two conductors connected with different ground points—that is, that there may be slight differences in ground potential. Such differences, although small, may have fatal consequences and must, therefore, be prevented. This may be accomplished by interconnecting the various ground points, or by grouping together at one point those that are connected with the same power service.

REFERENCES

1. Guld C, Rosenfalck A, Willison RG: Report of the committee on EMG instrumentation. Technical factors in recording electrical activity of muscle and nerve in man. Electroencephalogr Clin Neurophysiol 28:399, 1970

2. Rosenberg RN, White CL, Brown P, Gajdusek DC, Volpe JJ, Posner J, Dyck PJ: Precautions in handling tissues, fluids, and other contaminated materials from patients with documented or suspected Creutzfeldt-Jakob disease. Ann Neurol 19:75, 1986

3. Dorfman LJ, McGill KC, Cummins KL: Electrical properties of commercial concentric EMG electrodes. Muscle Nerve 8:1, 1985

4. Buchthal F, Guld C, Rosenfalck A: Action potential parameters in normal human muscle and their dependence on physical variables. Acta Physiol Scand 32:200, 1954

FURTHER READING

Dewhurst DJ: Physical Instrumentation in Medicine and Biology. Pergamon Press, Oxford, 1966

Geddes LA, Baker LE: Principles of Applied Biomedical Instrumentation. John Wiley & Sons, New York, 1968

Grob B: Basic Electronics. 2nd Ed. McGraw-Hill, New York, 1965

Reiner S, Rogoff JB: Instrumentation. p. 338. In Johnson EW (ed): Practical Electromyography. Williams & Wilkins, Baltimore, 1980

Rogoff JB, Reiner S: Electrodiagnostic apparatus. p. 24. In Licht S (ed): Electrodiagnosis and Electromyography. Elizabeth Licht, New Haven, CT, 1971

Starmer CF, McIntosh HD, Whalen RE: Electrical hazards and cardiovascular function. N Engl J Med 284:181, 1971

Strong P: Biophysical Measurements. Tektronix, Beaverton, OR, 1970

5

General Aspects of Electromyography

The description of the action potential given in Chapter 2 is based on data obtained by recording from an electrode placed inside the cell, but such a direct approach is not used in clinical electromyography. The electrical activity of muscle is recorded extracellularly and in situ, with the muscle fibers lying in a medium which, because it contains electrolytes, is able to conduct electricity and is, therefore, called a volume conductor. These differences in the recording situation will affect the nature of the potentials observed.

Although generated by the same physiologic events, action potentials recorded extracellularly from a single fiber in a volume conductor differ from those recorded intracellularly in terms of their electrical sign, their smaller size, and their triphasic or biphasic configuration (in contrast to a monophasic one), a phase being defined as a deflection to either side of the baseline. Several authors have provided detailed mathematical analyses of the relationship between action potentials recorded by these two means.[1,2] However, in the present context, such an approach is unnecessary, and the simpler explanation of Brazier is preferred.[3]

The direction of current flow is from positive to negative. It will be recalled from Chapter 2 that, during the propagation of an impulse, current flows in local circuits between active and inactive regions of the fiber. There is an inward flow of current at the active point, producing a so-called current sink there, and an outward flow of current through the volume conductor in adjacent regions. The propagated impulse can thus be regarded as a moving sink of current, preceded and followed by current sources. Such a concept clarifies the qualitative changes in potential that occur between an active electrode close to the fiber and a more remote reference electrode during the passage of an impulse.

If the region of the fiber in the pick-up zone of the active electrode is serving as a current source—that is, if current is flowing out from it—that region will be positive with respect to the reference electrode. Similarly, if the region is serving as a current sink, it will be negative in potential. When it is in its resting state, there will be no potential difference between the two electrodes. Accordingly, if the fiber is stimulated at a distance and the impulse is conducted toward the region under the active electrode, no change in potential is recorded until the current source preceding

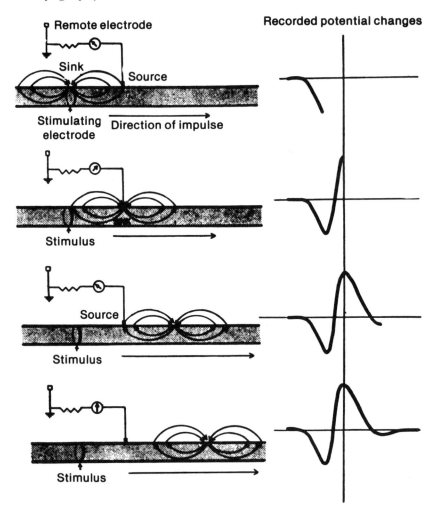

Fig. 5.1 Top to bottom, the sequential changes in potential recorded extracellularly from a single nerve or muscle fiber in a volume conductor, during the passage of an impulse. The active electrode is on the surface of the fiber, and the reference electrode is on inactive tissue having the property of an electrolytic conductor. (Brazier MAB: The Electrical Activity of the Nervous System. 3rd Ed. Pitman Medical, London, 1968.)

the impulse arrives there. At that time, the active electrode becomes positive with respect to the reference. In its turn, however, the impulse arrives, causing the active electrode to become negative, and this is succeeded by another positive phase as the impulse passes on and is followed by the current source behind it. Finally, this, too, passes on and there ceases to be a potential difference between the two electrodes.

These sequential changes in potential with the passage of an impulse are illustrated in Figure 5.1.

When the active electrode is placed over the region of the fiber at which the impulse is initiated, the recorded action potential does not contain an initial positive component and is, therefore, biphasic with a negative onset. The shape and dimensions of the action potential are influenced by a number of other factors relating to the precise arrangement of the electrodes, but for the present purposes only one requires emphasis. The amplitude of the action potential and the slope of its positive-negative component diminish as the distance is increased between the active electrode and the fiber from which it is recording. Further reference to this is made later in this chapter.

THE ELECTRICAL ACTIVITY RECORDED FROM MUSCLE

Relaxed, healthy muscle usually shows no spontaneous activity except in the region of its end-plates. However, activity can be provoked in healthy muscle by movement or insertion of an electrode, or voluntary contraction. In contrast, various types of spontaneous activity may be found in diseased muscle, and the insertion and voluntary activity of such muscle may differ in several respects from that found in normal muscle. Before the various types of potentials that can be recorded by electromyography are described, one general point must be made. The recording leads of the electromyographic system are usually connected in such a way that an upward deflection of the oscilloscopic trace signifies that the active electrode is negative with respect to the reference one. The reverse is true in the nonbiologic sciences.

Insertion Activity

When a needle electrode is inserted into a muscle or moved within it, a brief burst of electrical activity may be seen on the oscilloscope and heard over the loudspeaker. This *insertion activity* is caused by mechanical stimulation or injury of muscle fibers, and usually ceases in normal muscle as soon as the electrode movement stops or in the next 2 to 3 seconds. Kugelberg and

Petersen found that this activity normally consists of action potentials with an average amplitude and duration that are somewhat less than those of motor units but greater than those of fibrillation potentials.[4] Nevertheless, many insertion potentials are identical to either motor unit or fibrillation potentials with regard to these parameters.

Insertion activity is prolonged in a number of neuropathic and myopathic disorders. In denervated muscle, it usually consists of repetitively discharging fibrillation potentials and positive sharp waves. A similar pattern may be found, for example, in polymyositis, some forms of muscular dystrophy, and the myotonic disorders. In myotonic disorders, however, the discharge may wax and wane in amplitude and frequency, and may continue almost indefinitely after insertion of the electrode. Insertion activity may be diminished in certain metabolic disorders, such as hypokalemic periodic paralysis,[5] and is absent when there is no viable muscle tissue.

Spontaneous Activity

Spontaneous activity refers to the electrical activity that may be recorded from a fully relaxed muscle after cessation of insertion activity. Spontaneous activity may be normal or pathologic, depending upon the site from which it is recorded and the characteristics of the potentials comprising it.

END-PLATE NOISE

End-plate noise is found in the end-plate region of normal muscle and is of no pathologic significance. Two types of potentials have been described, and these may occur separately or together. The first type consists of monophasic, negative potentials that have an irregular, high-frequency pattern of discharge. Their duration is normally between 0.5 and 2 msec, and their amplitude is usually less than 100 μV, often being approximately 10 to 40 μV. These potentials are thought to correspond to the miniature end-plate potentials that can be recorded with microelectrodes in the end-plate region,[6] as discussed in Chapter 14.

The second type, which consists of biphasic potentials with an initial negative phase, have a duration of about 3 to 5 msec and an amplitude of 100 to 200 μV. Buchthal and Rosenfalck have postulated that these potentials represent the propagated action potentials of muscle fibers that are excited sporadically by spontaneous activity at the neuromuscular junction.[7] Others have suggested that these potentials originate from intramuscular nerve fibers. However, Brown and Varkey found that these potentials could be abolished by neuromuscular blocking drugs, and thus regarded them as postsynaptic muscle fiber action potentials, probably triggered by activity in presynaptic nerve fibers secondary to the mechanical irritation of the intramuscular electrode.[8]

The biphasic potentials of end-plate noise are sometimes mistaken for fibrillation potentials, but they may be distinguished from the latter by their initial negative phase and focal source. Moreover, when the recording electrode is in the end-plate region, the patient frequently complains of an unpleasant, boring pain which should alert the examiner to the possibility that the recording is being made from that region.

FIBRILLATION POTENTIALS

Fibrillation potentials arise spontaneously from either a single muscle fiber or a few muscle fibers, and are not associated with any visible contraction of the muscle, with the possible exception of when they occur in the tongue. The individual potentials have an amplitude that usually varies between 20 and 300 μV and a duration of

up to 5 msec, as shown in Figure 5.2. These potentials are biphasic or triphasic in configuration, with the initial phase being positive except in the end-plate region. This positive onset is helpful in distinguishing them from biphasic end-plate potentials. Their discharge rate is usually 2 to 20 per second, and their pattern of firing may be either regular or irregular. There does not appear to be any diagnostic significance to differences in firing pattern.[9] Fibrillations produce a characteristic, repetitive, sharp, high-pitched clicking sound over the loudspeaker, which facilitates their detection.

Fibrillation potentials can sometimes be found in an isolated, single site outside the end-plate region in normal muscle, although this is uncommon.[7] For this reason, their diagnostic significance should be questioned unless they are found in at least three separate sites within a muscle. Although they are characteristically found in denervated muscle, they are not pathognomonic of denervation, for they may also be found following muscle trauma; in certain myopathic disorders, such as the progressive muscular dystrophies and polymyositis; in metabolic disorders, such as acid maltase deficiency or hyperkalemic periodic paralysis;[10] and in botulism.[11] Buchthal and Rosenfalck, for example, found fibrillation potentials in 38 percent of patients with muscular dystrophy.[7]

As indicated above, fibrillation potentials are characteristically found in denervated muscle, in which they tend to be widespread, but they are not always seen. Indeed, between one-third and one-fourth of partially denervated muscles do not show fibrillations, which perhaps corresponds to the cyclic occurrence of fibrillations (with inactive periods of 2 to 3 days) in organ cultures of muscle.[9] Furthermore, fibrillations disappear when reinnervation occurs or when the denervated muscle has atrophied to such an extent that no viable tissue remains. They are found more commonly

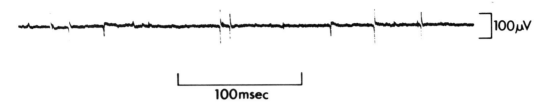

100 μV

100 msec

Fig. 5.2 Fibrillation potentials recorded in partially denervated muscle. In accordance with convention, an upward deflection in this and subsequent figures indicates that the active electrode is negative with respect to the reference one.

when the denervation is attributable to a peripheral nerve lesion than when it is a result of disease affecting the cell bodies of lower motor neurons. In the latter context, the incidence of fibrillation potentials is lower in the acute infantile forms of spinal muscular atrophy than in less progressive forms of the disease. Fibrillation potentials may not be found until 4 to 5 weeks after complete loss of functional continuity between nerve and muscle, and they do not develop until several days after insertion activity has increased. This interval is influenced by the distance between the nerve lesion and the muscle, with fibrillation potentials usually being detected sooner when the lesion is close to the muscle. However, in order for the potentials to be detected, the muscle must be warm.

The small size and simple configuration of fibrillation potentials imply that they arise from single muscle fibers, and their negative onset in the end-plate region suggests that this is where they originate, as has been shown more directly by Belmar and Eyzaguirre.[12] The mechanism by which they are generated is, however, uncertain. They are not due to mechanical stimulation from insertion of an electrode into the muscle because they can be recorded subcutaneously. Denny-Brown and Pennybacker suggested that fibrillation potentials are initiated in response to small amounts of circulating acetylcholine,[13] to which denervated muscle is supersensitive,[14] but the

failure of curare to prevent their occurrence[15] is against this view.

Li and associates demonstrated that the resting membrane potential of denervated skeletal muscle fibers tends to oscillate, generating a spike discharge when it reaches a critical level.[16] They tentatively attributed its instability to changes in muscle metabolism resulting from denervation. Such a basis for the origin of fibrillation potentials is provisionally accepted by some authorities, especially for fibrillation potentials that occur at a constant regular rate. However, those that discharge irregularly are thought to be triggered from non-propagated potentials in the former end-plate region.[9,17] The initiating events of both types of fibrillation are suppressed by tetrodotoxin or removal of external sodium ions, implying that they are related to changes in sodium conductance.[18]

The means by which fibrillation potentials are generated in myopathic disorders is equally obscure. One possibility is that the pathologic process isolates parts of muscle fibers from their end-plates, thereby leading to their functional denervation; another theory is that the fibers become hyperexcitable because of a decrease in intracellular potassium.[7,19]

Disuse or disease of upper motor neurons has sometimes been thought to produce fibrillation potentials in weak muscles, but in such cases, they may well have resulted in some instances from secondary peripheral nerve damage.

POSITIVE SHARP WAVES

Positive sharp waves are thought to arise from single muscle fibers that have been injured by the electrode; they are, therefore, an important component of prolonged insertion activity. They have a voltage similar to, or somewhat greater than, fibrillation potentials and usually last for longer than 10 msec, sometimes for up to 100 msec. They consist of an initial positive deflection of rapid onset, followed by a slower change of potential in a negative direction which may be prolonged into a negative phase of small amplitude, as shown in Figure 5.3. They occur repetitively with a rhythm that is often regular but is sometimes irregular, and their discharge frequency is usually about 5 to 10 per second, although it may range between 2 and 100 per second. They produce a rather dull sound over the loudspeaker.

Positive sharp waves have the same clinical significance as fibrillations. They occur spontaneously in denervated muscle, as do fibrillation potentials, and they may also be found in certain myopathic disorders, such as polymyositis and myotonic dystrophy. Buchthal and Rosenfalck found that, in denervated muscle, these potentials were prone to occur when the paresis was severe[7]—that is, when it was graded as 3 or less on the scale of the Medical Research Council.[20]

FASCICULATION POTENTIALS

Fasciculation potentials have the same dimensions as motor unit potentials and may be associated with a visible twitch or flicker of the muscle. They have been attributed to excitation of the muscle fibers comprising individual motor units,[13] but much doubt remains about their nature. Trojaborg and Buchthal[21] found that fasciculation potentials were not identical to the motor unit potentials that could be recorded at the same site in a muscle during weak or moderate contraction, or during passive stretch. Fasciculation potentials can occur either singly or repetitively. They are usually biphasic or triphasic, but up to 20 percent of them may be polyphasic. They produce a sudden, dull, thudding sound over the loudspeaker.

Fasciculation potentials may occur in normal muscle, sometimes in association with cramps; in such circumstances, they have no clinical significance. They are found in motor neuron disease and may also occur in other diseases affecting the lower motor neurons in the spinal cord, such as poliomyelitis and syringomyelia. Less commonly, they occur in motor radiculopathies or neuropathies, in thyrotoxic myopathy, and in patients with tetany or anticholinesterase toxicity. Unfortunately, the fasciculation potentials associated with these disorders cannot be distinguished morphologically from each other and from those sometimes found in normal muscles. Trojaborg and Buchthal found a difference in the frequency of their discharge, with the average interval between successive potentials being 3.5 seconds in a group of patients with motor neuron disease and 0.8 seconds in other subjects,[21] but there is too much overlap for this finding to have diagnostic relevance in individual patients.

Fasciculation potentials must be distin-

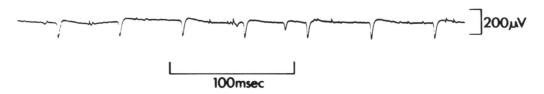

100msec

200μV

Fig. 5.3 Positive sharp waves recorded in partially denervated muscle.

guished from so-called contraction fasci-culations. The latter consist of regular, brief discharges of large motor units during weak voluntary or postural contraction, and are manifest clinically by a coarse twitching of part of the muscle. They may be found in normal elderly subjects and in patients with neurogenic atrophy of muscle, disappearing when complete relaxation of the muscle is achieved. The spontaneous motor unit potentials characterizing myokymic discharges and neuromyotonia are described separately on p. 58.

Fasciculation potentials may arise in both the central and the peripheral portion of the motor neuron. Wettstein used a collision technique to study the origin of fasciculations in patients with anterior horn cell involvement of diverse causes, and found that fasciculations could arise at multiple sites along the axons or somas of diseased motor neurons.[22] Using a similar technique, Roth studied the origin of 100 fasciculations in different disorders of the lower motor neurons and found that the potentials arose on the distal portion of the axon in 82 percent of the cases, irrespective of the severity of denervation or nature of the lesion.[23]

MYOTONIC DISCHARGES

Myotonic discharges are high-frequency discharges of action potentials that wax and wane in frequency and amplitude (Fig. 5.4), causing a sound resembling that of a dive-bomber on the loudspeaker. Many of these potentials resemble fibrillation potentials or positive sharp waves, suggesting that they are derived from single muscle fibers, whereas others look like motor unit potentials. The frequency of their discharge varies between 15 and 150 Hz.

Myotonic discharges are enhanced by cold and are evoked by insertion or movement of the electrode, percussion of the muscle, and electrical stimulation of the muscle or its motor nerve. They are also evoked by voluntary contraction but are reduced by repeated contractions. Myotonic discharges can be recorded by surface electrodes,[24] and so are not due simply to mechanical stimuli. They are found in patients with myotonia congenita, dystrophia myotonica, paramyotonia, and hyperkalemic periodic paralysis, and their occurrence is not restricted to those muscles with clinical evidence of myotonia—that is, those in which relaxation after a sustained contraction is delayed. They are also found in chondrodystrophic myotonia,[25,26] in occasional patients who have received diazocholesterol therapy,[27] in a few patients with chronic polyneuropathy[28] or neurogenic muscular wasting from other causes, and in patients with polymyositis or myopathy due to acid maltase deficiency.

Myotonic discharges are not prevented by neuromuscular blockade with curare.[24] Although the pathogenesis for all types of myotonia is unclear, the evidence that has been accumulated suggests that there is a disorder of the muscle fiber membrane in myotonia. A reduced permeability to chloride has been implicated in myotonia congenita and hereditary goat myotonia, whereas an increased permeability of the membrane to sodium has been incriminated in hyperkalemic periodic paralysis and paramyotonia congenita. The pathogenesis of

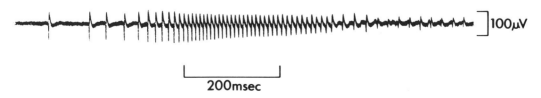

Fig. 5.4 A myotonic discharge evoked by electrode movement.

myotonia induced experimentally by dia-zocholesterol and of the myotonia in dys-trophia myotonica is controversial and re-mains to be clarified.[29]

COMPLEX REPETITIVE DISCHARGES

Complex repetitive discharges are high-frequency discharges of action potentials that occur spontaneously and in response to electrode movement or voluntary con-traction. They start and stop abruptly, but their amplitude and frequency remain con-stant (Fig. 5.5) rather than waxing and wan-ing as do myotonic discharges. In the older literature, they are sometimes referred to as pseudomyotonic discharges, but this term is ambiguous and, therefore, is best avoided. The individual potentials often have a polyphasic configuration. Their pre-cise origin is unclear, but they seem to arise in the muscle itself.[30,31]

Complex repetitive discharges may be found in the muscles of patients with mus-cular dystrophy, polymyositis, hyperka-lemic periodic paralysis, or chronic partial denervation. They may also occur in certain glycogen storage diseases, in Schwartz-Jampel syndrome (chondrodystrophic my-otonia), and occasionally in hypothyroid-ism.

SPONTANEOUS ACTIVITY OF MOTOR UNITS

Fasciculation potentials have already been described (p. 56). Motor unit activity may also occur spontaneously in a number of other clinical contexts, such as in my-okymia, nocturnal muscle cramps, tetany, neuromyotonia, and infantile spinal mus-cular atrophy.[32] The individual potentials have the same parameters as those de-scribed in the following section for normal motor units, but they fire involuntarily and repetitively.

In *tetany* and some cases of *myokymia*, potentials from the same unit fire with a consistent temporal relationship to each other so that double, triple, quadruple, or multiple discharges occur (Fig. 5.6). In-deed, the term *myokymic discharges* is probably best reserved for spontaneously occurring, grouped action potentials, each group being followed by a period of silence with subsequent semirhythmic recurrence of a grouped discharge of identical poten-tials.[33] The grouped discharges occurring in tetany resemble these myokymic dis-charges, but are under voluntary control. Double discharges may also occur as a nor-mal phenomenon at the beginning of a nor-mal voluntary contraction, as well as in pa-tients with anterior horn cell disorders, polyneuropathies, or radiculopathies.

Several features distinguishing the elec-trical activity associated with myokymia from that of fasciculation potentials have been described.[9] In particular, the activity associated with myokymia contains poten-tials that are of shorter duration than motor unit potentials, and usually have a discharge rate (up to 50 Hz) that is higher than that of fasciculation potentials. Myokymic dis-

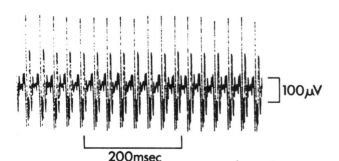

$100\mu V$

$200msec$

Fig. 5.5 Spontaneous, high-fre-quency repetitive discharge of ac-tion potentials in a partially dener-vated muscle.

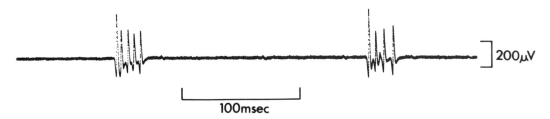

Fig. 5.6 Spontaneous, repetitive firing of a motor unit potential.

charges may also be enhanced after voluntary activity and reduced by phenytoin.

Myokymic discharges may be found in the limb muscles of patients with radiation-induced plexopathy or myelopathy. Less commonly, they are encountered in patients with chronic entrapment neuropathy, radiculopathy, or idiopathic plexopathy; demyelinative myelopathy; acute polyradiculoneuropathy or mononeuropathy;[33] and following gold therapy.[34] Myokymic discharges may also be found in facial muscles, especially in patients with intrinsic brain stem tumors, multiple sclerosis, or polyradiculoneuropathy. The discharges are generally restricted to one side in patients with brain stem neoplasms, they may occur on one or both sides of the face at different times in patients with multiple sclerosis,[35] or they may be bilateral in patients with polyradiculoneuropathy.[36]

The mechanism responsible for the generation of myokymic discharges is not clear. Abnormal excitability of anterior horn cells, peripheral nerves, neuromuscular junctions, or muscle fibers has been postulated, and the discharges may well be generated at several different sites, depending on the patient. In some instances, the underlying generator mechanism may be transaxonal ephaptic excitation at the site of focal peripheral nerve damage or development of a rhythmic, oscillating generator of action potentials within axons.[33]

The spontaneous activity found in many patients with *infantile spinal muscular atrophy* is unique. It consists of regular, spontaneously discharging motor unit activity at a frequency of 5 to 15 per second and is found in relaxed muscles, even during sleep.[32] The same units can also be activated volitionally.

In patients with *neuromyotonia*, spontaneous, long, high-frequency (up to 300 Hz) discharges of motor units are found. Discharges may occur continuously in severe cases, but vary in their configuration and dimensions, with some being especially short in duration. They may be increased transiently by voluntary activity; may become less evident after strenuous, continuous, voluntary activity; are unaffected by sleep or anesthesia; and are abolished by curare or succinylcholine. Neuromyotonia may occur in peripheral neuropathy of the axonal or demyelinative type, and has been attributed to repetitive discharges in motor nerves induced by afferent or efferent impulses passing along the nerve.[37] It may also occur without evidence of accompanying peripheral neuropathy, on either a sporadic or hereditary basis as discussed on p. 91 under the designation of Isaacs' syndrome.

Activity during Voluntary Contraction

MOTOR UNIT POTENTIALS

Excitation of a motor axon leads to the generation of action potentials in all of the muscle fibers that it innervates, and thus to their contraction. Since these fibers are scattered within the muscle, the motor unit potential only expresses the activity of that part of the unit that is within the recording range of the electrode. It is a compound potential, representing the sum of the individual potentials or spikes generated in the part under study, and the generators of these spikes are probably single muscle fibers rather than the groups of fibers proposed previously. Recent experimental studies in animals indicate that the fibers comprising a motor unit are normally arranged singly, rather than in groups, as discussed in Chapter 3, and the physicomathematical study of Rosenfalck[2] indicates that single fibers are capable of serving as a source of high-voltage spikes.

When recorded with a concentric needle electrode, motor unit potentials usually have a total duration of 2 to 15 msec, a peak-to-peak amplitude of 200 μV to 3 mV, and a biphasic or triphasic configuration, although in limb muscles, up to about 12 percent may be polyphasic.[38] Typical motor unit potentials are illustrated in Figure 5.7. They produce a dull, thumping sound over the loudspeaker when they are distant from the recording electrode, and a much sharper sound when close to it.

Duration

The duration of the motor unit potential is the time taken for the oscilloscope trace to return to the baseline after its original deflection from it at the beginning of that potential. The motor unit potential is longer than that of a single muscle fiber because the individual potentials of which it is the sum are temporally dispersed. Its duration is governed by the anatomic scatter of the end-plates of those muscle fibers that are within the recording range of the electrode and that belong to the unit under study. There are several possible reasons for this. The muscle fibers of the unit could be excited at different times by a nerve impulse because of differences in either the length or the diameter (and thus, the conduction velocity) of the terminal arborizations of the motor axon. Alternatively, the muscle fi-

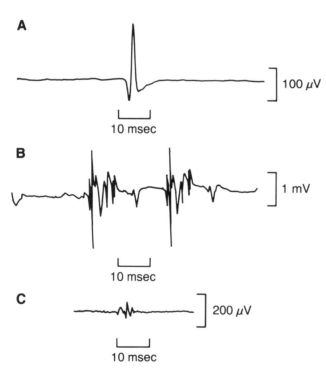

Fig. 5.7 Motor unit potentials. (**A**) Normal potential. (**B**) Long-duration polyphasic potential (shown twice). (**C**) Short-duration, low-amplitude, polyphasic potential.

bers themselves could conduct at different velocities. The most important reason, however, seems to be the different distances that separate the individual endplates and the recording electrode, and over which the muscle fiber action potentials are conducted before they reach the recording zone.[39,40]

Amplitude

Amplitude is measured between the greatest positive and negative deflections of the motor unit potential. The findings of Buchthal and associates suggest that the spike of the motor unit potential relates to the discharge of the single muscle fiber or few muscle fibers closest to the electrode, and that its amplitude is determined, to a considerable extent, by the distance between these fibers and the electrode, as shown in Figure 5.8.[41] They found, for example, that when the motor unit potential was recorded by means of a multielectrode containing 12 separate leads distributed over a length of 2.5 mm along a stainless steel cannula, the amplitude of its spike component decreased to 10 percent of its maximal value within a distance of 0.38 mm. The amplitude is also influenced by the number of active fibers lying close to the electrode, and by the temporal dispersion of their individual action potentials.

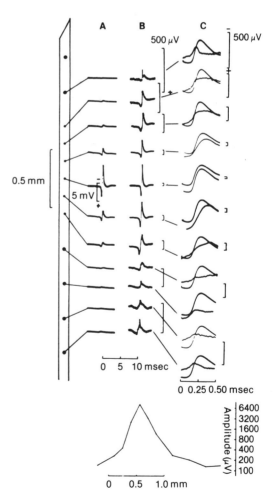

Fig. 5.8 The spike of a motor unit potential, recorded from different leads of a multielectrode. **(A)** The spike potential recorded with the same amplification on all leads; **(B)** the same potential recorded with adjusted amplification; **(C)** the same potential recorded at high sweep speed and with adjusted amplification for a detailed study of the positive-negative deflection. The potential from lead 6 was recorded simultaneously on the other beam of the oscilloscope for the purpose of comparison. The spike amplitude decreases markedly with increasing distance along the multielectrode from the lead with the greatest response. The curve in the lower part of the figure shows the relationship between spike amplitude and distance along the multielectrode. *Ordinate*, spike amplitude in microvolts, on a logarithmic scale; *abscissa*, distance along the multielectrode, expressed in millimeters. (Buchthal F, Guld C, Rosenfalck P: Volume conduction of the spike of the motor unit potential investigated with a new type of multielectrode. Acta Physiol Scand 38:331, 1957.)

These factors account, at least in part, for the wide variation in amplitude of different motor unit potentials that is found during electromyographic sampling of a muscle.

Shape

Motor unit potentials are usually biphasic or triphasic, but polyphasic ones, which are defined as having five or more phases, are occasionally seen as well. The shape of the motor unit potential depends particularly on the activity of the fibers closest to the electrode because of the marked decline in the amplitude of an action potential that occurs with increasing distance between its source and the recording electrode. Thus, the most prominent deflection consists of a negative spike that relates to the activity of these fibers. Except when recordings are made in the end-plate region, this spike is preceded by a low-amplitude, positive component which is most pronounced near the end-plate and which increases in duration as the distance between the end-plate and the site of the recordings increases. Another low-amplitude, positive component follows the spike and is believed to represent the re-polarization phase which can be recorded intracellularly. Activity in more distant fibers contributes mainly to these positive components of the potential.

Rise Time

The rise time of the negative spike (that is, the duration of the rapid inflection from the initial positive peak to the major negative peak following it, or the time taken from onset of the negative spike to its peak) depends on the distance from the recording electrode of the muscle fibers generating the spike. When these fibers are close to the electrode, the rise time of the spike is less than 500 μsec. A rise time of approximately 200 μsec indicates that the fibers generating

the spike are sufficiently close to allow the other characteristics of the motor unit potential to be evaluated usefully. In their multielectrode studies, Buchthal and co-workers found that the rise time of this component averaged 136 μsec when recorded at the site where the potential was of maximal amplitude, and increased by 100 μsec at a distance from there of 0.38 mm, when amplitude had fallen to 10 percent of its previous value.[41]

FACTORS INFLUENCING THE CONFIGURATION AND DIMENSIONS OF MOTOR UNIT POTENTIALS

When individual units are being characterized electrophysiologically, only the first few potentials recruited during a weak voluntary contraction and recorded from units with fibers close to the electrode should be studied in each of the sites explored within the muscle. A guide to the proximity of fibers contributing to the potential is provided by the amplitude of the potential and by the rise time of its positive-to-negative component, as discussed above.

The configuration and dimensions of individual motor unit potentials are normally constant provided that the position of the electrode is not altered. Even slight electrode movement leads to variation in the parameters of the potentials, causing their identity to be lost, because the spatial relationship between the electrode and the fibers of the unit is altered. A number of other factors may also influence these parameters and, therefore, merit careful consideration.

Physical Factors

As discussed in Chapter 4, the dimensions of motor unit potentials are influenced by the physical characteristics of the recording electrode and the amplifiers in the electromyographic system. The mean duration of these potentials is similar when recordings are made with concentric and monopolar needle electrodes, although potentials tend to be longer when the monopolar needle is used. (This is because there is no cancellation effect resulting from potentials also being recorded from the cannula of the electrode.) The mean duration of these potentials, as recorded with a bipolar needle electrode, is shorter than that recorded with a monopolar needle because distant activity arrives at the active and reference electrodes at the same time and is, therefore, cancelled. Furthermore, the mean amplitude of the potentials is greater with a monopolar than with a concentric needle electrode[42,43] because the recording area from the monopolar electrode is circular and thus not directional. These points must be borne in mind when results from different laboratories are compared.

Physiologic Factors

Motor unit potentials are affected by a number of physiologic factors. Their dimensions vary in *different muscles* so that, for example, their mean duration is 7.68 msec in the first dorsal interosseous muscle, 7.56 msec in the biceps brachii muscle, and 2.28 msec in the facial muscles.[42] The disparity of these values presumably relates to differences in the innervation ratios of these muscles, as well as to the spatial dispersion of their end-plates.

The dimensions of the potentials are influenced by *age*. Thus, their mean duration in the biceps brachii muscle was found by Buchthal and co-workers to have increased from 5.7 msec in children younger than 4 years of age to 10.4 msec in subjects between 70 and 80 years old.[44] This increase in duration with age has been attributed to widening of the end-plate region of the muscle by growth in persons up to the age of 20 years.[45] Subsequent increases in duration have been attributed to increasing fiber

density within the motor unit, due to a diminution in muscle volume, in older subjects. This permits a greater proportion of the initial and terminal components of the potentials to be distinguished from background noise. The duration of motor unit potentials increases much less with advancing age between 20 and 70 years in the extraocular and intrinsic hand muscles. This has been attributed to the greater fiber density of the fibers of the motor units in these muscles at all ages. Whether the change in duration also relates to loss of anterior horn cells (and so, the reinnervation of muscle) with aging is unclear. Mean amplitude of the potentials may also increase with age.[45]

Intramuscular *temperature* affects the parameters of motor unit potentials. Mean duration increases and mean amplitude declines as the temperature falls, and there is an increase in the number of polyphasic potentials. This presumably relates to increased temporal dispersion of individual muscle fiber action potentials with a reduction in temperature.

Fatigue is similarly associated with an increased incidence of polyphasic forms, but the mean duration and amplitude of the potentials are unaffected.[44] During fatigue, there is increased synchronization between discharges from different motor units, and the slight phase displacement of near-synchronous discharges from two or more motor units may then result in polyphasic potentials.

Pathologic Factors

In myopathic disorders, there is a reduction in the average number of functional muscle fibers per unit. As a result, the mean duration of motor unit potentials may be shortened due to loss of some of the distant fibers that previously contributed to the initial and terminal portions of the potentials. The shortening does not depend upon the type of myopathy, but is greater in patients with more advanced weakness and is more likely to be found in proximal than in distal muscles.[46] If the number of active fibers lying close to the electrode is reduced, the mean amplitude of the potentials may be diminished through loss of the contributions of fibers that have disappeared. Polyphasic potentials may also be encountered because the spikes generated by the surviving fibers are so widely separated in time that they do not summate to produce motor unit potentials of normal configuration.

In neuropathic disorders, there is a reduction in the number of functional motor units. The electrophysiologic changes that occur in surviving units are variable, however, and depend on a number of different factors, including the site of the lesion, the time that has elapsed since its onset, and whether or not regeneration has occurred. Nevertheless, it is instructive to consider the characteristic changes that may occur in certain typical situations.

First, the average number of muscle fibers per unit may be pathologically increased because denervated muscle fibers have been reinnervated by collateral branches from the neurons of surviving units. This leads to increased anatomic scatter of end-plates in the units so that the activity recorded by an electrode is temporally more dispersed than normal. The slower-than-normal velocity at which the immature collateral branches conduct impulses will contribute to this increased temporal dispersion, which results in motor unit potentials that are longer in duration than normal or are polyphasic, or both. The amplitude of the potentials may also be increased if the number of fibers lying close to the electrode is greater than normal. Potentials of this sort are often particularly prominent in disease affecting the cell bodies of the lower motor neurons in the spinal cord, such as motor neuron disease or poliomyelitis, but may also occur in peripheral neuropathies.

As reinnervation occurs after an acute neuropathic lesion, such as peripheral nerve transection, low-amplitude, short-duration, polyphasic motor unit potentials (often of variable configuration) are seen initially. These potentials subsequently give way to longer, somewhat larger, polyphasic potentials (that are nevertheless still smaller than normal) as increasing numbers of muscle fibers are reinnervated. The occurrence of potentials with an increased duration but normal or diminished amplitude, many of which are polyphasic, relates, at least in part, to reduced conduction velocity in the terminal branches of individual nerve fibers, and perhaps also to variations in endplate delay, so that there is greater temporal dispersion of the activity recorded by the electrode.[47]

Short-Duration and Low-Amplitude Potentials

From the points already made, it should be apparent that small or short-duration motor unit potentials may be found in a variety of myopathic disorders, in inflammatory disorders of muscle, in the early stages of reinnervation after severe peripheral nerve damage, and in disorders of neuromuscular transmission (see Ch. 14).

Long-Duration and High-Amplitude Potentials

Motor unit potentials with mean durations that are longer than normal and with increased amplitude are found in motor neuron disease and in disorders characterized by chronic partial denervation with subsequent reinnervation. Long-duration potentials may also be found late in the course of polymyositis and muscular dystrophies. Their occurrence reflects an increase in the number or density of fibers in motor units, or increased temporal dispersion of the activity picked up by the recording electrode as a result of greater anatomic scatter of end-plates or slowed conduction along the terminal branches of individual nerve fibers, or both.

Polyphasic Potentials

An increased incidence of polyphasic motor unit potentials may occur in myopathies and in weakness of neurogenic origin. Accordingly, the presence of excessive numbers of polyphasic potentials cannot, in itself, indicate the basis of weakness. In myopathic disorders, the polyphasic potentials are usually of short duration because of fiber loss (p. 63), but long-duration potentials may be found—in polymyositis or Duchenne type muscular dystrophy, for example—as a result of slowed conduction along regenerating muscle fibers.[46] In neuropathic disorders, both short- and long-duration polyphasic units may also be found, the former especially in the early stages of reinnervation and the latter at a somewhat later stage, as discussed earlier.

Motor Unit Variability

Although the dimensions of motor unit potentials are normally constant provided the position of the recording electrode remains unaltered, they may vary from moment to moment in a number of disorders, such as myasthenia gravis and the symptomatic myasthenic syndromes, in which there appears to be a defect of neuromuscular transmission. A similar variability may occur during the reinnervation of muscle after severe peripheral nerve injury or in patients with motor neuron diseases or myositis.

Late Components of Motor Units

Motor unit potentials may be followed after an interval of 15 msec or more by smaller, late potentials. The latter may relate to an ectopic end-plate or to delayed conduction along unmyelinated collateral nerve sprouts that supply previously denervated muscle fibers. Late potentials thus occur in neurogenic disorders.[48] Late potentials have also been reported in patients with advanced muscle diseases, such as polymyositis and muscular dystrophy, in which muscle fibers are presumed to become denervated by segmentation of existing fibers or by regeneration.[49]

THE RECRUITMENT PATTERN OF MOTOR UNITS

A concentric needle electrode inserted into one of the large muscles of the limbs probably picks up potentials from between 10 and 20 motor units during voluntary activity. This permits the recruitment pattern of these units during graded voluntary contractions to be studied.

With the onset of a weak contraction, a few scattered motor units begin firing irregularly at a low rate. As the force of contraction is increased, they begin to fire more regularly and rapidly, and additional units are activated (or "recruited"), as shown in Figure 5.9. In general, the units recruited first tend to be smaller in amplitude than those recruited with increasing force of contraction. The frequency at which a particular unit fires before another is recruited (that is, the *recruitment frequency*) is variable, depending, in part, on the muscle and unit being studied, but also on the number of units capable of firing and the tension that they can generate. When the number of functional units, or the tension that they can produce, is pathologically reduced, the units may fire at rates of about 50 per second during maximal effort. In the former instance, the reduction in number of functional motor units means that too few units are firing—that is, there is reduced recruitment. In the latter instance, the recruitment frequency of individual motor units and the

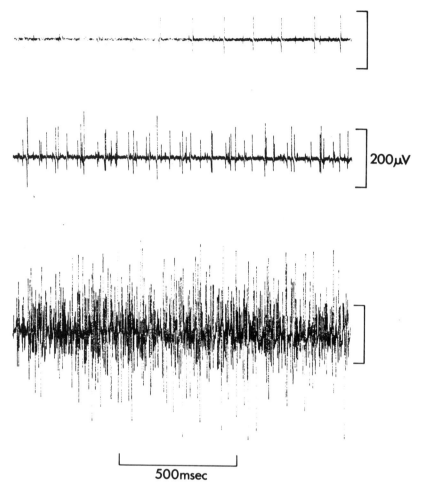

Fig. 5.9 Motor unit activity during increasing voluntary effort. The number of units activated increases with the force of contraction, and eventually (*bottom trace*), individual potentials can no longer be recognized.

rate at which units fire in relation to the number of units activated are both normal, but there is more rapid recruitment of units than normal in relation to the force generated.

As shown in Figure 5.9, with maximal effort so many units are normally active that individual potentials, which are occurring synchronously, can no longer be recognized. This pattern of electrical activity is called the *interference pattern,* and when it is full or complete, the baseline is usually interrupted continuously by the potentials. The interference pattern does, however, vary in different muscles and with the force of their contraction. Moreover, during strong contractions or fatigue, motor unit potentials may occur more synchronously than usual so that they appear in bursts, but these are of no clinical significance. Bursts of activity are also found in patients with nonorganic weakness, in whom muscular contraction occurs more tremulously than normal.

The interference pattern may be pathologically reduced so that, during a maximal voluntary contraction, the density of electrical activity recorded from the muscle is

Fig. 5.10 Electromyographic pattern of activity recorded during maximal voluntary contraction of a partially denervated muscle. Individual motor units can be recognized, and one is at least 10 mV in amplitude.

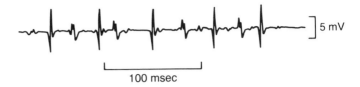

diminished and the baseline is not continually interrupted; the mean amplitude of the potentials may also be altered. If this reduction is so severe that individual motor units can be recognized, as in Figure 5.10, the pattern of activity is said to be discrete.

In myopathic disorders, the tension that individual motor units (with their reduced content of muscle fibers) are capable of generating is diminished, but the number of functional units remains unaltered until an advanced stage. Accordingly, there is a compensatory increase in their firing rates, and more motor units than normal are recruited for a given degree of voluntary contraction. The interference pattern therefore remains full, but of lower amplitude, until the disease is well advanced, and more potentials than normal are seen during contractions of weak or moderate strength. In neuropathic disorders, the number of intact motor units is diminished, and although surviving units fire at a faster rate than normal, the interference pattern is reduced.

If cooperation is limited because of pain, poor comprehension, or emotional overlay, the interference pattern during maximal effort may be reduced because only a small number of units is activated and they fire at a slow rate (for example, 10 to 20 times per second). However, the individual potentials will be normal in appearance.

PRACTICAL CONSIDERATIONS

Examination Procedure

When an electromyographic examination is performed, the time base of the oscilloscope is allowed to run freely so that it sweeps repetitively from left to right, with the sweep speed usually set at 10 msec/cm. Slower sweep speeds are helpful in characterizing firing patterns. In general, a gain of 50 or 100 μV/cm is convenient for the study of insertion and spontaneous activity, whereas a gain of 200 or 500 μV/cm is suitable for the examination of motor unit activity. Lower gains may be required when high-amplitude potentials are to be studied. Filter settings of 20 Hz (low-frequency filter) and 10,000 Hz (high-frequency filter) are convenient, but a low-frequency filter of 2 Hz is preferable when the duration of motor unit potentials is to be determined. The loudspeaker is used to facilitate the detection of increased insertion activity, the identification of abnormal spontaneous activity, and the recognition of short duration or polyphasic motor unit potentials.

The ground lead is placed over a bony surface on the same limb as the muscle that is to be examined. The patient is asked to contract the muscle so that its surface markings can be confirmed, and the skin overlying a suitable portion of the muscle belly is cleaned with a sterile spirit swab. The electrode is then inserted into the relaxed muscle, and the nature of any insertion and spontaneous activity is noted. Muscle relaxation may be facilitated by gently manipulating or repositioning the limb under study or, in anxious patients who have difficulty relaxing, by requesting the slight voluntary activation of a muscle that is an antagonist to the one being examined. Once the muscle is fully relaxed, the electrode is then used to search the muscle carefully for the presence of spontaneous activity. This may be achieved without subjecting the patient to the discomfort of multiple skin punctures by systematically exploring, in turn, each of the four quadrants surrounding the point at which the electrode was first inserted. In each case, the electrode is abruptly advanced some 2 to 3 mm at a time and then allowed to remain undisturbed for up to about 1 minute to permit any spontaneous activity to be detected. After three or four different depths have been examined in one quadrant, the electrode is withdrawn from the muscle, angulated to face another quadrant, and reinserted. The nature and duration of the insertion activity provoked by the electrode movement is noted, as is the presence and character of any spontaneous activity in each of the areas examined.

The patient is then asked to contract the muscle very slightly while the electrode is left within it, so that a single motor unit starts firing repetitively. After the dimensions and configuration of this unit have been noted, the patient is asked to increase gradually the strength of this contraction so that the firing rate of the active unit increases and other units, which are recognized by their different appearance, begin to fire. After these motor units have been studied, power is further increased so that more units are activated, and the interference pattern is compared to the strength of contraction until maximal power is being exerted. As indicated earlier, in defining the character of individual potentials, attention should be concentrated on those potentials that represent the activity of units with fibers close to the electrode and that are recruited early during weak voluntary activity.

Motor unit activity should be examined in this way in several parts of the muscle. Many electromyographers rely on subjective visual impressions in reaching conclusions from this part of the examination. This approach has the practical advantage of being much less time-consuming than precise analysis of motor unit potentials by direct measurement from photographs, but

the latter is the more reliable procedure provided a sufficient number of individual units (preferably, more than 20) are studied. A number of other quantitative techniques have also been developed over the years, but these are generally not used in routine clinical practice. They are considered briefly in Chapter 8.

The examination is undertaken in a warm, quiet room. The muscles to be examined must be warm in order to prevent distortion of the configuration and dimensions of the motor unit potentials, and to ensure that fibrillation potentials are not missed. The muscles that are examined depend on the patient's symptoms and signs and on the clinical diagnosis. If abnormalities suggestive of denervation are found, an attempt should be made to determine whether they are attributable to a spinal cord, radicular, or peripheral nerve lesion by studying their distribution in different muscles and measuring nerve conduction velocity. When muscle biopsy is contemplated, however, the proposed operative site should be avoided, as histologic changes may result from the electromyographic sampling procedure.

Electromyography is more difficult in children because they generally do not tolerate the discomfort of the procedure very well, and they may be too young to cooperate with the examiner. The examination is best undertaken without parents being present, with a nurse or technician providing reassurance and, if necessary, restraint. When a particular muscle has to be examined in infants or very young children, its contraction can sometimes be prevented by holding it in its anatomically shortest position. Conversely, its contraction can be encouraged by noxious stimuli or by gently shortening its antagonist.[50] In searching for spontaneous activity in infants, it may also be helpful to examine muscles that are known to be relatively inactive at the particular developmental stage of the patient. In evaluating motor unit activity in infants up to about 3 or 4 months old, however, it is often useful to take advantage of reflex patterns of movement in the extremities.[51] If nerve conduction studies are required, they should be performed before muscles are sampled electromyographically because the latter procedure usually causes more distress.

Reporting Electromyographic Findings

In reporting electromyographic results, a factual account is first provided, specifying the type of electrode used, the degree of cooperation by the patient, and the findings in each of the muscles examined. Specific comments should be made concerning the character and duration of insertion activity; the nature of any spontaneous potentials and the extent to which they are encountered; and the dimensions, configuration, firing frequency, and recruitment pattern of motor unit potentials. In the interest of brevity, such data are best presented in tabular form. The amount of fibrillation encountered can be graded numerically as follows: 0 = no fibrillations; 1+ = single trains in at least 3 areas; 2+ = moderate numbers of fibrillations in 3 or more areas; 3+ = many fibrillations in all areas; and 4+ = fibrillation potentials filling the baseline in all areas. Nonspecific terms, particularly those such as "dystrophic potentials", to which diagnostic implications might mistakenly be attributed, should be avoided.

An account is then given of any further procedures, such as nerve conduction studies, that were undertaken, and the results obtained. The manner in which these are best recorded is discussed in Chapter 7.

Finally, the findings are interpreted in pathophysiologic terms and related to the clinical problem. Thus, it may be possible to indicate whether weakness is myopathic or neuropathic in origin and, in the latter

case, whether it is secondary to, for example, a root or peripheral nerve lesion. Taken alone, however, the electromyographic findings cannot be used to provide a clinical diagnosis for they are not pathognomonic of specific etiologic factors. Comment on this aspect of the clinical problem is, therefore, not justified.

REFERENCES

1. Lorente de No R: A study of nerve physiology. p. 384. In Studies from the Rockefeller Institute for Medical Research. Vol. 132 (part 2). Rockefeller Institute for Medical Research, New York, 1947
2. Rosenfalck P: Intra- and extracellular potential fields of active nerve and muscle fibres. Acta Physiol Scand, suppl. 321, 1969
3. Brazier MAB: The Electrical Activity of the Nervous System. 3rd Ed. Pitman Medical, London, 1968
4. Kugelberg E, Petersen I: "Insertion activity" in electromyography. With notes on denervated muscle response to constant current. J Neurol Neurosurg Psychiatry 12:268, 1949
5. Shy GM, Wanko T, Rowley PT, Engel AG: Studies in familial periodic paralysis. Exp Neurol 3:53, 1961
6. Wiederholt WC: "End-plate noise" in electromyography. Neurology 20:214, 1970
7. Buchthal F, Rosenfalck P: Spontaneous electrical activity of human muscle. Electroencephalogr Clin Neurophysiol 20:321, 1966
8. Brown WF, Varkey GP: The origin of spontaneous electrical activity at the end-plate zone. Ann Neurol 10:557, 1981
9. Buchthal F: Fibrillations: Clinical electrophysiology. p. 632. In Culp WJ, Ochoa J (eds): Nerves and Muscles as Impulse Generators. Oxford University Press, Oxford, 1982
10. Morrison JB: The electromyographic changes in hyperkalaemic familial periodic paralysis. Ann Phys Med 5:153, 1960
11. Petersen I, Broman AM: Electromyographic findings in a case of botulism. Nord Medicin 65:259, 1961

12. Belmar J, Eyzaguirre C: Pacemaker site of fibrillation potentials in denervated mammalian muscle. J Neurophysiol 29:425, 1966
13. Denny-Brown D, Pennybacker JB: Fibrillation and fasciculation in voluntary muscle. Brain 61:311, 1938
14. Brown GL: The actions of acetylcholine on denervated mammalian and frog's muscle. J Physiol 89:438, 1937
15. Rosenblueth A, Luco JV: A study of denervated mammalian skeletal muscle. Am J Physiol 120:781, 1937
16. Li C-L, Shy GM, Wells J: Some properties of mammalian skeletal muscle fibres with particular reference to fibrillation potentials. J Physiol 135:522, 1957
17. Thesleff S, Vyskocil F, Ward MR: The action potential in end-plate and extrajunctional regions of rat skeletal muscle. Acta Physiol Scand 91:196, 1974
18. Purves D, Sakmann B: Membrane properties underlying spontaneous activity of denervated muscle fibres. J Physiol 239:125, 1974
19. Norris FH, Chatfield PO: Some electrophysiological aspects of muscular dystrophy. Electroencephalographr Clin Neurophysiol 7:391, 1955
20. Medical Research Council: Aids to the Investigation of Peripheral Nerve Injuries. War Memorandum No. 7. Her Majesty's Stationery Office, London, 1943
21. Trojaborg W, Buchthal F: Malignant and benign fasciculations. Acta Physiol Scand, 41:suppl. 13, 251, 1965
22. Wettstein A: The origin of fasciculations in motoneuron disease. Ann Neurol 5:295, 1979
23. Roth G: The origin of fasciculations. Ann Neurol 12:542, 1982
24. Landau WH: The essential mechanism in myotonia: An electromyographic study. Neurology 2:369, 1952
25. Aberfeld DC, Hinterbuchner LP, Schneider M: Myotonia, dwarfism, diffuse bone disease and unusual ocular and facial abnormalities (a new syndrome). Brain 88:313, 1965
26. Aberfeld DC, Namba T, Vye MV, Grob D: Chondrodystrophic myotonia: Report of two cases. Arch Neurol 22:455, 1970
27. Somers JE, Winer N: Reversible myopathy and myotonia following administration of a hypocholesterolemic agent. Neurology 16:761, 1966
28. Worster-Drought C, Sargent F: Muscular fasciculation and reactive myotonia in polyneuritis. Brain 75:595, 1952
29. Furman RE, Barchi RL: 20, 25-Diazocholesterol myotonia: An electrophysiological study. Ann Neurol 10:251, 1981
30. Emeryk B, Hausmanowa-Petrusewicz I, Nowak T: Spontaneous volleys of bizarre high frequency potentials (b.h.f.p.) in neuromuscular diseases. 1. Occurrence of spontaneous volleys of b.h.f.p. in neuro-muscular diseases. Electromyogr Clin Neurophysiol 14:303, 1974
31. Stoehr M: Low frequency bizarre discharges: A particular type of electromyographic spontaneous activity in paretic skeletal muscle. Electromyogr Clin Neurophysiol 18:147, 1978
32. Buchthal F, Olsen PZ: Electromyography and muscle biopsy in infantile spinal muscular atrophy. Brain 93:15, 1970
33. Albers JW, Allen AA, Bastron JA, Daube JR: Limb myokymia. Muscle Nerve 4:494, 1981
34. Mitsumoto H, Wilbourn AJ, Subramony SH: Generalized myokymia and gold therapy. Arch Neurol 39:449, 1982
35. Radu EW, Skorpil V, Kaeser HE: Facial myokymia. Eur Neurol 13:499, 1975
36. Daube JR, Kelly JJ, Martin RA: Facial myokymia with polyradiculoneuropathy. Neurology 29:662, 1979
37. Warmolts JR, Mendell JR: Neuromyotonia: Impulse-induced repetitive discharges in motor nerves in peripheral neuropathy. Ann Neurol 7:245, 1980
38. Caruso G, Buchthal F: Refractory period of muscle and electromyographic findings in relatives of patients with muscular dystrophy. Brain 88:29, 1965
39. Buchthal F, Guld C, Rosenfalck P: Innervation zone and propagation velocity in human muscle. Acta Physiol Scand 35:174, 1955
40. Buchthal F, Guld C, Rosenfalck P: Multielectrode study of the territory of a motor unit. Acta Physiol Scand 39:83, 1957

41. Buchthal F, Guld C, Rosenfalck P: Volume conduction of the spike of the motor unit potential investigated with a new type of multielectrode. Acta Physiol Scand 38:331, 1957

42. Petersen I, Kugelberg E: Duration and form of action potential in the normal human muscle. J Neurol Neurosurg Psychiatry 12:124, 1949

43. Buchthal F, Guld C, Rosenfalck P: Action potential parameters in normal human muscle and their dependence on physical variables. Acta Physiol Scand 32:200, 1954

44. Buchthal F, Pinelli P, Rosenfalck P: Action potential parameters in normal human muscle and their physiological determinants. Acta Physiol Scand 32:219, 1954

45. Sacco G, Buchthal F, Rosenfalck P: Motor unit potentials at different ages. Arch Neurol 6:366, 1962

46. Buchthal F: Electromyography in the evaluation of muscle diseases. Neurol Clin 3:573, 1985

47. Buchthal F, Pinelli P: Action potentials in muscular atrophy of neurogenic origin. Neurology 3:591, 1953

48. Borenstein S, Desmedt JE: Range of variations in motor unit potentials during reinnervation after traumatic nerve lesions in humans. Ann Neurol 8:460, 1980

49. Desmedt JE, Borenstein S: Regeneration in Duchenne muscular dystrophy: Electromyographic evidence. Arch Neurol 33:642, 1976

50. Johnson EW: Electromyographic examination. p. 352. In Licht S (ed): Electrodiagnosis and Electromyography. Elizabeth Licht, New Haven, CT, 1971

51. Johnson EW: Examination for muscle weakness in infants and small children. JAMA 168:1306, 1958

MEM

To: *Cl*

From:

Date:

6

Clinical Aspects of Electromyography

Electromyography is an important means of evaluating the function of motor units, and it is particularly helpful in determining whether weakness is myopathic or neurogenic in origin. In patients with neurogenic weakness, the pattern of involved muscles is helpful in determining the level of the lesion—that is, whether it involves the nerve roots, limb plexus, or peripheral nerves—and the electromyographic findings also provide a guide to prognosis. The electromyographic findings must, however, be considered collectively and in their clinical context, with some understanding of the limitations of the technique. In an attempt to improve the objectivity and accuracy of conventional electromyography, various quantitative or computerized techniques (including single-fiber electromyography) have been developed, and these are considered briefly in Chapter 8.

DISORDERS OF MUSCLE

Increased insertion activity and abnormal spontaneous activity may be found in myopathic as well as neuropathic disorders. The electromyographic features that most typify a myopathy, therefore, relate to the form, dimensions, and recruitment pattern of the motor unit potentials. There is an increased incidence of polyphasic forms, and many potentials are shorter in duration (1 to 4 msec) or lower in amplitude than normal. The recognition of such potentials is facilitated by the characteristic crackling sound that they produce on the loudspeaker. The number of potentials occurring during weak contractions is excessive. Although the interference pattern during maximal effort is usually full, in myopathy it is lower in amplitude than in healthy muscle, and it contains more spikes. The interference pattern may, however, be reduced in advanced myopathy, thereby resembling the pattern found in neuropathic disorders, because the entire fiber content of some units is lost. The pathophysiologic basis of these changes was discussed in Chapter 5.

The electromyographic changes just described do not, in themselves, establish conclusively that the underlying disorder is myopathic in nature. Engel has cogently argued on theoretical grounds that several hypothetical neurogenic mechanisms could lead to similar abnormalities.[1] Certainly, during the reinnervation of muscle after a severe neuropathic lesion, electromyographic findings may be similar to that found in myopathic disorders.[2] This does not detract from the practical usefulness of electromyography, however, provided the findings are evaluated in their clinical context and in relation to the results of other investigations.

In some cases of myopathy, electromyography may reveal no significant abnormality. In other instances, however, it may provide information of diagnostic significance when histologic examination of muscle biopsy specimens is unrewarding. These two procedures should, therefore, be regarded as complementary rather than alternatives to each other. Such discrepancies presumably arise because the muscle involvement is patchy in distribution, and affected areas may, therefore, be missed by the exploring electrode or may not be contained in the biopsy specimen. Engel and Warmolts have also stressed, however, that motor unit potentials may be normal in appearance if type 2 muscle fibers are selectively involved by the pathologic process since it is the type 1 units that fire during weak contractions and thus it is their parameters that are studied in detail during the electromyographic examination.[3]

Buchthal and Kamieniecka compared electromyographic, histologic, and histochemical findings in 264 patients with neuromuscular disorders that were categorized according to history and to clinical and other laboratory findings.[4] They found that muscle histology, histochemistry, or both, and electromyographic findings were in accord with the clinical findings in 77 percent of 188 patients with myopathy and in 91 percent of 64 patients with neurogenic lesions. The electromyographic findings were in accord with the clinical classification in 87 percent of patients with myopathy and 91 percent of patients with neurogenic lesions, whereas the corresponding figures for the findings on muscle biopsy were 79 percent and 92 percent, respectively.

Sometimes, the results of properly performed electromyographic and histologic examinations are completely contradictory, with the findings being suggestive of a myopathy in one case and of neurogenic atrophy in the other. The basis for this contradiction can be understood if one appreciates that chronically denervated muscle may, for example, show electrical and structural changes suggestive of a secondary myopathy.[5] It can be exceedingly difficult, therefore, to distinguish with certainty between these two pathologic processes, no matter which investigative procedure is favored— hence the need for a dual approach.

The following discussion stresses the manner in which the electromyographic abnormalities found in individual myopathic disorders differ from those described above. Brief clinical details are provided for the benefit of readers without formal neurologic training, but a comprehensive clinical account is beyond the scope of the present work and must therefore be obtained from standard textbooks.

The Muscular Dystrophies

The muscular dystrophies are a group of inherited disorders characterized by a progressive, primary, degenerative myopathy that is manifested clinically by weakness and wasting. Several different types of muscular dystrophy have been recognized, varying in the pattern of inheritance, age at onset, distribution of affected muscles, and rate of progression.

The X-linked recessive type of muscular dystrophy occurs in males but is transmitted to the next generation by females. Severe (Duchenne) and mild (Becker) forms have been distinguished, and in both, there is progressive weakness and wasting of the pelvic and shoulder girdle muscles. In the former, the muscles often show hypertrophy or pseudohypertrophy in early stages, the disease progresses rapidly from its onset in the first 5 years of life, and death usually occurs before the second decade as a result of respiratory infection or heart failure. In patients with the Becker variety, the onset is later, progression is slower, and the life span may be normal.

Muscular dystrophy may also be inherited in either sex in an autosomal recessive manner. The limb girdle type begins between the ages of 10 and 30 years by affecting the muscles of the shoulder or pelvic girdle, and spreads over some years until both are involved. Another less common variety that is inherited in the same way resembles the Duchenne type in its distribution, but is less severe, usually appears later in life, and progresses more slowly. Walton and Gardner-Medwin[6] have emphasized that many cases once considered to be of this sort may well have been spinal muscular atrophy of the type described by Kugelberg and Welander.[7]

Facioscapulohumeral muscular dystrophy has an autosomal dominant mode of transmission, occurs in either sex, and can become manifest at any age. It initially affects the muscles of the face and shoulder girdle, spreading later to involve the muscles of the pelvic girdle and legs. Rarer forms of the disorder with dominant inheritance include the distal variety, which involves the muscles in the hands and those below the knees (eventually spreading proximally), and the ocular and oculopharyngeal varieties.

Recent studies have suggested that there may also be a neurogenic basis for the clinical features of many cases previously regarded as examples of limb girdle, facioscapulohumeral, distal, or ocular muscular dystrophy. The muscular dystrophies can usually be distinguished from neurogenic atrophy by electromyography and by pathologic examination of muscle biopsy specimens. However, as indicated earlier, discrepancies occasionally arise between the electrical and pathologic findings. Patients with suspected muscular dystrophy should therefore undergo both types of investigation before a definitive diagnosis is made.

The usual electromyographic findings in muscular dystrophy conform to those described earlier as being characteristic of myopathic disorders in general. The incidence of short-duration, low-amplitude, and polyphasic motor unit potentials is increased, and the interference pattern is full, spiky, and of low amplitude. Polyphasic potentials of long duration may also be found with Duchenne muscular dystrophy, and have been attributed to slowed conduction along regenerating muscle fibers. Insertion activity is increased in a few cases, and abnormal spontaneous activity—consisting of fibrillation potentials, positive sharp waves, and complex repetitive discharges—may be present.

Electromyographic abnormalities are sometimes inconspicuous, however, despite a careful search of the muscle. Pinelli and Buchthal, for example, found that the mean duration of motor unit potentials was decreased in only about two-thirds of the 32 patients with muscular dystrophy whom they studied, and even then, not all of the muscles sampled were abnormal in this respect.[8] Indeed, Buchthal has emphasized that, in 50 percent of patients with relatively benign forms of muscular dystrophy, such as the limb girdle or facioscapulohumeral type, the mean duration of motor unit potentials is normal.[9]

Attempts have been made to identify female carriers of the gene for the sex-linked type of muscular dystrophy by electromyography. The parameters of motor unit potentials[10,11] and the refractory period of muscle fibers[12] have been measured, and the changes in potential that occur in a muscle in response to a given load have been analyzed,[13] but the success rate with these techniques is variable and their practical usefulness is limited.

Inflammatory Disorders of Muscle

There are a number of inflammatory my-opathies, and these are generally divided into those resulting from viral, bacterial, protozoal, or other infective agents, and those in which no such infective agents can be identified. Inflammatory infiltrates are present in skeletal muscle, and are usually associated with the destruction of muscle fibers.

POLYMYOSITIS

The term *polymyositis* is used to refer to a group of disorders of uncertain etiology in which there is destruction of muscle fibers and inflammatory infiltration of the muscles. In some instances, the muscle pathology may relate to immunologically mediated vascular damage. Polymyositis occurs at all ages, progresses at a variable rate, and leads to weakness and then to wasting, especially of the proximal and girdle muscles. The neck muscles are frequently involved, but the facial and ocular muscles are rarely affected. Muscle pain and tenderness, dysphagia, and Raynaud's phenomenon are other features of the disorder that are frequently troublesome. There may be accompanying cutaneous manifestations (dermatomyositis), or an association with malignant disease (usually a carcinoma) or with one of the collagen disorders. Polymyositis has thus been reported in association with systemic lupus erythematosus, scleroderma, rheumatic fever, rheumatoid arthritis, polyarteritis nodosa, and Sjögren's syndrome. The association with malignant disease is especially common in patients older than 55 years who have dermatomyositis.

It is important to distinguish polymyositis from the muscular dystrophies since patients may recover from it spontaneously or may respond to treatment with steroids or a cytotoxic immunosuppressive drug. The electromyographic changes that occur in polymyositis are patchy in distribution and vary with the stage of the disease. Nevertheless, the motor unit potentials usually conform in character to those seen in other myopathies. Thus there is an increased incidence of polyphasic and short-duration potentials,[14] and an electrically full interference pattern at reduced effort. In contrast to the muscular dystrophies, however, prolonged insertion activity and abnormal spontaneous activity are often conspicuous features, with the latter usually consisting of fibrillation potentials and positive sharp waves. Lambert and associates found such activity in 80 percent of the 80 patients with polymyositis or dermatomyositis that they studied. They related it to the timing of the examination, with spontaneous activity becoming less conspicuous as the disease regressed.[15] Complex repetitive discharges may also be found, occurring in about 15 to 20 percent of cases.[15] DeVere and Bradley reported that only 11 percent of patients had normal findings at electromyography, this percentage being higher than the proportion of patients with an elevated erythrocyte sedimentation rate or serum creatine kinase, or with an abnormality on muscle biopsy.[16]

Some researchers have reported large, long-duration, polyphasic potentials with loss of motor units and increased motor unit territory in the chronic phase of the disorder after muscle fiber regeneration, and increased jitter and fiber density may be detected by single fiber electromyography. The latter technique is discussed in Chapter 8.

Repetitive electrical stimulation of the nerves to affected muscles sometimes provides electrophysiologic evidence of impaired neuromuscular transmission (as discussed in Chapter 14), but nerve conduction velocity remains normal.

The earliest electromyographic sign of

improvement is the disappearance of fibrillation potentials,[17] but electromyography is of limited value in assessing the response to treatment. When a deterioration of muscle strength occurs in patients who are receiving steroids and who have a normal serum creatine kinase, electromyography may help to differentiate a reactivation of the myositis from a steroid-induced myopathy.

INCLUSION BODY MYOSITIS

Inclusion body myositis is a rare, slowly progressive, painless, chronic myopathy that involves both proximal and distal muscles and shows little response to treatment with steroids or immunosuppressive drugs. Electrophysiologically, either myopathic or neuropathic changes, or both, are found.[18,19]

POSTINFLUENZAL MYOSITIS

Postinfluenzal myositis is characterized by muscle pain and tenderness, sometimes accompanied by swelling, that develops within a week following a bout of influenza. It is especially common in children, but occasionally occurs in older persons. Symptoms generally settle over a week or so, but during the active phase, electromyography may show abnormalities suggestive of a multifocal, myopathic process.[20]

ECHOVIRUS MYOSITIS

Electromyographic changes suggestive of myopathy have been reported in cases of myositis that are associated with infection of the central nervous system by echovirus in the context of agammaglobulinemia.[21,22]

TRICHINOSIS

Trichinosis is contracted by ingesting infested meat, usually pork, and its incidence is still relatively high in the United States. Its clinical manifestations are variable, but the most common is a myositis. In patients with trichinosis, motor unit potentials and their recruitment pattern are often of the myopathic type, but excessive insertion activity, profuse fibrillation potentials, and positive sharp waves may also be found.[23,24] The electromyographic pattern is, therefore, similar to that seen in polymyositis. Treatment with steroids and a benzimidazole drug is useful, and marked clinical improvement may be accompanied by reversion of the electromyogram to normal. In some patients, however, the electromyographic findings are normal at all times, presumably because of the patchy nature of the underlying pathology.

TOXOPLASMOSIS

Muscle pain and weakness may occur in patients with the clinical features of toxoplasmosis. Muscle involvement by *Toxoplasma gondii* may lead to typical myopathic changes in the electromyogram, accompanied in some cases by abnormal spontaneous activity.[25,26]

POLYMYALGIA RHEUMATICA

Polymyalgia rheumatica occurs more commonly in women than in men and rarely affects patients younger than 50 years of age. It is characterized by muscle pain and stiffness, and the erythrocyte sedimentation rate is increased. Neither electromyography nor muscle biopsy usually reveals any abnormality. However, if quantitative analysis is performed (see Ch. 8), myopathic changes may be revealed by electromyography in 61 percent of cases and by muscle biopsy in 35 percent.[27]

SARCOID MYOPATHY

The muscles may coincidentally be involved in patients with systemic sarcoidosis, or they may show generalized involvement in patients without symptoms of involvement elsewhere. Patients with the latter clinical profile develop progressive muscle weakness and wasting, similar to that of a primary disorder of muscle, and motor unit potentials are of a myopathic type.[28] Abnormal spontaneous activity is usually not present. The electromyographic findings may be more difficult to interpret if, for example, the peripheral nerves are involved (see Ch. 11), but they are then especially valuable in determining the extent to which the neuropathy is contributing to symptoms.[29]

Endocrine Myopathies

Myopathy may occur in patients with thyrotoxicosis, myxedema, hyperparathyroidism, hypoparathyroidism, hypopituitarism, acromegaly, or Cushing's syndrome, or in patients undergoing treatment with steroids. It may also occur in Conn's syndrome.[30] In general, the electrophysiologic changes are characteristic of a myopathy, and abnormal spontaneous activity is not found, but normal findings are common in steroid myopathy. The muscle involvement that occurs in patients with thyroid disorders, however, may be atypical in some respects.

In thyrotoxicosis, weakness, muscle atrophy, and electromyographic abnormalities occur more commonly in proximal than in distal muscles, and involve the arms more often than the legs. Fasciculation potentials may be present, but other types of spontaneous activity are not found. Motor unit potentials are similar to those occurring in other myopathies, with an increased incidence of short-duration potentials and increased polyphasia. Some authors have reported evidence of denervation in the distal muscles of the legs despite a paucity of clinical signs there and in the presence of normal motor conduction velocity in the peripheral nerves.[31] Histologic examination generally reveals little or no loss of muscle fibers, but there may be a reduction in the diameter of the muscle fibers.[32] This, together with the clinical and electromyographic improvement that accompanies successful treatment of the thyroid disorder,[33,34] suggests that the myopathy is attributable to a disturbance in function of the muscle fibers. An acquired variety of periodic paralysis, of hypokalemic type, may also occur in association with thyrotoxicosis (p. 79).

The clinical manifestations of muscle involvement in cases of myxedema are varied and do not parallel the hypothyroidism in terms of severity.[35] The delay in muscular relaxation that sometimes occurs has occasionally been mistaken for myotonia, but the electromyogram does not show the characteristic repetitive discharges of true myotonia. Slowness of contraction and relaxation has been reported in association with muscle hypertrophy and weakness in adults (Hoffman's syndrome) and cretinous children (Debré-Sémélaigne syndrome). In other cases of hypothyroidism, a girdle myopathy, characterized by mild, proximal muscle weakness and wasting, has been described.[36] There is no general agreement on the electromyographic findings associated with this clinical entity, but several authors have reported an increase in insertion activity.[37–39] Spontaneous fibrillation and fasciculation potentials, as well as trains of complex repetitive discharges, are sometimes found,[39] but this is probably uncommon unless there is concomitant neuropathy. In 20 unselected patients, Rao and associates found no abnormal spontaneous activity,[40] confirming earlier studies that used quantitative techniques.[41] The appearance and recruitment pattern of motor unit potentials either show changes consistent with a myopathy or they are normal.

Some of the endocrine disturbances that give rise to a myopathy may be associated with other types of neuromuscular disorders, and these may complicate interpretation of the electromyographic findings. For example, various types of neuropathy may occur in diabetics, patients with myxedema or acromegaly are liable to develop carpal tunnel syndromes or polyneuropathies, hypoparathyroidism may cause tetany, and myasthenia gravis or hypokalemic periodic paralysis sometimes occurs in association with thyrotoxicosis. Episodic weakness similar to that which occurs in hypokalemic periodic paralysis also occurs in Conn's syndrome. These disorders are considered in other sections of this book.

Metabolic Myopathies

Clinical and electromyographic features of a myopathy may be found in patients with osteomalacia or chronic renal failure. Hypokalemic myopathy often occurs in association with drug therapy (p. 80). Rarer metabolic disorders associated with a myopathy include lysine cystinuria, in which the electromyogram may be normal,[42] and xanthinuria, in which short-duration, polyphasic motor unit potentials are found.[43]

In carnitine deficiency myopathy, the electromyogram may reveal motor unit potentials of low amplitude and brief duration, with an increased incidence of polyphasic forms.[44,45] Muscle stiffness and myoglobinuria after exercise may occur with carnitine palmityl transferase deficiency, and needle electromyography is reportedly normal in such patients.[46]

A number of other metabolic disorders affect muscle function, but their electrophysiologic characteristics require more detailed description.

THE PERIODIC PARALYSIS SYNDROMES

Periodic paralysis syndromes, which may be familial or acquired, are characterized by episodes of flaccid weakness or paralysis, often occurring in association with abnormalities of the plasma potassium level. In hypokalemic periodic paralysis, impulse propagation by the muscle fiber membrane is blocked for reasons that are uncertain. There is an influx of potassium ions into the muscle fiber from the extracellular fluid, but the membrane becomes not hyperpolarized[47] but depolarized.[48] In hyperkalemic periodic paralysis, the muscle fiber membrane becomes depolarized to a variable degree, but this cannot be accounted for by an efflux of potassium ions from the fiber. Creutzfeldt and co-workers have suggested that this depolarization is a result of an increased permeability of the membrane to sodium,[48] which may also occur in the periodic paralysis that is associated with normal plasma potassium levels.[49] The paralysis itself has been attributed by some to muscle fiber inexcitability secondary to inactivation of the regenerative sodium conductance system,[49] but the precise pathophysiologic mechanism remains uncertain.

In the hypokalemic variety, attacks often occur upon awakening or after exercise or a heavy meal, and they may last for several days. Electromyographic studies obtained during attacks reveal no abnormal insertion or spontaneous activity, but the motor unit potentials are of short duration and are reduced in number so that the interference pattern is diminished. In severe cases, there is complete electrical silence during attempted voluntary contraction of the muscle.[47] Between attacks, there is either no abnormality or, less commonly, there is clinical and electromyographic evidence of a proximal myopathy.

Attacks associated with an elevated plasma potassium level (adynamia episodica hereditaria) tend to occur after exercise and usually last for less than an hour, whereas those accompanied by normal potassium levels last longer and are more severe. Electromyographic findings may or may not be normal between attacks, but during attacks, insertion activity is increased; spontaneous fibrillation potentials, myotonic discharges, and complex repetitive discharges may be evident; and motor unit potentials are reduced in duration and number.[50,51]

GLYCOGEN STORAGE DISEASES

Several of the glycogen storage diseases affect muscle, the main ones in this respect being attributable to deficiencies of acid maltase (Pompe's disease), debrancher enzyme (Cori's disease), phosphorylase (McArdle's disease), or phosphofructokinase. With regard to their muscular manifestations, both Pompe's and Cori's disease may lead to hypotonia and muscle weakness. Although Pompe's disease often has a rapidly progressive course leading to death from cardiac or respiratory failure before the age of 2 years, mild cases survive for much longer and sometimes simulate muscular dystrophy; cases presenting in the adult years have also been described.[52] The electromyogram of affected patients is myopathic in type, but abnormal spontaneous activity consisting of fibrillation potentials, positive sharp waves, myotonic discharges, and complex repetitive potentials may be found.[52-54] Deficiency of debrancher enzyme may also present in adults with slowly progressive weakness, and there may be distal wasting. However, clinical myopathy does not seem to affect all patients with this disorder. The subject has been reviewed by DiMauro and associates[55] who reported that electromyography may reveal "a mixed pattern" with abnormal spontaneous activity (fibrillations, positive waves, complex repetitive discharges, and sometimes fasciculations) and short, polyphasic motor unit potentials of reduced or normal amplitudes in some patients and long or high-voltage polyphasic potentials in other patients.

In phosphorylase or phosphofructokinase deficiency, muscle stiffness, pain, and weakness occur during exertion, and a contracture develops if exercise is continued. Electromyography of resting muscle is usually normal, and no electrical activity can be recorded during the period of contracture.[56,57]

Myopathy Secondary to Drugs or Alcohol

A number of drugs cause weakness of myogenic origin.[58] The myopathy induced by steroids is perhaps the most widely recognized in this context. In that disorder, electromyography may reveal changes consistent with a diffuse myopathic process, without abnormal spontaneous activity, or the findings may be normal.

Drugs that cause hypokalemia may lead to myopathic changes, which are often accompanied by fibrillation potentials and other evidence of muscle fiber irritability.

Chloroquine occasionally leads to progressive, proximal muscle weakness that begins in the legs. The presence of increased numbers of short-duration or polyphasic motor unit potentials in the electromyogram is suggestive of a myopathy. However, in other sites, the number of functional units may be reduced. These changes, together with the reduced conduction velocity of peripheral nerves that is sometimes noted, indicate that there are both myogenic and neurogenic components of the weakness induced by chloroquine.[59]

Clofibrate may cause a myopathy with typical electromyographic changes, whereas myopathy secondary to epsilon aminocaproic acid, emetine, and certain beta blocker drugs may be characterized in addition by an increase in insertion activity and spontaneous fibrillations. Experimental and pathologic studies indicate that vincristine may occasionally lead to a myopathy, but the electrophysiologic abnormalities found in patients receiving this drug are usually those of a neuropathy.[60] Rare cases of a myopathy caused by colchicine[61] and accompanied by appropriate electromyographic changes have also been described. Myotonic discharges are sometimes found in the muscles of patients receiving diazocholesterol, but motor unit potentials are normal in configuration and weakness is unusual in these cases.[62]

D-pencillamine may cause a disorder resembling polymyositis, and can also induce myasthenia gravis. A number of other drugs may similarly cause a myasthenic syndrome, as described in Chapter 14.

Several types of muscle disorders may occur in chronic alcoholics.[32] Acute, reversible muscle necrosis may occur shortly after acute intoxication and is characterized by muscle pain, swelling, and tenderness,[63] sometimes accompanied by myoglobinuria. Needle examination may reveal spontaneous fibrillation and positive sharp waves, as well as small, short-duration motor unit potentials suggestive of a myopathy. A somewhat similar electromyographic appearance occurs in patients with acute alcoholic hypokalemic myopathy. This is a disorder that develops during an alcoholic binge and in which progressive limb weakness occurs without muscle pain, swelling, or tenderness and without myoglobinuria.[64] In other instances, progressive, proximal muscle weakness and wasting may develop over several weeks, accompanied by electromyographic signs of a myopathy. Similar electrical abnormalities may also be found in patients without clinical evidence of myopathy.[65]

Congenital Myopathies of Unknown Etiology

Congenital myopathies of unknown origin are primary myopathies that present in early life and are usually nonprogressive. Microscopic examination reveals degenerative or structural changes that, in some cases, have permitted distinct entities to be recognized. *Central core disease* is characterized by large muscle fibers with abnormal and probably nonfunctional central cores, whereas *nemaline myopathy* may be distinguished by the presence of subsarcolemmal rods that are thought to result from Z-band degeneration. *Mitochondrial myopathy* is characterized by the presence of abnormal or excessive numbers of mitochondria (megaconial and pleoconial forms, respectively), and *centronuclear myopathy* is distinguishable by the presence of fibers containing central nuclei rather than fibrils. These disorders lead to hypotonia and weakness of the limb muscles, although additional clinical features are associated with some of them. For instance, weakness of the extraocular and facial muscles is common in centronuclear myopathy, and skeletal changes may accompany nemaline myopathy. The electromyogram is normal or myopathic in type, but abnormal spontaneous activity may be seen in the nemaline and centronuclear varieties. In the latter, the abnormal spontaneous activity may include myotonic discharges.[66]

Another group of congenital myopathies is characterized by abnormalities in the distribution of muscle fiber types. Congenital fiber type disproportion may take several histologic forms, but patients are clinically similar, presenting with hypotonia at birth, weakness, developmental delay, and commonly, skeletal abnormalities. Functional performance improves with age. At electromyography, insertion and spontaneous activity are usually normal, but the mean amplitude and duration of motor unit potentials are reduced, the incidence of polyphasic motor unit potentials is increased, and the number of motor units recruited for a given degree of voluntary activity is excessive.[66]

A number of other congenital myopathies have been described in recent years, but do not merit consideration here.

Myopathy and Malignant Disease

Polymyositis or dermatomyositis may develop in patients who have, or are developing, a malignant tumor, as may a proximal, noninflammatory myopathy. A myopathy may also occur as a result of the metabolic or endocrine disturbances that are sometimes associated with malignant disease. The electromyographic findings are as described earlier, but they may be complicated by concomitant neuropathy or myasthenic syndrome associated with the malignant disease, or by denervation secondary to metastases.

Myotonic Disorders

CLINICAL FEATURES

Myotonic disorders are characterized by a delay in the ability of affected muscles to relax following a contraction, due probably to an abnormality of the muscle fiber membrane. Patients complain of muscle stiffness, and myotonia can usually be demonstrated clinically by a difficulty in relaxing handgrip or by the response of an affected muscle to percussion of its belly.

Dystrophia myotonica is a slowly progressive, dominantly inherited disorder that usually appears in the third or fourth decade but may develop in early childhood. Myotonia is accompanied, and often overshadowed, by weakness and wasting of the facial, sternomastoid, and distal limb muscles. Other associated features include cataracts, frontal baldness in men, gonadal atrophy and other endocrine disturbances, cardiac involvement, and intellectual changes.

Myotonia congenita may have either a dominant or a recessive mode of transmission. The dominant form (Thomsen's disease) is usually present from birth, but may not appear until early childhood. The only symptom is muscle stiffness, which is enhanced by cold and inactivity and relieved by exercise. The muscles are diffusely hypertrophied, but are not weak. In contrast, the recessive form, which has a rather late onset, is associated with mild weakness and atrophy of distal muscles.

Paramyotonia congenita is a dominantly inherited disorder in which myotonia and generalized weakness of the voluntary muscles occur in response to cold and are exacerbated by rest after exercise, or by sleep. Controversy surrounds its precise relationship to the periodic paralysis syndromes.

Chondrodystrophic myotonia, or the *Schwartz-Jampel syndrome,* is a disorder that is probably inherited in an autosomal recessive manner and is characterized by stiff muscles, abnormal gait, dwarfism, skeletal deformities, and developmental anomalies of the face and orbit.[67,68] Fariello and associates recently summarized the previously published cases of this syndrome and described the findings in a patient of their own.[69] It appears that it is not a homogeneous disorder, and that its only consistent feature is the unusual muscle physiology.

ELECTROMYOGRAPHIC FEATURES

The characteristic electromyographic feature of the myotonic disorders is the occurrence of high-frequency discharges of potentials that wax and wane in frequency and amplitude, producing a sound like that of a dive-bomber over the loudspeaker. These potentials are evoked by electrode movement and by percussion or voluntary contraction of the muscle, as described in Chapter 5. In the Schwartz-Jampel syndrome, complex repetitive discharges may occur, as may high-frequency discharges of a relatively constant frequency, which may be present both at rest and during activity. The latter discharges are referred to as *neuromyotonia* (p. 59) and, unlike classical myotonia, can be abolished by curare.[70] Motor unit potentials are generally normal in appearance except in dystrophia myotonica and the recessive type of myotonia congenita, in which they show myopathic features. Low-voltage, short-duration potentials may also be found in the Schwartz-Jampel syndrome.[69] In dystrophia myotonica, there may be a mild slowing of motor conduction velocity and a reduction in the number of functional motor units.[71] The electrical response of muscles to repetitive nerve stimulation commonly shows a decrement in the myotonic disorders, but this is not invariable. The occurrence of a decrement is unrelated to disease severity or precise diagnosis, and is not related consistently to the presence of weakness.[72]

In paramyotonia congenita, but not myotonia congenita, profuse fibrillations may be found in muscles after exercise, and cold (20°C) induces a marked reduction in the size of the compound muscle action potential. Cold may also increase or induce a decrement to repetitive (2 Hz) stimulation, and markedly diminishes or abolishes myotonic discharges and voluntary recruitment of motor unit potentials on needle examination.[73]

Dystrophia myotonica is believed to result from a single dominant gene, but the nature, severity, and age of onset of its clinical manifestations vary widely. For prognostic and genetic purposes, therefore, at-tention has been devoted to identifying carriers of the gene among asymptomatic subjects presumed to be at risk for the disorder because of their family history. Polgar and colleagues found that the most useful procedure for detecting carriers of the gene was a physical examination, but concluded that, in clinically normal subjects, electromyography was the most helpful ancillary procedure.[74] Bundey and associates similarly reported that electromyographic abnormalities were present in asymptomatic subjects, although they found that slit lamp examination for the presence of lenticular abnormalities was even more productive in identifying carriers of the gene.[75] These studies thus suggest that electromyography has a definite place in the investigation of asymptomatic relatives to determine whether they, too, are at risk for developing dystrophia myotonica.

NEUROPATHIC DISORDERS

Electromyography has no practical role in the diagnosis of upper motor neuron lesions, and further reference to such disorders is deferred to Chapter 15. The following discussion is concerned only with those conditions in which there is lower motor neuron involvement. In such circumstances, weakness is accompanied by wasting, and sometimes fasciculation, of affected muscles, and the tendon reflexes are depressed or absent if their arc is interrupted. The electromyographic findings are variable, depending as they do on a number of different factors.

Immediately after the onset of an acute neuropathic lesion, motor unit potentials are normal in appearance but reduced in number. A complete interference pattern is not seen during maximal effort despite a significant increase in the firing rate of individual units, and in severe cases, no units may remain under voluntary control. If denervation has occurred, insertion activity increases after several days, and spontaneous fibrillation, positive sharp waves, fasciculation, and complex repetitive discharges may eventually be found. The earliest time at which abnormal spontaneous activity is encountered depends very much on the site of the lesion, as described in Chapter 5, but it may not be for as long as 5 to 6 weeks. As reinnervation occurs, spontaneous activity becomes less conspicuous and low-amplitude, short- or long-duration motor unit potentials are seen, some of which have a complex polyphasic form. The interference pattern during maximal effort is still incomplete, and units fire at fast rates. With further recovery, however, the number of motor unit potentials seen during voluntary activity increases and many potentials revert to a normal appearance. The extent of any residual electromyographic abnormalities depends on the completeness of recovery.

In disorders causing chronic partial denervation, long-duration motor unit potentials of increased amplitude are found when the underlying lesion involves the anterior horn cells. With more peripheral lesions, motor units of long duration are also seen, but their amplitude is usually increased only slightly or even decreased. With lesions in either situation, the incidence of polyphasic potentials is excessive, the interference pattern is reduced and the motor unit firing rate is increased during maximal contractions, and abnormal insertion and spontaneous activity is usually present. The pathophysiologic basis of these changes has already been considered in Chapter 5 and need not be reiterated.

The distribution of clinical and electromyographic abnormalities in patients with neurogenic weakness depends on the site of the underlying pathology. Further details regarding the findings in various disorders are provided below.

Spinal Cord Disorders

LOCALIZED MYELOPATHIES

The spinal cord may be involved by tumors or developmental anomalies, and compressive, spondylotic, traumatic, ischemic, and inflammatory myelopathies may also occur. Weakness is often accompanied by sensory or sphincter disturbances, and pain is a conspicuous feature of some disorders. In addition to signs of lower motor neuron involvement at the level of the lesion, there is usually clinical evidence of a pyramidal deficit below it. These clinical features, supplemented by information obtained from radiologic contrast procedures, usually permit the lesion to be localized to the cord. Electromyography is sometimes helpful in defining the severity and segmental distribution of any lower motor neuron involvement, but it cannot be used to distinguish between the various possible causes of the lesion. The changes found are similar to those accompanying motor neuron disease (described later in the chapter), but are more restricted in their distribution.

POLIOMYELITIS

In poliomyelitis, the cells in the anterior horns of the spinal cord are invaded by poliovirus and degenerate. Weakness is of rapid onset, often begins in association with clinical evidence of aseptic meningitis, frequently follows a general systemic illness, and is not accompanied by sensory loss. Any of the muscles of the limbs, trunk, or lower cranial nerves may be affected, but the motor deficit is commonly restricted to one limb. Progression of the deficit occurs for 3 to 4 days, after which it stabilizes.

The electromyographic findings in affected muscles depend on the timing of the examination after onset of the weakness. During the first month or so, the only abnormality may be a reduction in the number of motor unit potentials occurring during attempted voluntary contraction; the interference pattern is reduced, and in severe cases, there is complete electrical silence. After this, however, insertion activity increases, and spontaneous fibrillations and fasciculation potentials and positive sharp waves are found. An increase occurs in the mean amplitude and duration of motor unit potentials, as well as in the number of motor unit potentials that are polyphasic. The presence of profuse fibrillation potentials in a muscle retaining no motor units under voluntary control is generally indicative of a poor prognosis for recovery. As reinnervation occurs, fibrillation potentials become less conspicuous, but often persist to a mild degree. Long-duration, "giant" motor unit potentials are seen, some of which may have an amplitude of more than 10 mV. Years after the illness, such evidence of reinnervation may be found in muscles that clinically appear normal.[76] Nerve conduction velocity is normal, but the size of the compound muscle action potential elicited from clinically involved muscles may be reduced, depending on the severity of denervation. Sometimes there is also a defect of neuromuscular transmission, as evidenced by a decrement in the amplitude of the action potential recorded from the surface of the muscle during repetitive stimulation of its motor nerve.

POSTPOLIOMYELITIS SYNDROME

Progressive muscle weakness and wasting may occur many years after poliomyelitis in occasional patients. Electromyography may reveal some spontaneous fibrillations, and fasciculation, but this is usually sparse; there is reduced recruitment of motor units, and an increased incidence of large motor unit potentials. These electromyographic findings do not predict clinical progression of the disorder. When progression occurs, it does so very gradually, unlike amyotrophic lateral sclerosis. The pathogenesis of the disorder is unknown. There is no evidence of reinfection with—or reactivation of—poliovirus. Some attribute the progressive deficit to the effect of aging, with loss of anterior horn cells from a pool that was previously depleted by the original infection,[76,77] whereas others believe it represents a special, more restricted and benign form of amyotrophic lateral sclerosis.[78]

NONHEREDITARY DEGENERATIVE DISORDERS OF ANTERIOR HORN CELLS

Motor neuron disease is a degenerative disorder characterized clinically by signs of mainly lower motor neuron involvement of the spinal cord (progressive spinal muscular atrophy) or brain stem (progressive bulbar palsy), by signs of a predominantly upper motor neuron deficit in the cord or brain stem (primary lateral sclerosis or pseudobulbar palsy, respectively), or by mixed upper and lower motor neuron signs (*amyotrophic lateral sclerosis*). There is no sensory loss.

A primary degeneration of anterior horn cells, without sensory or conspicuous corticospinal tract involvement, also occurs in a number of other disorders, and these frequently have a hereditary basis. In the past, they were often mistaken for one or another of the muscular dystrophies because of their familial nature, the distribution of the weakness and wasting to which they eventually lead, and their occurrence in infants and children.

The typical electromyographic findings in these degenerative motor disorders are of chronic partial denervation with increased insertion activity; spontaneous occurrence of fasciculations, fibrillation potentials, positive sharp waves, and complex repetitive discharges; and impaired recruitment of motor units with a reduced interference pattern. The mean duration and amplitude of the motor unit potentials are increased, "giant" potentials may be encountered (as in other disorders in which the anterior horn cells are involved), and there is an increased incidence of polyphasic potentials. Stimulation techniques reveal that sensory action potentials and conduction velocity are normal, that motor conduction velocity is usually normal but may be slightly reduced because the fastest conducting fibers have degenerated, and that there may be electrophysiologic evidence of a neuromuscular transmission defect (see Ch. 14).

At least in amyotrophic lateral sclerosis and progressive spinal muscular atrophy, variation in the amplitude and morphology of motor unit potentials over brief periods of time signifies active disease and indicates a poor prognosis.[79] Similarly, a decrement in the size of the compound muscle action potential in response to repetitive stimulations of its motor nerve at slow rates (see Ch. 14) has also been thought to suggest active disease and a poor prognosis.[80]

Two general points of practical importance require emphasis. First, the electromyographic examination of patients suspected of having one of these irremediable disorders should be planned so that the information obtained excludes other conditions that might be more amenable to treatment. The number of muscles sampled should, therefore, be sufficient to provide evidence of more widespread denervation than could occur with a single, localized cord lesion. Abnormal spontaneous activity is found most readily in weak, wasted muscles. After the clinically involved limbs have been examined, the muscles in other limbs or those supplied by the cranial nerves should be examined to determine whether there is more widespread involvement. Nerve conduction studies should always be performed to exclude a peripheral nerve disorder. Especially if compound muscle action potentials are recorded from muscles that are markedly wasted as a result of neurogenic atrophy, the responses to supramaximal stimulation of motor nerves will be abnormally small, reflecting the severity of axonal loss. Maximal motor conduction velocity may be slightly reduced (because of loss of the fastest conducting fibers) or normal, and F wave latencies may be slightly increased. Sensory conduction studies are normal. Unfortunately, it is not possible to distinguish between anterior horn cell disease and pathology involving multiple anterior nerve roots by these means.[81]

Second, although fasciculation potentials are encountered in most cases of motor neuron disease, they may also be found in some normal subjects and in a number of patients with other neuromuscular disorders. As Lambert has stressed, the significance of these potentials can only be assessed by reference to clinical and other electromyographic findings.[82]

In patients with pure upper motor neuron deficits, no abnormalities may be found at electromyography.[83] However, there may be poor activation of motor units so that only a few fire, and then only at low rates, despite maximal voluntary effort.

Juvenile spinal muscular atrophy simulating the Kugelberg-Welander syndrome may occur in association with hexosaminidase deficiency[84,85] that can be recognized in the course of Tay-Sachs screening. Motor neuron disease of the classic variety may also be simulated by pure lower motor neuron syndromes occurring in association with paraproteinemias,[81,86,87] and these are responsive to cytotoxic drugs and plasmapheresis. A fascinating case of a pure motor syndrome clinically resembling progressive spinal muscular atrophy and associated with an IgM gammopathy was recently reported. At autopsy, the syndrome was found to be caused by pathology affecting primarily the anterior nerve roots.[81]

FOCAL FORMS OF SPINAL MUSCULAR ATROPHY

Focal forms of spinal muscular atrophy, usually involving one of the upper limbs, have been described. A series of 71 cases reported from Japan has permitted delineation of this disorder. It occurs more commonly in men than women,[88] and it is characterized by a juvenile onset, with a restricted distribution of muscle atrophy in the hand and forearm. There is no definite sensory or cranial nerve involvement. The tendon reflexes are usually depressed in the affected limb. Onset is insidious, with rapid progression for the first 2 years or so and slow progression thereafter. The electrophysiologic findings are of chronic partial denervation similar to that described above, except that it is more restricted in distribution. Needle examination of non-atrophic muscles on the clinically unaffected side, however, reveals similar abnormalities in most patients, suggesting bilateral involvement.[88] Motor conduction velocity in the nerves of the arm is normal.

HEREDITARY SPINAL MUSCULAR ATROPHY

Several varieties of hereditary spinal muscular atrophy may be distinguished by the pattern of inheritance, age of onset, and muscles affected.[89] Similar disorders may also occur on an apparently sporadic basis.

Predominant Involvement of Proximal Muscles

When spinal muscular atrophy begins in infancy, the clinical presentation is with weakness and hypotonia. The disorder often progresses rapidly, leading to a fatal outcome before about 5 years of age (Werdnig-Hoffmann disease). This clinical course is not invariable, however, and the disease sometimes progresses more slowly, despite an early age of onset. In either case, inheritance is usually as an autosomal recessive trait.

When onset occurs in later childhood or adolescence, the disease generally follows a progressive but more benign course, again having an autosomal recessive mode of inheritance (Kugelberg-Welander disease). Similar cases with a benign course may begin in adulthood. Less commonly, progressive spinal muscular atrophy affecting the limbs diffusely, but with a proximal emphasis, occurs with a dominant mode of inheritance.

Needle electromyography may be helpful in distinguishing this group of disorders from a myopathy, with which it is sometimes confused because of the conspicuous involvement of the proximal muscles. In Werdnig-Hoffmann disease, spontaneously occurring motor unit potentials may also be found, even during sleep.[90] Motor conduction velocity is generally normal or reduced only slightly.

Conspicuous Involvement of Distal Muscles

The form of hereditary spinal muscular atrophy that primarily involves the distal muscles may be inherited as either an autosomal dominant or a recessive trait, with onset during either childhood or adult life. Although the motor deficit is usually more conspicuous in the legs than in the arms, in some instances the converse is true. The disorder is usually gradually progressive with a relatively benign prognosis, although at least one variety follows a more rapid downhill course. This group of progressive distal spinal muscular atrophies represents one form of Charcot-Marie-Tooth disease, or peroneal muscular atrophy. Such hereditary cases usually are fairly symmetric clinically. Needle electromyography provides evidence of chronic partial denervation in affected muscles. Maximal motor conduction velocity is usually normal or reduced only slightly, and sensory conduction studies are similarly normal.

Other Varieties

Other hereditary varieties of progressive spinal muscular atrophy have been described. In particular, there may be involvement distally in the legs and proximally in the arms, with either a dominant or recessive mode of inheritance. Such a scapuloperoneal distribution may mimic myopathic disorders, and definitive diagnosis may only be possible on the basis of electromyography, muscle biopsy, or both. Bulbospinal involvement, inherited on an X-linked recessive basis, and rare hereditary forms are described in a recent review by Harding.[89]

The results of quantitative electromyography in a large number of patients with the infantile or juvenile forms of spinal muscular atrophy have recently been reported. Spontaneous, rhythmic firing of motor units was found in patients with Werdnig-Hoffmann disease and in intermediate forms of spinal muscular atrophy, but not in Kugelberg-Welander disease. Fibrillations and fasciculations, by contrast, were more common in Werdnig-Hoffmann disease. Complex repetitive discharges were never seen in children younger than about 6 years of age, and became increasingly common with advancing age and duration of disease. Motor unit parameters also differed in the different forms of the disease. In Werdnig-Hoffmann disease, some of the motor units were small and of short duration, whereas others were large and of long duration. The mean amplitude and duration of potentials was increased to a greater extent in Kugelberg-Welander disease than in intermediate forms of proximal spinal muscular atrophy, and this was attributed to the presence of hypertrophic muscle fibers and of signs of reinnervation. Furthermore, mean duration of the potentials increased with age in these patients to a much greater extent than in age-matched controls. Such differences suggest that, in the early stages of spinal muscular atrophy, the electromyographic findings may have prognostic as well as diagnostic value.[91]

Root Lesions

A clear understanding of the anatomy of the spinal nerve roots is an essential prerequisite to the electromyographic examination of patients suspected of having a radiculopathy. Anterior and posterior roots emerge from the spinal cord at each segmental level, uniting just lateral to the posterior root ganglia to form the spinal nerves that pass out through the intervertebral foramina. Each nerve divides into anterior and posterior primary rami, the former innervating the limbs and the lateral and anterior aspects of the trunk and the latter supplying the back. Only the anterior primary rami, therefore, contribute to the brachial and lumbosacral plexuses from which the nerves to the limbs arise, and the main limb nerves contain contributions from several different spinal roots.

The most common causes of an isolated radiculopathy are spondylosis and prolapse of an intervertebral disc. Other causes include trauma; metastasis; myelomatosis; vertebral osteitis; extramedullary spinal tumors, such as neurofibromas or meningiomas; and developmental anomalies. A more widespread radiculopathy may result from neoplastic, infective, inflammatory, or toxic causes.

Patients with an isolated root lesion often experience pain, and may have segmental muscle weakness, wasting, and sensory disturbances. Depending on the level of the lesion, sphincter function may also be impaired. Electromyographic examination may reveal signs of chronic partial denervation in the muscles supplied by the affected root, but motor unit potentials do not often reach an amplitude comparable to that found in myelopathic disorders. The paraspinal muscles generally show abnormalities sooner than the limb muscles and should, therefore, be examined with particular care in patients in whom the duration of symptoms has been brief. Even so, abnormalities may not be found until 7 to 10 days after onset of the lesion. No conclusions should be reached concerning the segmental level of the lesion based on findings in the paraspinal muscles, however, because there is considerable overlap in the territory supplied by each of the posterior primary rami.

The number of limb muscles examined must be sufficient to demonstrate that the distribution of electromyographic abnormalities conforms to a radicular rather than a peripheral nerve distribution. For the convenience of readers, some of the limb muscles that can easily be examined electromyographically are tabulated in Chapter 13, where they are arranged according to the spinal segments and peripheral nerves that supply them. If a peripheral nerve lesion is suspected, motor conduction velocity should always be measured in nerves supplying the affected muscles. It may be slow if the nerve is, indeed, affected, but it is normal when the root is involved because fibers in the nerve that originate from other roots continue to conduct at normal velocities. The size of the compound muscle action potential elicited by supramaximal nerve stimulation of weak, wasted muscles may, however, be reduced, indicating that there has been axonal loss. Sensory action potentials, recorded peripherally, are normal unless there is coexisting disease affecting the sensory root ganglia or fibers distal to this point. The distinction between a root and plexus lesion is discussed below.

Because of the frequency with which radiculopathies are encountered in clinical practice, the comprehensive electrophysiologic investigation of these lesions is considered in detail in Chapter 13.

Plexus Lesions

Brachial plexus lesions are often related to developmental anomalies or minor variations in the anatomy of the cervicobrachial region. They may also result from other compressive lesions, neoplastic infiltration, irradiation, or trauma, as do lesions of the lumbosacral plexus. A brachial neuritis without obvious cause (termed neuralgic amyotrophy) may also occur, in some cases developing a few days after surgical procedures, infective illnesses, or injections of serum or vaccine. The distribution of clinical signs and electromyographic abnormalities depends on the site and extent of the lesion, as discussed in Chapter 13. Depending on their precise location, lesions of the lumbosacral plexus may cause weakness and sensory symptoms in a polyradicular or peripheral nerve distribution in the legs (see Ch. 13).

Electromyographic sampling of affected muscles may reveal signs of partial denervation but, as already indicated, the timing of the examination is important in this respect. Myokymic discharges may also be present in patients with radiation-induced plexopathy. Since only the anterior primary rami contribute to the plexuses, a proximal radiculopathy can be distinguished from a plexus lesion by sampling the muscles supplied by the posterior primary rami. Signs of denervation in the paraspinal as well as the limb muscles indicate that the lesion involves both anterior and posterior primary rami, thereby suggesting a root lesion. Root and plexus lesions can also be differentiated by recording appropriate sensory action potentials in the extremities. These potentials are lost or attenuated if the lesion is beyond the posterior root ganglion and causes wallerian degeneration of afferent fibers, but they are preserved when the lesion is proximal, as in a radiculopathy, because peripheral sensory fibers do not then degenerate.

In distinguishing a lesion involving the plexus from a peripheral nerve lesion, the history and physical signs are of paramount importance. However, electrophysiologic assessment may also be useful as it permits the distribution of affected muscles to be delineated and enables conduction velocity to be measured in the nerve in question. Little help in distinguishing between these two types of lesion is provided by techniques in which the trunks of the brachial plexus are stimulated percutaneously at Erb's point while the responses of the proximal muscles of the arm are recorded. This is because the latency of the responses may be normal or prolonged in either case. For example, Gassel found that, in patients with brachial neuritis or a brachial plexus injury, latencies were prolonged in some wasted muscles and normal in others, and this presumably depends on whether all of the fastest conducting nerve fibers to a particular muscle are affected.[92]

The electrophysiologic evaluation of plexopathies includes the application of a number of techniques other than needle electromyography. Accordingly, further details of these lesions and their electrophysiologic characterization are presented in Chapter 13.

Peripheral Nerve Lesions

Disorders of the peripheral nerves may occur as a result of trauma or for a variety of other reasons, and reference has already been made to the abnormalities that may be found when affected muscles are sampled electromyographically. The distribution of these changes may be helpful in confirming that there is isolated peripheral nerve involvement and in distinguishing between this type of lesion and a lesion that is located more proximally (for example, at the level of the limb plexus or the individual nerve roots). The pathologic site may also be localized more precisely to a particular level of the peripheral nerve or one of its main nerve trunks by determining the pattern of muscles in which abnormalities are detected on needle examination. In patients known to have an isolated mononeuropathy, as may follow injury, for example, the electromyographic findings may help to indicate the severity and completeness of the lesion, may provide a guide to prognosis, and can be used to follow the course of recovery. In patients with polyneuropathies, electromyographic abnormalities are present in limb muscles and have a predominantly distal distribution. If the neuropathy is of the demyelinative variety, abnormal insertion and spontaneous activity is often relatively inconspicuous, but there is poor recruitment of motor units in weak muscles. In axonal polyneuropathies, by contrast, both conspicuous abnormal spontaneous activity and reduced recruitment of motor units may be found, and large, long-duration, polyphasic units may be present if reinnervation has occurred.

Motor and sensory conduction velocity, as well as the amplitude of sensory action potentials, can be measured in individual nerves, and the information obtained thereby is of particular importance in determining the nature of nerve involvement and the site of any localized lesion. Such studies are usually done in conjunction with needle electromyography. Further discussion of peripheral nerve lesions is therefore deferred to the following chapters, in which their clinical and electrophysiologic features are considered in detail.

Miscellaneous Disorders

Cramps are characterized clinically by the involuntary, painful shortening of a muscle. Electromyographic examination shows that they are associated with intermittent bursts of repetitive, high-frequency motor unit discharges in different parts of the muscle.[93] Cramps may occur on a familial basis and in a number of generalized, metabolic disorders, but their pathogenesis and site of origin are unknown.[94] Most people experience occasional cramps, and these are of no clinical relevance.

A *contracture* also involves a painful, involuntary shortening of a muscle but, unlike a cramp, it is electrically silent and not accompanied by motor unit action potentials.

Isaacs' syndrome of continuous muscle fiber activity[95] is characterized clinically by muscle stiffness and spasms, difficulty in muscle relaxation, cramps, muscle twitching, and hyperhidrosis. The syndrome may develop spontaneously, may be hereditary, or may be associated with peripheral neuropathy.[96–100] Needle electromyography may reveal fasciculations and spontaneous discharges of doublets, triplets, or even multiplets. There are also continuous, high-frequency discharges (neuromyotonia) of motor unit potentials and shorter potentials which are increased by, and immediately following, voluntary contraction. These discharges are abolished by curare but persist during sleep, spinal or general anesthesia, or nerve block. This activity is thought to arise in the peripheral nerves. Administration of phenytoin or carbamazepine may be helpful.

Tetany is characterized clinically by typical abnormal postures (carpal, pedal, or carpopedal spasms) that are associated with hypocalcemia, hypomagnesemia, or hyperventilation (alkalosis). During the spasms of tetany, the electromyogram resembles that of voluntary activity, but motor unit potentials may be seen to fire repetitively in doublets, triplets, or multiplets.[101]

Tetanus is caused by a toxin, produced by *Clostridium tetani*, that affects the central nervous system. The disease is characterized primarily by muscle stiffness and by reflex and spontaneous muscle spasms that may be either localized or generalized. During the spasms, sudden, simultaneous contractions of both agonists and antagonists occur, often triggered by sensory stimuli, emotion, or movement. Particularly well known are the spasms known as trismus (lockjaw) and risus sardonicus (facial grimacing). Electromyography reveals continuous excessive motor unit activity, the precise origin of which is unclear; however, there is evidence of both a peripheral and a major central source. Diazepam may help to control the spasms, but neuromuscular blockade is sometimes necessary.

Stiff-man syndrome or *Moersch-Woltman syndrome* is a disorder of uncertain nature that is presumed to have a central basis and that affects persons of either sex. It is of unknown etiology. Electromyographic examination shows normal-appearing but continuous motor unit activity that disappears in sleep, after general or spinal anesthesia, or after peripheral nerve block.

Myasthenia gravis is described in Chapter 14, where its electrophysiologic features, as well as those of other disorders of neuromuscular transmission, are described in detail. It is convenient, however, to summarize here the electromyographic findings evident upon voluntary contraction of an affected muscle. There is marked variation in amplitude of individual motor unit potentials, and during sustained contractions, the number of active units declines. Those that remain functional tend to fire in bursts. Particularly at the end of a sustained contraction when power has weakened, many potentials are polyphasic or of short duration, or both. In rare cases, increased insertion activity, as well as spontaneous fibrillation potentials and positive sharp waves, may also be present.[102] The characteristic electrophysiologic feature of the disorder, however, is the decrement in size of the muscle action potential that occurs in response to repetitive stimulation of the motor nerve.

Arthrogryposis multiplex congenita is the name given to a congenital syndrome characterized by joint deformities and muscle involvement. Pathologic and electrophysiologic studies have suggested that its origin is often neurogenic but sometimes myogenic, whereas Dastur and co-workers have advanced the view that many cases are due to defective embryonic development of muscle.[103] Bharucha and associates reported that the electromyographic findings were suggestive of denervation in 8 of 13 cases and of a myopathy in 2 cases; the findings were normal in the remaining 3 cases.[104]

The term *myokymia* has been used clinically to refer to involuntary, relatively slow, repetitive contractions that occur independently in different parts of a muscle so that the surface appearance resembles "the movement of an army of parallel earthworms."[105] Many different skeletal muscles may be involved in affected patients. There is often an associated impairment of muscular relaxation (Isaacs' syndrome), but this is not accompanied by electrical evidence of true myotonia. The electromyographic findings associated with myokymia are prolonged bursts of repetitive potentials resembling those of motor units, or repetitive multiplets containing 2 to more than 200 potentials with intervals of about 20 msec between component spikes.

Facial myokymia may occur in patients with multiple sclerosis or brain stem tumors, and presumably is central in origin. In patients with multiple sclerosis, Hjorth and Willison found that single or double discharges of individual motor units occurred spontaneously and regularly at intervals of 100 to 200 msec, and that some of the affected units could not be activated voluntarily.[106] In their electromyographic study of patients with brain stem tumors, however, Lambert and colleagues found that facial myokymia was accompanied by intermittent firing of motor units for up to 900 msec at intervals of 2 to 4 seconds and at

rates of 30 to 40 per second.[107] The alternating activity of neighboring units was thought to produce the vermicular clinical appearance. The term myokymia has also been used to describe the flickering of an eyelid or part of a muscle that is sometimes seen during fatigue, but this movement actually consists of a series of twitches rather than the activity described above.

Hemifacial spasm was also studied by Hjorth and Willison.[106] Two types of abnormal movement were distinguished. The first consisted of brief twitches, occurring spontaneously or in association with blinking, that affected several different muscles simultaneously. The second type involved a prolonged, irregular, fluctuating contraction. The former movement is characterized electromyographically by isolated bursts of repetitive, high-frequency, motor unit discharges, with each burst consisting of discharges from the same unit. In the latter type of movement, units fire irregularly at lower frequencies, but bursts of activity identical to those just described may also be found.

If one branch of the facial nerve on the affected side is stimulated, the direct muscle response elicited is followed by a late response that arises from muscles supplied by other branches of the facial nerve.[108] Impulses conducted antidromically along the branch that was stimulated appear to cross to other branches, and are then conducted orthodromically to excite other muscles. The site of this "cross-talk" is controversial. Some authors believe that ephaptic transmission and ectopic excitation occur in the intracranial, extra-axial segment of the facial nerve[108,109] which is commonly compressed by an anomalous blood vessel. Others believe that they arise at the level of the facial nerve nucleus.[110] The work of Nielsen has clarified many of these issues, and the evidence that he has accumulated provides strong support for the theory that the lesion is peripheral to the facial nerve nucleus, although this does not exclude the possibility of some involvement of the nucleus as well. Certainly, there is slowing in some facial nerve axons in patients with hemifacial spasms,[109] and this is a prerequisite for ephaptic transmission to occur. Intraoperative recordings of nerve action potentials from above and below the site of microvascular compression, as well as recordings of facial muscle action potentials elicited by intraoperative stimulation of the intracranial portions of the facial nerve above and below this site,[110] provide eloquent evidence of focal demyelination and slowing of conduction at the site of the lesion. Direct evidence in support of the peripheral site of "cross-talk" may be derived from collision studies in which orthodromic impulses of the blink reflex collide with antidromic impulses generated by direct stimulation of facial nerve branches.[111]

The Floppy Infant

Needle electromyography is an important means of evaluating the floppy infant to determine whether the underlying pathology is a peripheral neuromuscular disorder or whether disease of the central nervous system or other conditions are involved. Among peripheral neuromuscular disorders, hypotonia can be caused by spinal muscular atrophy, motor neuropathy, peripheral neuropathy, neonatal or congenital myasthenia, or various myopathic disorders. Electromyographic findings help to distinguish between these various possibilities, especially when the results are combined with those of nerve conduction studies (see Ch. 7) and repetitive nerve stimulation (see Ch. 14).

ELECTROMYOGRAPHY OF THE SPHINCTER MUSCLES

The anal sphincter receives its somatic innervation from the anterior divisions of the S2, S3, and S4 roots through the pudendal nerve, whereas the urethral sphincter is innervated through the perineal nerve. Electromyography may be helpful in evaluating sphincteric disturbances. The electrophysiologic principles involved are the same as those that apply to the examination of limb muscles and the nerves that supply them. Preoperative needle electromyography may help to determine whether the anal sphincter muscle is present and to evaluate its functional capacity in patients with imperforate anus.[112] When the muscle is damaged—for example, by surgery—needle electromyography may permit the extent of such damage to be defined. The urethral sphincter can also be evaluated by this means, but such an examination is best undertaken in conjunction with other urologic investigations. Nevertheless, recent studies suggest that urethral sphincter electromyography is the most effective means of assessing damage to vesicourethral innervation caused by pelvic surgery.[113] When such damage is suspected after surgery, urodynamic assessment may also be helpful. However, the findings of an open bladder neck and loss of the voiding reflex are nonspecific, as they may occur in a variety of neurogenic and non-neurogenic causes of bladder dysfunction.[113] Needle electromyography may also be helpful in excluding a neurologic lesion in patients with a long history of incontinence or urinary retention.[114]

When needle electromyography is to be performed, the resting muscle of the sphincter is examined and the activity that occurs in response to maximal voluntary contraction is then noted. The reflex responses of the sphincter muscles can also be recorded. Reflex activity of the sphincter muscles may be elicited by digital examination of the anus, by the bulbocavernous reflex, or by coughing or crying.[115]

Recording needle electrodes (concentric or monopolar) are placed in the external urethral sphincter in women by inserting them about 1 cm to the side of the urethral meatus and guiding them toward the midline. In men, an electrode is placed through the perineum in the midline, 1 or 2 cm in front of the anus, and the tip is guided toward the apex of the prostate by a finger in the rectum (Fig. 6.1). The anal sphincter may be examined by inserting a needle electrode through the skin just to the side of the mucocutaneous junction. A ground electrode (and reference electrode for monopolar recording) can be placed on either thigh, and the patient can be examined in either the lateral decubitus or modified lithotomy position.

Electromyography of the sphincteric muscles generally shows low-frequency, small-amplitude (less than 500 μV) tonic activity at about 1 to 4 Hz, even when these muscles are "at rest."[116,117] This activity varies according to the position and state of arousal of the subject, being somewhat diminished during sleep. If electrical activity does not persist, the possibility of displacement of the needle electrode should be considered.[115] However, as the bladder fills, the number and firing rate of motor unit potentials increase until, just before or upon voiding, or just after the onset of bladder contraction, complete electrical silence occurs.

Voluntary contraction of the sphincter muscles (elicited by asking the patient to

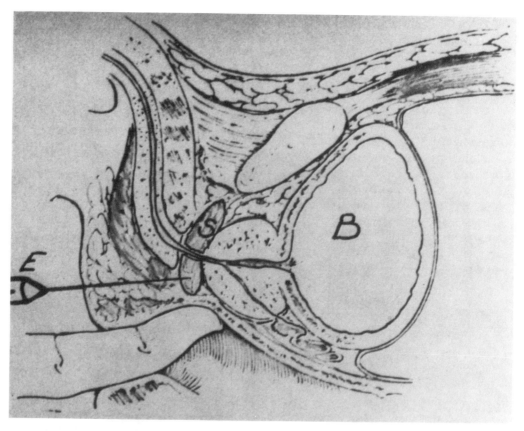

Fig. 6.1 Preliminary technique for examining the urethral sphincter in the male. B, bladder; E, electrode; S, urethral sphincter. (Chantraine A: EMG examination of the anal and urethral sphincters. p. 423. In Desmedt JE (ed): New Developments in Electromyography and Clinical Neurophysiology. Vol. 2. S. Karger AG, Basel, 1973.)

"squeeze," for example) usually generates potentials that range between 200 μV and 1 mV, but which occasionally are twice this size. In adults, the mean duration of these potentials in the urethral and anal sphincters is 5.5 msec and 5.6 msec, respectively.[117] Up to about 10 percent of the motor units may be polyphasic. With increasing effort, or in response to stimuli eliciting a reflex response, a full interference pattern is normally evident in patients who are 1 year of age or older. However, the completeness of the interference pattern depends on the position of the electrode tip within the muscle.

In patients with lower motor neuron lesions or an autonomous bladder, spontaneous fibrillation and positive sharp waves may be found, but these are hard to distinguish from the activity found in normal resting muscle. Complex repetitive discharges may also be encountered. The recruitment of motor units is reduced and the interference pattern is incomplete. There may also be an increased incidence of long-duration or large-amplitude motor unit potentials, or both,[114] and many potentials may be polyphasic. In patients with upper motor neuron lesions and a reflex bladder, the findings may be normal unless the patient is examined during bladder filling and voiding. When voiding begins, an increase rather than a decrease in activity in the sphincter muscles may be seen. Mixed upper and lower motor neuron patterns are present in some patients, especially those with anterior spinal artery syndrome; congenital malformations, such as spina bifida with meningomyelocele; and trauma.

Nerve conduction studies of the pudendal and perineal nerves may be helpful in distinguishing cord involvement from more peripheral involvement. Technical details of the methods that can be used for this purpose, which involve a digitally directed, intrarectal, stimulating technique, are provided by Snooks and associates.[118] Significant increases in the distal motor latencies in the pudendal and perineal nerves have been noted in patients with fecal incontinence or double incontinence, as compared to control subjects.[118]

In patients with anorectal incontinence, conventional electromyography can provide information about the pattern of voluntary control of the external sphincter, especially if there is a cauda equina lesion.[116] Single fiber electromyography (see Ch. 8) has also been used to study the function of the external anal sphincter, and especially, to measure fiber density. In incontinent subjects, the mean fiber density is reportedly increased compared to that of normal subjects, which is consistent with the belief that the loss of sphincter control has a neurogenic basis.[119]

ELECTROMYOGRAPHY OF THE EXTRAOCULAR MUSCLES

Electromyographic examination of the extraocular muscles is generally conducted by or in conjunction with ophthalmologists. In view of its potential hazards, the procedure should only be undertaken by persons who are familiar with the detailed regional anatomy of the eye. A particularly useful summary of the technique and its clinical applications has been provided by Breinin.[120] The technique has been used to distinguish between denervation of the extraocular muscles, ocular myopathy, and myasthenia gravis, and it is also of importance in differentiating extraocular palsies from pseudopalsies secondary to mechanical limitations of the globe.

The needle electrodes that are used for the investigation of extraocular muscles are much finer than those used for examining the peripheral skeletal muscles. The preparation of these electrodes is described by Breinin.[120]

The motor unit potentials recorded from the extraocular muscles are smaller in size than those recorded from limb muscles.

Their normal amplitude is up to about 600 μV, averaging 200 μV in the primary position, and their normal duration ranges from 1 to 2 msec.[121] These findings reflect the smaller diameter of the extraocular muscle fibers and their low innervation ratio compared to those of motor units in limb muscles. Most potentials are biphasic or triphasic in form, but occasionally polyphasic units are encountered. The motor unit potentials generally have a high discharge rate, sometimes firing several hundred times per second.

Unlike the peripheral limb muscles, tonic activity is present in the extraocular muscles of alert subjects with the eye in the primary position. If the eye is rotated out of the field of action of a given muscle, however, the discharge rate declines from the high rate found otherwise.

The electromyographic findings in patients with disease involving the extraocular muscles are similar to those found in the limb muscles. In patients with *neurogenic extraocular palsies,* fibrillation potentials may be present, but they are hard to distinguish from motor unit potentials because their dimensions are similar. However, they fire spontaneously without relation to volitional activity, and fail to recruit with effort. If the eye is moved out of the field of the muscle under examination, recognition of these potentials is facilitated. Neurogenic lesions are also characterized by poor recruitment of motor units, poorly sustained discharges, and a reduced interference pattern. In a totally paralyzed muscle, there may be very few motor units under voluntary control. However, complete electrical silence is encountered only rarely, except in diabetic neuropathy.[121] Large motor unit potentials may accompany aberrant regeneration of the oculomotor nerve.[121]

In patients with *ocular myopathy,* the interference pattern remains full, and abnormal spontaneous activity is generally absent. The motor unit potentials may, however, be small in amplitude and short in duration. Somewhat similar changes may be found in patients with pseudotumor of the orbit.[121] In thyroid ophthalmoplegia, myopathic changes may also be noted, but in other instances there are high-amplitude, high-frequency discharges that may be difficult to distinguish from normal.[121]

In *myasthenia gravis,* motor unit potentials may vary in amplitude and configuration over time. Moreover, a sustained maximal voluntary contraction may be accompanied by a progressive decline in the number of discharging motor unit potentials.

REFERENCES

1. Engel WK: Brief, small, abundant motor-unit action potentials: A further critique of electromyographic interpretation. Neurology 25:173, 1975
2. Kugelberg E: Electromyograms in muscular disorders. J Neurol Neurosurg Psychiatry 10:123, 1947
3. Engel WK, Warmolts JR: The motor unit. Diseases affecting it in toto or in portio. p. 141. In Desmedt JE (ed): New Developments in Electromyography and Clinical Neurophysiology. Vol. 1. S. Karger AG, Basel, 1973
4. Buchthal F, Kamieniecka Z: The diagnostic yield of quantified electromyography and quantified muscle biopsy in neuromuscular disorders. Muscle Nerve 5:265, 1982
5. Gath I, Sjaastad O, Loken AC: Myopathic electromyographic changes correlated with histopathology in Wohlfart-Kugelberg-Welander disease. Neurology 19:344, 1969
6. Walton JN, Gardner-Medwin D: Progressive muscular dystrophy and the myotonic disorders. p. 561. In Walton JN (ed): Disorders of Voluntary Muscle. 3rd Ed. Churchill Livingstone, London, 1974
7. Kugelberg E, Welander L: Heredofamilial juvenile muscular atrophy simulating muscular dystrophy. Arch Neurol Psychiatry 75:500, 1956
8. Pinelli P, Buchthal F: Muscle action po-

tentials in myopathies with special regard to progressive muscular dystrophy. Neurology 3:347, 1953

9. Buchthal F: The electromyogram. Its value in the diagnosis of neuromuscular disorders. World Neurol 3:16, 1962

10. van den Bosch J: Investigations of the carrier state in the Duchenne type dystrophy. p. 23. Members of the Research Committee of the Muscular Dystrophy Group (eds): Research in Muscular Dystrophy. The Proceedings of the Second Symposium on Current Research in Muscular Dystrophy. Pitman Medical, London, 1963

11. Gardner-Medwin D: Studies of the carrier state in the Duchenne type of muscular dystrophy. 2. Quantitative electromyography as a method of carrier detection. J Neurol Neurosurg Psychiatry 31:124, 1968

12. Caruso G, Buchthal F: Refractory period of muscle and electromyographic findings in relatives of patients with muscular dystrophy. Brain 88:29, 1965

13. Willison RG: Quantitative electromyography. The detection of carriers of Duchenne dystrophy. p. 123. In Barbeau A, Brunette J-R (eds): Progress in Neuro-Genetics. Proceedings of the Second International Congress of Neuro-Genetics and Neuro-Ophthalmology of the World Federation of Neurology. Vol. 1. Excerpta Medical International Congress Series No. 175. Excerpta Medica Foundation, Amsterdam, 1967

14. Buchthal F, Pinelli P: Muscle action potentials in polymyositis. Neurology 3:424, 1953

15. Lambert EH, Sayre GP, Eaton LM: Electrical activity of muscle in polymyositis. Trans Am Neurol Assoc 79:64, 1954

16. DeVere R, Bradley WG: Polymyositis: Its presentation, morbidity and mortality. Brain 98:637, 1975

17. Bohan A, Peter JB: Polymyositis and dermatomyositis. N Engl J Med 292:403, 1975

18. Eisen A, Berry K, Gibson G: Inclusion body myositis (IBM): Myopathy or neuropathy? Neurology 33:1109, 1983

19. Lacy JR, Simon DB, Neville HE, Ringel SP: Inclusion body myositis: Electrodiagnostic and nerve biopsy findings. Neurology 32(2):A202, 1982

20. Ruff RL, Secrist D: Viral studies in benign acute childhood myositis. Arch Neurol 39:261, 1982

21. Bardelas JA, Winkelstein JA, Seto DSY, Tsai T, Rogol AD: Fatal ECHO 24 infection in a patient with hypogammaglobulinemia: Relationship to dermatomyositis-like syndrome. J Pediatr 90:396, 1977

22. Mease PJ, Ochs HD, Wedgwood RJ: Successful treatment of echovirus meningoencephalitis and myositisfasciitis with intravenous immune globulin therapy in a patient with X-linked agammaglobulinemia. N Engl J Med 304:1278, 1981

23. Waylonis, GW, Johnson EW: The electromyogram in acute trichinosis: Report of four cases. Arch Phys Med Rehabil 45:177, 1964

24. Gross B, Ochoa J: Trichinosis: Clinical report and histochemistry of muscle. Muscle Nerve 2:394, 1979

25. Rowland LP, Greer M: Toxoplasmic polymyositis. Neurology 11:367, 1961

26. Buchthal F, Rosenfalck P: Electrophysiological aspects of myopathy with particular reference to progressive muscular dystrophy. p. 193. In Bourne GW, Golarz MN (eds): Muscular Dystrophy in Man and Animals. S. Karger AG, Basel, 1963

27. Trojaborg W: Electrodiagnosis in the rheumatic diseases. Clin Rheum Dis 7:349, 1981

28. Crompton MR, MacDermot V: Sarcoidosis associated with progressive muscular wasting and weakness. Brain 84:62, 1961

29. Douglas AC, MacLeod JG, Matthews JD: Symptomatic sarcoidosis of skeletal muscle. J Neurol Neurosurg Psychiatry 36:1034, 1973

30. Sambrook MA, Heron JR, Aber GM: Myopathy in association with primary hyperaldosteronism. J Neurol Neurosurg Psychiatry 35:202, 1972

31. Ludin HP, Spiess H, Koenig MP: Neuromuscular dysfunction associated with thyrotoxicosis. Eur Neurol 2:269, 1969

32. Layzer RB: Neuromuscular Manifestations of Systemic Disease. F.A. Davis, Philadelphia, 1985

33. Sanderson KV, Adey WR: Electromyographic and endocrine studies in chronic thyrotoxic myopathy. J Neurol Neurosurg Psychiatry 15:200, 1952

34. Ramsay ID: Electromyography in thyrotoxicosis. Q J Med 34:255, 1965
35. Wilson J, Walton JN: Some muscular manifestations of hypothyroidism. J Neurol Neurosurg Psychiatry 22:320, 1959
36. Astrom K-E, Kugelberg E, Muller R: Hypothyroid myopathy. Arch Neurol 5:472, 1961
37. Ross GT, Scholz DA, Lambert EH, Geraci JE: Severe uterine bleeding and degenerative skeletal-muscle changes in unrecognized myxedema. J Clin Endocrinol Metab 18:492, 1958
38. Waldstein SS, Bronsky D, Shrifter HB, Oester YT: The electromyogram in myxedema. Arch Intern Med 101:97, 1958
39. Ozker RR, Schumacher OP, Nelson PA: Electromyographic findings in adults with myxedema: Report of 16 cases. Arch Phys Med Rehabil 41:299, 1960
40. Rao SN, Katiyar BC, Nair KRP, Misra S: Neuromuscular status in hypothyroidism. Acta Neurol Scand 61:167, 1980
41. Scarpalezos S, Lygidakis C, Papageorgiou C, Maliara S, Koukoulommati AS, Koutras DA: Neural and muscular manifestations of hypothyroidism. Arch Neurol 29:140, 1973
42. Clara R, Lowenthal A: Familial and congenital lysine-cystinuria with benign myopathy and dwarfism. J Neurol Sci 3:433, 1966
43. Chalmers RA, Johnson M, Pallis C, Watts RWE: Xanthinuria with myopathy. Q J Med 38:493, 1969
44. Engel AG, Siekert RG: Lipid storage myopathy responsive to prednisone. Arch Neurol 27:174, 1972
45. Engel AG, Angelini C: Carnitine deficiency of human skeletal muscle with associated lipid storage myopathy: A new syndrome. Science 179:899, 1973
46. Bank WJ, DiMauro S, Bonilla E, Capuzzi DM, Rowland LP: A disorder of muscle lipid metabolism and myoglobinuria. N Engl J Med 292:443, 1975
47. Shy GM, Wanko T, Rowley PT, Engel AG: Studies in familial periodic paralysis. Exp Neurol 3:53, 1961
48. Creutzfeldt OD, Abbott BC, Fowler WM, Pearson CM: Muscle membrane potentials in episodic adynamia. Electroencephalogr Clin Neurophysiol 15:508, 1963
49. McComas AJ, Mrozek K, Bradley WG: The nature of the electrophysiological disorder in adynamia episodica. J Neurol Neurosurg Psychiatry 31:488, 1968
50. Buchthal F, Engbaek L, Gamstorp I: Paresis and hyperexcitability in adynamia episodica hereditaria. Neurology 8:347, 1958
51. Layzer RB, Lovelace RE, Rowland LP: Hyperkalemic periodic paralysis. Arch Neurol 16:455, 1967
52. Engel AG: Acid maltase deficiency in adults: Studies in four cases of a syndrome which may mimic muscular dystrophy or other myopathies. Brain 93:599, 1970
53. Smith HL, Amick LD, Sidbury JB: Type II glycogenosis. Am J Dis Child 111:475, 1966
54. Swaiman KF, Kennedy WR, Sauls HS: Late infantile acid maltase deficiency. Arch Neurol 18:642, 1968
55. DiMauro S, Hartwig GB, Hays A, Eastwood AB, Franco R, Olarte M, Chang M, Roses AD, Fetell M, Schoenfeldt RS, Stern LZ: Debrancher deficiency: A neuromuscular disorder in 5 adults. Ann Neurol 5:422, 1979
56. McArdle B: Myopathy due to a defect in muscle glycogen breakdown. Clin Sci 10:13, 1951
57. Layzer RB, Rowland LP, Ranney HM: Muscle phosphofructokinase deficiency. Arch Neurol 17:512, 1967
58. Lane RMJ, Mastaglia FL: Drug-induced myopathies in man. Lancet 2:562, 1978
59. Whisnant JP, Espinosa RE, Kierland RR, Lambert EH: Chloroquine neuromyopathy. Proc Mayo Clin 38:501, 1963
60. Casey EB, Jellife AM, LeQuesne PM, Millett YL: Vincristine neuropathy: Clinical and electrophysiological observations. Brain 96:69, 1973
61. Kontos HA: Myopathy associated with chronic colchicine toxicity. N Engl J Med 266:38, 1962
62. Somers JE, Winer N: Reversible myopathy and myotonia following administration of a hypocholesterolemic agent. Neurology 16:761, 1966
63. Hed R, Lundmark C, Fahlgren H, Orell S: Acute muscular syndrome in chronic alcoholism. Acta Med Scand 171:585, 1962
64. Rubenstein AE, Wainapel SF: Acute hy-

pokalemic myopathy in alcoholism. A clinical entity. Arch Neurol 34:553, 1977

65. Ekbom K, Hed R, Kirstein L, Astrom KE: Muscular affections in chronic alcoholism. Arch Neurol 10:449, 1964

66. Wiechers D: Congenital myopathies. p. 29. Syllabus, Symposium on Muscle. Twenty-sixth Annual Meeting, American Association of Electromyography and Electrodiagnosis, 1979

67. Schwartz O, Jampel RS: Congenital blepharophimosis associated with a unique generalized myopathy. Arch Ophthalmol 68:52, 1962

68. Aberfeld DC, Namba T, Vye MV, Grob D: Chondrodystrophic myotonia: Report of two cases. Arch Neurol 22:455, 1970

69. Fariello R, Meloff K, Murphy EG, Reilly BJ, Armstrong D: A case of Schwartz-Jampel syndrome with unusual muscle biopsy findings. Ann Neurol 3:93, 1978

70. Taylor RG, Layzer RB, Davis HS, Fowler WM: Continuous muscle fiber activity in the Schwartz-Jampel syndrome. Electroencephalogr Clin Neurophysiol 33:497, 1972

71. Panayiotopoulos CP, Scarpalezos S: Dystrophia myotonica: Peripheral nerve involvement and pathogenetic implications. J Neurol Sci 27:1, 1976

72. Aminoff MJ, Layzer RB, Satya-Murti S, Faden AI: The declining electrical response of muscle to repetitive nerve stimulation in myotonia. Neurology 27:812, 1977

73. Subramony SH, Malhotra CP, Mishra SK: Distinguishing paramyotonia congenita and myotonia congenita by electromyography. Muscle Nerve 6:374, 1983

74. Polgar JG, Bradley WG, Upton ARM, Anderson J, Howat JML, Petito F, Roberts DF, Scopa J: The early detection of dystrophia myotonica. Brain 95:761, 1972

75. Bundey S, Carter CO, Soothill JF: Early recognition of heterozygotes for the gene for dystrophia myotonica. J Neurol Neurosurg Psychiatry 33:279, 1970

76. Hayward M, Seaton D: Late sequelae of paralytic poliomyelitis: A clinical and electromyographic study. J Neurol Neurosurg Psychiatry 42:117, 1979

77. Wiechers DO, Hubbell SL: Late changes in the motor unit after acute poliomyelitis. Muscle Nerve 4:524, 1981

78. Mulder DW, Rosenbaum RA, Layton DD: Late progression of poliomyelitis or forme fruste amyotrophic lateral sclerosis? Mayo Clin Proc 47:756, 1972

79. Daube JR: Electrophysiologic studies in the diagnosis and prognosis of motor neuron diseases. Neurol Clin 3:473, 1985

80. Bernstein LP, Antel JP: Motor neuron disease: Decremental responses to repetitive nerve stimulation. Neurology 31:204, 1981

81. Parry GJ, Holtz SJ, Ben-Zeev D, Drori JB: Gammopathy with proximal motor axonopathy simulating motor neuron disease. Neurology 36:273, 1986

82. Lambert EH: Electromyography in amyotrophic lateral sclerosis. p. 135. In Norris FH, Kurland LT (eds): Motor Neuron Diseases: Research on Amyotrophic Lateral Sclerosis and Related Disorders. Grune & Stratton, New York, 1969

83. Russo LS: Clinical and electrophysiological studies in primary lateral sclerosis. Arch Neurol 39:662, 1982

84. Johnson WG, Wigger HJ, Karp HR, Glaubiger LM, Rowland LP: Juvenile spinal muscular atrophy: A new hexosaminidase deficiency phenotype. Ann Neurol 11:11, 1982

85. Parnes S, Karpati G, Carpenter S, Ng Ying Kin NMK, Wolfe LS, Suranyi L: Hexosaminidase-A deficiency presenting as atypical juvenile-onset spinal muscular atrophy. Arch Neurol 42:1176, 1985

86. Patten BM, Onderdonk KJ: Neuromuscular disorders associated with monoclonal gammopathy. Neurology 31(2):156, 1981

87. Engel WK, Hopkins LC, Rosenberg BJ: Fasciculating progressive muscular atrophy (F-PMA) remarkably responsive to antidysimmune treatment (ADIT)—A possible clue to more ordinary ALS? Neurology 35:suppl. 1, 72, 1985

88. Sobue I, Saito N, Iida M, Ando K: Juvenile type of distal and segmental muscular atrophy of upper extremities. Ann Neurol 3:429, 1978

89. Harding AE: Inherited neuronal atrophy and degeneration predominantly of lower motor neurons. p. 1537. In Dyck PJ, Thomas PK, Lambert EH, Bunge R (eds):

Peripheral Neuropathy. Vol. 2. W.B. Saunders, Philadelphia, 1984

90. Buchthal F, Olsen PZ: Electromyography and muscle biopsy in infantile spinal muscular atrophy. Brain 93:15, 1970

91. Hausmanowa-Petrusewicz I, Karwanska A: Electromyographic findings in different forms of infantile and juvenile proximal spinal muscular atrophy. Muscle Nerve 9:37, 1986

92. Gassel MM: A test of nerve conduction to muscles of the shoulder girdle as an aid in the diagnosis of proximal neurogenic and muscular disease. J Neurol Neurosurg Psychiatry 27:200, 1964

93. Denny-Brown D, Foley JM: Myokymia and the benign fasciculation of muscular cramps. Trans Assoc Am Phys 61:88, 1948

94. Layzer RB: Motor unit hyperactivity states. p. 295. In Vinken PJ, Bruyn GW (eds): Handbook of Clinical Neurology. Vol. 41. North-Holland, Amsterdam, 1979

95. Isaacs H: A syndrome of continuous muscle-fibre activity. J Neurol Neurosurg Psychiatry 24:319, 1961

96. McGuire SA, Tomasovic JJ, Ackerman N: Hereditary continuous muscle fiber activity. Arch Neurol 41:395, 1984

97. Auger RG, Daube JR, Gomez MR, Lambert EH: Hereditary form of sustained muscle activity of peripheral nerve origin causing generalized myokymia and muscle stiffness. Ann Neurol 15:13, 1984

98. Lance JW, Burke D, Pollard J: Hyperexcitability of motor and sensory neurons in neuromyotonia. Ann Neurol 5:523, 1979

99. Rowland LP: Cramps, spasms, and muscle stiffness. Rev Neurol 41:261, 1985

100. Lutschg J, Jerusalem F, Ludin HP, Vassella F, Mumenthaler M: The syndrome of 'continuous muscle fiber activity.' Arch Neurol 35:198, 1978

101. Kugelberg E: Activation of human nerves by ischemia. Trousseau's phenomenon in tetany. Arch Neurol Psychiatry 60:140, 1948

102. Simpson JA: The defect in myasthenia gravis. p. 345. In Bittar EE, Bittar N (eds): The Biological Basis of Medicine. Vol. 3. Academic Press, New York, 1969

103. Dastur DK, Razzak ZA, Bharucha EP: Arthrogryposis multiplex congenita. Part 2. Muscle pathology and pathogenesis. J Neurol Neurosurg Psychiatry 35:435, 1972

104. Bharucha EP, Pandya SS, Dastur DK: Arthrogryposis multiplex congenita. Part 1. Clinical and electromyographic aspects. J Neurol Neurosurg Psychiatry 35:425, 1972

105. Gardner-Medwin D, Walton JN: Myokymia with impaired muscular relaxation. Lancet 1:127, 1969

106. Hjorth RJ, Willison RG: The electromyogram in facial myokymia and hemifacial spasm. J Neurol Sci 20:117, 1973

107. Lambert EH, Love JG, Mulder DW: Facial myokymia and brain tumor: Electromyographic studies. News Letter, Am Assoc Electromyogr Electrodiagn 8:8, 1961

108. Nielsen VK: Pathophysiology of hemifacial spasm: 1. Ephaptic transmission and ectopic excitation. Neurology 34:418, 1984

109. Nielsen VK: Pathophysiology of hemifacial spasm: 11. Lateral spread of the supraorbital nerve reflex. Neurology 34:427, 1984

110. Moller AR, Jannetta PJ: Hemifacial spasm: Results of electrophysiologic recording during microvascular decompression operations. Neurology 35:969, 1985

111. Soso MJ, Nielsen VK: The lesion of hemifacial spasm is peripheral to the facial nucleus. Muscle Nerve 7:578, 1984

112. Archibald KC, Goldsmith EI: Sphincteric electromyography. Arch Phys Med Rehabil 48:387, 1967

113. Kirby RS, Fowler CJ, Gilpin SA, Gosling JA, Milroy EJG, Turner-Warwick RT: Bladder muscle biopsy and urethral sphincter EMG in patients with bladder dysfunction after pelvic surgery. J R Soc Med 79:270, 1986

114. Fowler CJ, Kirby RS, Harrison MJG, Milroy EJG, Turner-Warwick R: Individual motor unit analysis in the diagnosis of disorders of urethral sphincter innervation. J Neurol Neurosurg Psychiatry 47:637, 1984

115. Chantraine A: EMG examination of the anal and urethral sphincters. p. 421. In Desmedt JE (ed): New Developments in Electromyography and Clinical Neurophysiology. Vol. 2. S. Karger AG, Basel, 1973

116. Jesel M, Isch-Treussard C, Isch F: Electromyography of striated muscle of anal and urethral sphincters. p. 406. In Desmedt JE (ed): New Developments in Electromyography and Clinical Neurophysiology. Vol. 2. S. Karger AG, Basel, 1973

117. DiBenedetto M, Yalla SV: Electrodiagnosis of striated urethral sphincter dysfunction. J Urol 122:361, 1979

118. Snooks SJ, Barnes PRH, Swash M: Damage to the innervation of the voluntary anal and periurethral sphincter musculature in incontinence: An electrophysiological study. J Neurol Neurosurg Psychiatry 47:1269, 1984

119. Neill ME, Swash M: Increased motor unit fibre density in the external anal sphincter muscle in ano-rectal incontinence: A single fibre EMG study. J Neurol Neurosurg Psychiatry 43:343, 1980

120. Breinin GM: The Electrophysiology of Extraocular Muscle. With Special Reference to Electromyography. American Ophthalmological Society, University of Toronto Press, Toronto, 1962

121. Breinin GM: Ocular electromyography. p. 305. In Goodgold J, Eberstein A (eds): Electrodiagnosis of Neuromuscular Diseases. 3rd Ed. Williams & Wilkins, Baltimore, 1983

7

Nerve Conduction Studies: Basic Principles and Pathologic Correlations

The introduction into routine practice of laboratory procedures for studying nerve conduction has aroused considerable interest in peripheral nerve disorders and has provided an objective method for evaluating patients in whom these disorders are suspected. The principles and basic technical aspects of these procedures are discussed in this chapter; their clinical application is described in the following chapters, in which the various electrode placements used for studying the function of individual nerves are discussed, together with the electrophysiologic findings in various disorders of the peripheral nervous system.

PRINCIPLES AND TECHNICAL ASPECTS

Nerve conduction studies are best conducted with the patient reclining comfortably in warm, quiet surroundings. The nature of the procedure should be explained to the patient, and the patient should be reassured and encouraged to relax as much as possible. When electromyographic sampling procedures are also to be undertaken, they should be deferred, if possible, until the nerve conduction studies have been completed, as they are often more distressing to the patient.

Nerve conduction studies involve the use of stimulation techniques, and the patient should always be warned before stimulation is commenced. The stimuli should be of short duration—0.05 to 0.2 msec is usually adequate—and may conveniently be applied at a repetition rate of 1 per second. Nerves are stimulated at sites where they are relatively superficial, with the stimulating electrodes being positioned so that the cathode is closest to the recording electrodes, because stimulation normally occurs at the cathode rather than the anode. The stimulator is made to trigger the sweep of the oscilloscope before the stimulus is delivered so that the directly conducted stimulus artifact can be seen on the trace in full. A time marker should also be made to appear on the screen. A ground electrode, which is attached to the limb being examined, should be placed between the stimulating and recording electrodes. This helps to reduce excessive stimulus artifact, as do the use of short leads and surface electrodes that are clean, the maintenance of low skin impedances, the assurance that the skin between electrodes is clean and dry, the optimal positioning and adequate separation of the stimulating and recording electrodes, the avoidance of stimuli of excessive intensity, the separation of leads from the stimulating and recording electrodes, and the adjustment, if necessary, of the filter setting of the recording amplifier. Further technical details are given in the following sections.

Motor Conduction Studies

If the motor fibers of a peripheral nerve are stimulated electrically, a response is evoked in the muscles that they supply. This potential, which is called the direct or M response, can be recorded with needle or surface electrodes, observed on the oscilloscope, and recorded photographically. The interval of time between the onset of the stimulus and that of the response is called the *conduction time,* or *latency.* It represents the time the impulse takes to travel along the nerve fibers and their fine terminal branches from the point of stimulation, the delay that occurs at the neuromuscular junction before the muscle fibers are excited, and the time that the impulse takes to travel along the muscle fibers to the pick-up zone of the recording electrode.

The velocity at which the impulse is propagated along the fastest conducting motor fibers in a nerve can be determined by stimulating the nerve at two separate points and recording the evoked responses of a muscle that it supplies (Fig. 7.1). The conduction time from the most distal site of stimulation is then referred to as the *distal* or *terminal latency* (Fig. 7.2). The time taken for the impulse to travel between the two points of stimulation is equal to the difference in latency of the two responses. If this time (in milliseconds) is divided into the distance (in millimeters) between the two sites of stimulation, the conduction velocity (in meters per second) in the intervening segment of nerve may be calculated.

Either surface or needle electrodes can be used for stimulation. The former are less distressing for patients, less time-consuming, and are adequate for routine clinical use except when a deeply situated nerve, such as the sciatic nerve at the gluteal fold, is to be stimulated. Surface electrodes may, however, necessitate the use of higher-intensity stimuli than needle electrodes, which is sometimes uncomfortable. The stimulating cathode must be placed as close to the nerve as possible, and this is the position at which the stimulus intensity required to evoke a muscle response is lowest. If bipolar stimulation of the nerve is to be employed using surface electrodes, both cathode and anode are placed along the nerve, with the cathode distal to the anode. For monopolar stimulation, a small cathode is positioned over the nerve and a large anode is placed more proximally at a distance from it.

The latency of a submaximal response may be longer than that of a maximal one. Any results based on a submaximal response may, therefore, be misleading. Moreover, with an inadequate stimulus, an H reflex (p. 108) may be elicited and mistaken for a direct motor response of prolonged latency, especially when evoked by proximal stimulation. The stimulus must, therefore, be of sufficient intensity to evoke a maximal motor response; to ensure its adequacy in practice, it should be somewhat greater in intensity than is actually required for this purpose.[1] This is accomplished by gradually increasing the stimulus intensity until the response obtained is maximal in size, and then increasing the intensity by an additional 30 percent. Care must be taken to ensure that the intensity of the stimulus is no greater than this, however, because an adjacent nerve may be excited by stimulus spread, and the resultant response

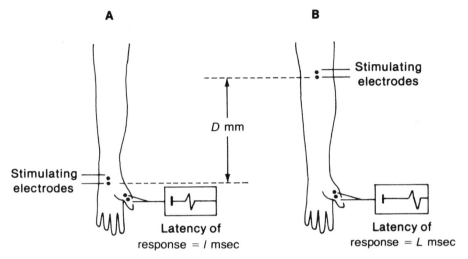

Fig. 7.1 Arrangement for measuring motor conduction velocity in the forearm segment of the median nerve. The nerve is stimulated distally (**A**) and proximally (**B**), and the evoked potentials are recorded from the abductor pollicis brevis muscle. (Ground electrode not shown.) Maximal motor conduction velocity (m/sec) between the proximal and distal sites of stimulation is calculated by dividing the distance between these sites by the difference in latency of the responses.

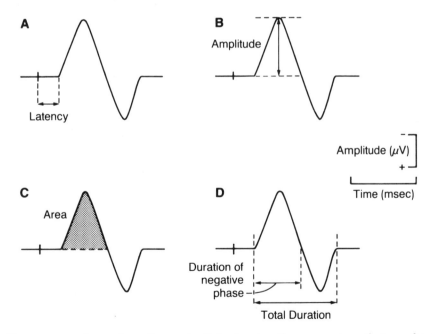

Fig. 7.2 The compound muscle action potential, showing the parameters that can be measured. (**A**) Latency of the response. (**B**) Amplitude of the negative component of the response. (**C**) Area of the negative component of the response. (**D**) Duration of the response.

will complicate the findings if picked up by the recording electrode.

The active recording electrode should be positioned close to the end-plate region of the muscle, and in this site the response is usually biphasic, with a negative onset. If recordings are made from further away, the response will have an initial positive deflection, and its latency will be increased by the time necessary for activity to be conducted along the muscle fibers to the pick-up zone of the electrode. This additional delay is small, and will not affect the calculated conduction velocity between the two points at which the nerve is stimulated because both proximal and distal latencies are increased equally by it.[1] Nevertheless, the electrode should be repositioned.

Recordings can be made with surface electrodes, the active electrode (G1) being placed over the muscle belly and the reference electrode (G2) positioned over its tendon. The first deflection from the baseline then indicates the latency of the fastest conducting motor fibers. Surface electrodes have a wide pick-up range, and the *amplitude of the main negative component* (Fig. 7.2) of the recorded potential therefore provides an indication of the number of muscle fibers activated by the stimulus. The amplitude also depends on the muscle being studied and the placement of the recording electrodes, and it may vary widely among different subjects and in response to repetitive stimulation in patients with defective neuromuscular transmission. The amplitude of the negative component of the compound muscle action potential is usually slightly reduced when the nerve is stimulated proximally rather than distally. This is attributable to temporal dispersion of the action potentials in the individual nerve fibers comprising the nerve, which occurs as a result of their differing conduction velocities. Greater variation in the amplitude of the responses of individual muscles to stimulation of their nerve supply at different sites occurs if the stimulus is supramaximal

at one site but submaximal in another, if the motor axons follow an anomalous course (p. 165), or in patients with peripheral nerve disorders when conduction is blocked or delayed because of a localized lesion. This change in amplitude may be of diagnostic significance. For example, in patients with an ulnar nerve lesion at the elbow, the size of the response recorded over the abductor digiti minimi muscle in the hand after supramaximal stimulation of the ulnar nerve above the elbow may be markedly diminished compared to the response to stimulation below the elbow. The amplitude may also vary if movement causes a change in the distance between the electrode and the muscle.

The *area* of the negative component of the compound muscle action potential (Fig. 7.2) elicited by a supramaximal stimulus also provides an indication of the number of muscle fibers activated, but more technically sophisticated equipment is required for its measurement than for the amplitude of the response. It, too, depends on the distance between the muscle and the recording electrode, declining as the conduction distance increases.

Subcutaneously inserted needle electrodes are sometimes preferred to surface electrodes. These subcutaneous electrodes are placed over the muscle and its tendon, and although their use is more distressing for the patient, they are less likely to lead to movement artifacts than are surface electrodes.

There are certain other disadvantages to the use of surface electrodes. It may be difficult to determine the precise time of onset of the response unless the amplifier is set at high gain. Again, the precise origin of the response may be uncertain, and it will then be necessary to insert a needle electrode directly into the muscle it is intended to study. Furthermore, it may not be possible with surface electrodes to pick up a response from severely wasted muscle. In such circumstances, a needle electrode will have to be inserted directly into the muscle to search for surviving units that are responsive to nerve stimulation.

The most convenient, intramuscularly inserted, needle electrode for clinical purposes is the concentric needle electrode, the features of which have been described earlier (p. 41). This type of electrode has a restricted pick-up zone; by adjusting its position, the activity of different motor units can be examined. Its position can also be adjusted until motor responses have a sharp onset or "take-off," thereby facilitating the accurate measurement of latency. The latency and configuration of the responses will vary, however, with the units whose activity is being recorded, and thus, with the position of the needle. Care must be taken, therefore, not to move the recording electrode while the nerve is stimulated at different points along its course because the responses must be comparable if estimates of conduction velocity are to be valid. A further disadvantage of the concentric needle electrode is that, as a consequence of its restricted pick-up zone, the amplitude of the potential recorded with it has much less significance than that recorded with surface electrodes.

In order to calculate conduction velocity, the length of the nerve between the proximal and distal sites of stimulation is determined by surface measurement while the limb is maintained in exactly the same position as when it was stimulated. Measurements are consistently made to the position occupied either by the center or, less commonly, the leading edge of the stimulating cathode, and this site should be marked on the skin with a pencil before the electrode is removed. The distance between the two points of stimulation—which, in the interest of accuracy, should be greater than 10 cm— is then divided by the difference in latency of the responses evoked by stimulation of the nerve at these sites. To prevent any bias when measurements of latency are made, it is advisable to leave unchanged the gain of the amplifier while responses to stimulation of the nerve at both sites are recorded.[2]

Inaccuracies in the calculated conduction velocity may occur because of observer error in making any of these measurements, because the length of nerve between the two points of stimulation differs from that determined by surface measurements, or because the actual point at which the nerve is excited does not correspond with the position of the stimulating cathode on the skin. Henriksen found that motor conduction velocity in the ulnar nerve of normal subjects could vary by up to 7.5 m/sec when measurements were made on different days,[3] and Simpson emphasized that even greater discrepancies could occur if the different factors considered above should happen to operate in the same direction.[1] Calculations of conduction velocity will also be inaccurate if the nerve fibers under study have an aberrant course.

The values for conduction velocity obtained while using the technique described above and recording with surface electrodes refer only to the most rapidly conducting fibers in the nerve. There is no satisfactory method in routine use for systematically determining conduction velocity in fibers that conduct at a slower rate. Some of the normal values obtained for maximal conduction velocity in the motor fibers of the individual nerves in the limbs are given in Chapters 9 and 10. It should be noted, however, that these values are influenced by a number of biologic and technical factors, as discussed in the following sections.

The *duration* of the muscle action potential (Fig. 7.2) recorded by surface electrodes in response to nerve stimulation relates, at least in part, to the range of conduction velocities in the fibers constituting the nerve, and increases with an increase in the conduction distance. Dispersion of the potential may result from slowing of conduction in some of these fibers, as occurs in the demyelinative neuropathies, but it may also be caused by other factors.[4] When dispersion is so pronounced that the compound muscle action potential is broken up into multiple spike components, abnormalities of the myelin of the nerve are responsible.

Brief mention must be made of certain potentials, other than the direct or M response, which can sometimes be recorded from muscle in response to nerve stimulation. These may otherwise cause some confusion when motor conduction studies are being performed.

The *H reflex* is a monosynaptic reflex response to electrical stimulation of spindle afferent (Ia) fibers. In relaxed, normal adults, it can be recorded with surface electrodes from the soleus or flexor carpi radialis muscles in response to stimulation of their motor nerves. It is facilitated by slight contraction or stretching of the muscle, and it is inhibited by active contraction of its antagonists. It cannot usually be elicited in other muscles by stimulation of their nerves, except in infants or in patients with pyramidal lesions. Its latency, which is approximately 30 msec for the soleus muscle and 16 msec for the flexor carpi radialis, depends on the site of stimulation, decreasing as the stimulating electrode is moved proximally. The stimulus should be of a lower intensity than is required to elicit a maximal M response, otherwise the H reflex will be blocked. Blocking occurs because antidromic impulses evoked in motor axons by direct stimulation collide with orthodromic impulses evoked reflexly in these axons in response to stimulation of the spindle afferent fibers,[5] as shown in Figure 7.3. The H reflex has a role in the neurophysiologic evaluation of certain clinical disorders, further details of which are provided in Chapter 8.

The *F wave* is another potential that is evoked in muscle by electrical stimulation of the peripheral nerve from which it is supplied. The F wave has a latency similar to that of the H reflex, but it requires a more intense stimulus and is not blocked if the stimulus evokes a maximal M response in the muscle. It is best recorded from the small muscles of the hands or feet. It is variable in size and latency, is smaller than the M response, and may not be elicited by every stimulus that is applied, even if they are of the same intensity. The F wave occurs as a result of a motor neuron discharge elicited by antidromic activation, rather than by any reflex phenomenon.[6] It can thus be elicited in the deafferented muscles of experimental animals[7] or humans,[8] and its latency decreases as the stimulating electrode is moved proximally. Further technical details are provided in Chapter 8, where the clinical utility of recording F waves is also considered.

Late potentials secondary to *axon reflexes* are sometimes found in patients with chronic partial denervation. These potentials have a constant latency that is greater than that of the M response but shorter than that of the H reflex or F wave. Fullerton and Gilliatt, in recording them from the small muscles of the hand in patients with peripheral nerve pathology, found that the impulse initiated by a stimulus at the wrist appeared to ascend the arm for a certain distance and then return to the hand.[9] They suggested that branching had occurred in motor fibers in the arm, and that the impulses ascended to the point of branching and then returned by passing down the other branch to the muscle.

If the muscle action potential is recorded at high gain, it is sometimes preceded by a small negative wave. This wave seems to arise mainly from *sensory intramuscular nerve fibers*,[10] and should be neglected when the latency of the response is measured.

Sensory Conduction Studies

Dawson and Scott described a technique for recording nerve action potentials in which the median or ulnar nerve was stim-

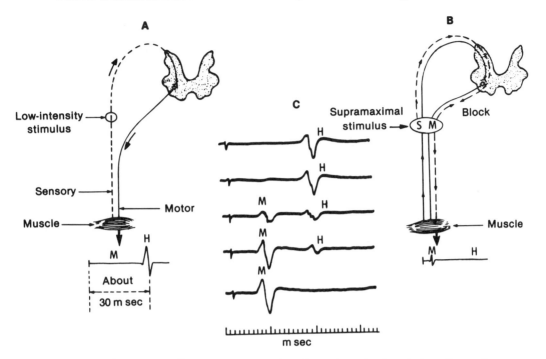

Fig. 7.3 The H reflex. (**A**) Reflex response to a low-intensity stimulus that excites only sensory fibers. (**B**) Response to a supramaximal stimulus that excites both motor and sensory fibers. Antidromic impulses in the motor fibers collide with orthodromic impulses evoked reflexly in the motor fibers, thereby blocking the H reflex. (**C**) Responses to increasing intensity of stimulation. (Smorto MP, Basmajian JV: Clinical Electroneurography. © 1972. The Williams & Wilkins Co., Baltimore.)

ulated at the wrist and action potentials were recorded over the nerve more proximally.[11] These potentials included not only orthodromic impulses in sensory fibers but also antidromic motor impulses. In order to eliminate the latter, Dawson subsequently stimulated the purely sensory, digital fibers of these nerves in the fingers while recording from the nerve trunk more proximally.[12] This technique was subsequently applied in a clinical context by Gilliatt and Sears.[13] Since that time, the recording of action potentials from the various nerves in the limbs has become a routine investigative procedure, with both the conduction time or velocity and the amplitude and configuration of the evoked nerve action potentials being of clinical significance. Meticulous attention to technical detail is necessary, how-

ever, because the potentials to be recorded are much smaller than those evoked from muscle by stimulation of its motor nerve.

The nerves are stimulated with electrodes similar to those used for motor conduction studies, but ring electrodes are convenient when digital fibers are to be activated in the fingers. A cutaneous nerve can be stimulated while the response is recorded further along the same nerve or the mixed nerve trunk from which it branches, or vice versa.

Recordings can be made using a pair of electrodes placed over the nerve, so that the impulses pass under each in turn ("bipolar recording"). Alternatively, a single electrode can be placed over the nerve and measurements made of the change in potential that occurs with respect to a second electrode placed at a distance from the nerve on the other side of the limb ("mono-polar recording"). The potential recorded in a bipolar manner represents the difference between the potential changes that can be recorded individually at each of the two electrodes with respect to a remote one. Its shape, size, and duration are influenced by the distance between the electrodes and between the stimulating and recording sites, as well as by the conduction velocity. Bipolar recording is, nevertheless, employed for routine clinical purposes by the majority of neurophysiologists because random activity from muscle affects both electrodes similarly and is, therefore, rejected by the differential amplifier. This technique provides a stable baseline and a relatively robust response. Surface electrodes are usually satisfactory, and the saddle-shaped ones described by Dawson and Scott[11] are particularly convenient because their shape ensures that the effect of small, lateral displacements is minimized. Needle electrodes are preferred by some workers, however, especially when the potentials to be recorded are of particularly low amplitude. The recording of sensory action potentials by a needle electrode placed close to the nerve has advantages over surface recordings in that the size of the response is considerably larger and the noise from the electrode-tissue surface is less. Consequently, the signal-to-noise ratio is approximately five times higher than that achieved with surface electrodes, and the averaging time is considerably shorter.[14] However, the needle cannot always be positioned at a constant distance from the nerve, and the distance between nerve and electrode influences the amplitude of the potential. Indeed, repeated studies of the same nerve in the same subject show that the amplitude of the potential recorded with a needle electrode varies by up to about one-third, due in part to differing distances between electrode and nerve.[14] Moreover, the amplitudes recorded with surface electrodes are more frequently abnormal than those

recorded with needle electrodes in patients with peripheral nerve pathology, at least in the experience of Andersen.[15]

The position of the mixed nerve trunk is determined for recording purposes by using a stimulating electrode to activate its motor fibers and then finding the point at which the stimulus threshold for evoking a muscle action potential is lowest.

Subjects must be encouraged to relax as much as possible during the recording procedure because nerve action potentials are of relatively low amplitude and they are obscured by muscle activity. In this regard, it is often helpful to provide patients with feedback from the loudspeaker of the electromyographic system of their muscle contractions. Similarly, stimulus artifacts must be kept to a minimum so that they do not obscure the potentials of interest. The ground electrode should be positioned between the stimulating and recording electrodes, and the skin between the various electrodes should be kept clean and dry. When surface electrodes are used for recording, they should have a clean surface and the impedance between them and the skin should be reduced by washing the skin with ether or acetone, abrading it with pumice or sandpaper, and applying electrode paste, as discussed in Chapter 4. Both stimulating and recording electrodes must be placed optimally, and stimuli of excessive intensity avoided. It is useful, however, to record a small stimulus artifact in the sweep of the oscilloscope, as this indicates the precise time at which the stimulus is applied and thus permits accurate measurement of the interval between stimulus and response. It should, therefore, appear in its entirety on the oscilloscope trace, and this is achieved by triggering the horizontal sweep of the oscilloscope with the stimulator before the stimulus is delivered.

The detection of small nerve action potentials is facilitated by using an electronic averaging technique, or by photographically superimposing a number of traces on the same piece of film so that a potential occurring at a constant time in the sweep of the oscilloscope is emphasized (Fig. 7.4).

If a nerve is stimulated at one point, the potential recorded from another point along the course of the nerve is typically triphasic with a positive onset. An estimate of maximal *conduction velocity* is obtained by dividing the conduction distance by the conduction time, or latency. The value obtained is, to some extent, an approximation because the conduction time includes the time taken to excite the nerve, and any spread of current from the stimulating cathode may alter the conduction distance. These factors may be avoided by recording from two or more separate points along the course of the nerve; conduction velocity in the intervening segment is then estimated from the difference in conduction time to these points. However, the results of the comparative study by Gilliatt and coworkers suggest that the former technique does not introduce any significant error in practice, with the possible exception of when very strong stimuli are used, and it is, therefore, satisfactory for clinical purposes.[16]

The *latency* of nerve action potentials is generally measured from the onset of the stimulus artifact to the onset of the main negative deflection of the potential (Fig. 7.5), since this coincides with the arrival of the impulse at the nearest recording electrode. Measurements to this point are unreliable, however, if action potentials are very small; in such circumstances, latency is more satisfactorily measured to the peak of the negative deflection. Estimates of conduction velocity based on the peak-latency value will not relate to the fastest conducting fibers, and such values can never be used to calculate conduction velocity when recordings are made from two separate points along the nerve because different axons will then be responsible for the peak at each of the two sites. In fact, if measurements have to be made to the peak rather than to the onset of the negative deflection, the value so obtained is best left as a measure of latency rather than being converted into conduction velocity.

The *peak-to-peak amplitude* of the potentials should also be measured (Fig. 7.5). The amplitude relates to the number of fibers activated, the distribution of their conduction velocities, and the distance of the nerve from the recording electrodes. The rise time of the potential is directly related to this distance. Potentials may be small or unrecordable because of axonal degeneration or conduction block, or because of

Fig. 7.4 Response to stimulation of the middle finger, recorded from the median nerve at the forearm. Top tracing (1), single response; middle tracing (20), photographic superimposition of 20 responses; bottom tracing (500), electronic average of 500 responses. (Buchthal F, Rosenfalck A: Evoked action potentials and conduction velocity in human sensory nerves. Brain Res 3:1, 1966.)

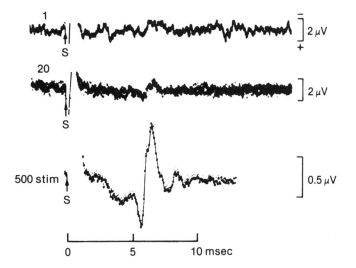

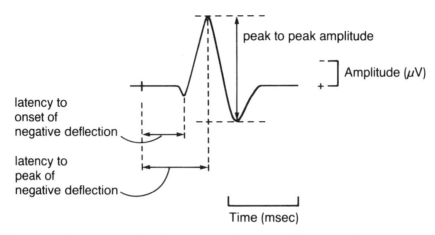

Fig. 7.5 Diagrammatic representation of a sensory action potential showing latency to onset, latency to peak, and peak-to-peak amplitude of the response.

marked slowing of conduction velocity (such as occurs in demyelinated or remyelinating fibers, or regenerating axons). Nonpathologic factors may also influence the size of the sensory action potential. In particular, a stimulus that is insufficient to excite all of the large myelinated fibers in the nerve will produce an attenuated potential. Response amplitude diminishes as the distance between the nerve and recording electrode increases, so that responses recorded with surface electrodes are smaller than those obtained with needle electrodes. The response also becomes more dispersed (i.e., smaller in amplitude and longer in duration) as the distance between recording and stimulating electrodes increases, and it is influenced by the recording technique, as described on p. 110. There is a progressive reduction in size, duration, and area of the response as temperature increases over the physiologic range, but the reason for this is not clear. This reduction has been related, at least in part, to a reduction in duration of the action potential of single myelinated fibers with increasing temperature.[17] The human sensory action potential may also vary with sex, being greater in women than in men. This is probably because men generally have somewhat larger digits and

wrists than women, so that a surface recording electrode is at a greater distance from the subjacent nerve.[18]

Reduced conduction velocity of the sensory action potential may be attributable to conduction along demyelinated, remyelinated, or regenerating nerve fibers. Dispersion of the response may occur for the same reason, but may not be apparent unless needle electrodes are used for recording. The earliest sign of nerve dysfunction is often a change in the configuration of the sensory action potential, and this is sometimes the sole abnormality.

In entrapment lesions, the diagnostic yield from recording sensory action potentials is generally greater than that achieved with motor conduction studies. However, to localize the lesion, the sensory action potentials must be recorded along the segment of nerve in question, and also both distal and proximal to the site of the lesion. It must be shown either that there is disproportionate slowing along that segment or that the potential is dispersed or attenuated when recorded after impulses have traversed the segment.

Dispersion of nerve action potentials is sometimes the sole abnormality and may indicate a disorder of sensory conduction, but this finding must be interpreted with caution because the configuration of potentials is influenced to such an extent by the recording arrangements.

Some of the normal values that have been obtained for these parameters in the various nerves of the limbs are given in Chapters 9 and 10. However, it must be appreciated that these values are influenced by the physiologic factors to be discussed in the following sections.

ERRORS IN THE PERFORMANCE OF NERVE CONDUCTION STUDIES

Nerve conduction studies may lead to erroneous conclusions for a variety of reasons. Many of these have already been mentioned, but are conveniently summarized here.

Biologic Factors

Motor conduction velocity or distal latency may seem abnormal because axons follow an anomalous course to the muscle from which the response is being recorded, so that measurements of conduction distance are incorrect. An anomalous communication occurs commonly between the median and ulnar nerves in the forearm. Further description of this anomaly and the consequences of its presence are given on p. 165. In the legs, the extensor digitorum brevis may be supplied anomalously by the accessory deep peroneal nerve; the electrophysiologic recognition of this anomaly is discussed on p. 207.

When motor conduction studies are performed, it is important that the direct response of muscle to stimulation of its motor nerve be identified correctly. As already indicated, other responses may be encountered, including the H reflex, the F wave, late potentials related to axon reflexes, and intramuscular nerve action potentials. If these are mistaken for the direct motor response, the latency used for determining conduction velocity will be incorrect.

The responses obtained by proximal and distal stimulation must be similar in configuration if the difference in their latencies is to be used to determine conduction velocity. If they are not similar, they may relate to conduction in different subpopulations of nerve fibers, either because of some anomaly of innervation, inappropriate stimulus intensities (at one or both sites), or some pathologic change in the nerve between the two sites of stimulation.

A number of physiologic factors influence nerve conduction velocity, but these do not necessarily produce erroneous values and so are considered separately.

Technical Factors

Technical errors are common and if unrecognized may lead to spurious values for nerve conduction velocity. If a submaximal stimulus is used, for instance, some of the fastest-conducting fibers may not be stimulated, and this in turn will lead to prolonged latency values or a reduced conduction velocity. The stimulus should, therefore, be approximately 30 percent greater than that which is required to elicit a maximal response. However, inappropriately high stimulus intensities should not be used since this can lead to spread of the stimulating current to a point at some distance from the stimulating cathode, or to a nerve or muscle not being tested. This is especially likely when two or more nerves run closely together, such as in the axilla where the median and ulnar nerves are in close proximity. Finally, if the stimulating cathode is inadvertently reversed with the anode, the conduction distance will be measured incorrectly.

Errors in the measurement of conduction distance can occur for other reasons. It is very important that the position of the stimulating cathode be marked with care before the electrode is removed. Measurements must also be made with the limb in an appropriate position, as this can influence the apparent conduction distance, and so may alter the calculated conduction velocity. For example, when measurements of the conduction distance are made across the elbow segment with the arm extended rather than flexed at this joint, low values for ulnar conduction velocity are obtained.[19,20] Finally, inaccuracies of measurement may be inevitable when the course taken by nerve fibers can only be plotted imprecisely on the body surface, as in the case of fibers traversing the brachial plexus.

Observer error may occur, not only in the measurement of the distance between stimulating and recording sites, but also when the latency of the response is measured. To avoid this, the response should have a well-defined take-off point, and the beam of the cathode ray oscilloscope should be focused properly. An appropriate sweep duration should be selected and the accuracy of the time marker checked periodically. The equipment should be inspected at regular intervals to ensure that it is functioning properly and, in particular, that the sweep is always triggered correctly. The importance of leaving the gain of the amplifier unchanged when responses to stimulation of the nerve at two sites are recorded has been mentioned previously. As indicated by Gassel,[2] this will prevent any bias when latency measurements are made.

PHYSIOLOGIC FACTORS AFFECTING NERVE CONDUCTION VELOCITY

Age

Motor conduction velocity in the ulnar nerve of newborn infants is about half the adult value, reaching the adult level between the ages of 2 and 5 years.[21] Comparable figures for motor conduction velocity in the median, ulnar, and peroneal nerves of the neonate have been obtained,[22] with the values increasing during childhood, as shown in Figure 7.6. Similar changes in sensory conduction velocity have been reported to occur during infancy and childhood.[23] Sensory action potentials were small and difficult to record in subjects younger than 3 months of age, but in older children were similar in size to those of adults.

Although it is commonly accepted that no functional changes occur in the peripheral nerves during later childhood, Lang and associates have recently reported slight but significant changes in motor and sensory conduction velocity during this period.[24] Velocity reportedly increased slightly in the arms and decreased in the legs, regardless of sex.

Conduction velocity—at least in motor fibers—in premature infants is even slower than that of full-term neonates. It correlates with body weight and thus, presumably, with the degree of maturity.[25]

Conduction velocity may decline with advancing age, as reported by Wagman and Lesse, who found that motor conduction velocity may be reduced by about 10 percent in subjects older than 60 years of age.[26] Sensory conduction in the median and ulnar nerves is normally about 10 m/sec slower (i.e., about 15 percent slower) in subjects between 70 and 88 years old than in those between 18 and 25 years of age. Moreover, the amplitude of sensory action potentials recorded at the wrist in the older subjects is about one-third of that in the younger age group.[27] The reduction in amplitude of median sensory action potential is associated with an increased duration of the potential, implying that the change in amplitude with age is not attributable to fiber loss but rather to slowing of conduction velocity (at least until the seventh decade).[28,29]

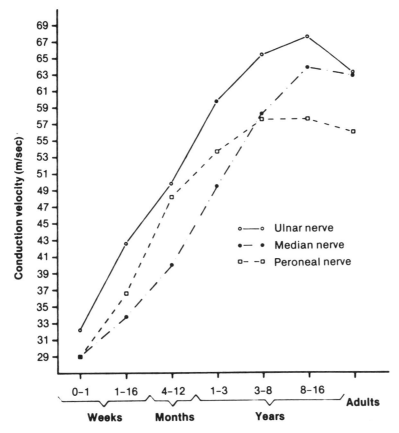

Fig. 7.6 Mean motor conduction velocity in the ulnar, median, and peroneal nerves in different age groups. (Gamstorp I: Normal conduction velocity of ulnar, median and peroneal nerves in infancy, childhood and adolescence. Acta Paediatr suppl. 146:68, 1963.)

Temperature

A progressive decline in latency, duration, amplitude, and area of sensory nerve action potentials and compound muscle action potentials accompanies a physiologic temperature rise.[30,31] Not surprisingly, then, the conduction velocity of peripheral nerves depends on the temperature. Henriksen, for example, found a reduction of 2.4 m/sec in the maximal motor conduction velocity of the human ulnar nerve for each degree Celsius that the intramuscular temperature declines.[3] Similarly, conduction velocity in sensory fibers of the human median nerve decreases by 2 m/sec with each degree Celsius that the temperature declines near the nerve.[27]

In disease of the peripheral nerves, these temperature effects are altered. In abnormal nerve, the rate of change accompanying a rising temperature tends to be less for amplitude, and greater for latency.[31] Thus, the rate of decrease in amplitude and area of the sensory action potential and the compound muscle action potential has been found to be about half that in normal nerve. In compressive neuropathy, the rate of decline of distal motor latency (msec/°C) is greater than normal, and in polyneuropathy, the F-wave latency declines at a much greater rate than in normal nerves.[31]

It is, therefore, important to ensure that the limbs are warm before nerve conduction is studied, particularly when they are likely to be cooler than normal, as in patients with peripheral vascular disease or wasted muscles. The surface temperature of the limb is best checked routinely by means of a thermistor, and should certainly be checked if the limb feels cold. If the temperature is less than about 34°C, the extremity should be warmed. This can be achieved rapidly by immersing the extremity in warm tap water for about 5 minutes, after which the limb should be dried rapidly and then kept covered with toweling to diminish heat loss. Radiant heating appliances can also be used, as can electrical warming blankets. Rather than warming the limb, some authors have used correction factors when the temperature in the extremities has been low. However, these factors are based on the response of normal nerves to changes in temperature, and their application to diseased nerves may be misleading.[31]

Location of the Nerve Fibers Under Study

In general, conduction velocity is greater in proximal segments of nerves than in their more distal portions. This may relate to differences in temperature, in the diameter of axons, or in internodal distances in different parts of limbs. Maximal conduction velocity in both motor and sensory fibers is lower in the legs than in the arms, but the reasons for this have not yet been established with certainty.

LIMITATIONS OF CONVENTIONAL NERVE CONDUCTION STUDIES

Conventional nerve conduction studies have several limitations. First, conduction velocity is easily measured only in the fastest-conducting fibers in the nerve, and the values obtained in the laboratory refer only to this subpopulation of fibers. Second, nerves that are not placed superficially are not easily studied. Third, the nerve roots, limb plexuses, and proximal portions of the peripheral nerves are relatively inaccessible because of their proximal location, and conduction through these segments can only be studied by rather specialized techniques, as discussed in Chapter 8. Fourth, sensory-conduction studies fail to assess the function of sensory receptors or the most distal portions of sensory axons, and these are the very regions where dysfunction may first occur in certain neuropathic disorders. Finally, it may not be possible, by electrophysiologic means, to distinguish between a neuronopathy (in which the primary pathologic process is at the level of the cell bodies) and an axonopathy (in which the peripheral axon is the primary site of involvement).

CORRELATION OF ELECTROPHYSIOLOGIC FINDINGS WITH UNDERLYING PATHOLOGY

Peripheral nerve lesions may lead to axonal degeneration, to abnormalities in conduction along preserved axons, or to both. As Waxman has recently emphasized, several different types of conduction abnormality may occur.[32] Conduction velocity may be reduced in some fibers, resulting in temporal dispersion or loss of coherence of nerve impulses. In such circumstances, maximal motor conduction velocity may be reduced only slightly despite a marked reduction in the size of nerve action potentials. Conduction may be blocked at the site of the lesion, and the block may affect either some or all of the fibers in a nerve. Moreover, the block may be complete or it may be a frequency-related phenomenon. In more subtle disturbances, abnormal temporal patterns or sequences of impulse trains may occur without actual failure of any single impulse. Other abnormalities include ephaptic interactions between fibers, as well as impulse reflections at the sites of axonal injury.

Acute Compressive Nerve Lesions

The pathologic and electrophysiologic changes that occur in focal nerve lesions have been studied experimentally, with special reference to the compressive lesions produced by pneumatic tourniquets. This has been one of the major areas of interest of Gilliatt and co-workers in London.[33,34] An acute compressive lesion may lead to a rapidly reversible conduction block as a result of ischemia of the compressed nerve fibers. More severe and sustained compression leads to localized structural damage to the nerve fibers or to axonal degeneration, both of which cause weakness or paralysis of the muscles supplied by these fibers. With mild lesions, pathologic change is usually limited to the region under the tourniquet, and occurs especially toward the edges of the compressed region, with the more central section being spared. Demyelination occurs in the region of the nodes of Ranvier. Electron microscopy of single, teased fibers viewed in longitudinal section reveals displacement of the nodes along each fiber so that the paranodal myelin is stretched on one side of the node and invaginated on the other. Invagination always occurs away from the cuff and toward the uncompressed tissue. The stretched myelin lamellae are damaged and may rupture, and degeneration then leads to the appearance of paranodal demyelination. Large myelinated fibers appear to be more liable to such injury than fibers having an external diameter of less than 5 μm, and afferent and efferent fibers of comparable size seem to be equally susceptible.

Electrophysiologic studies show that such lesions are associated with conduction block in many nerve fibers, and that this occurs near the edges of the length of the nerve previously compressed. In other words, there are two areas of partial conduction block. At these sites, conduction velocity in unblocked fibers is markedly reduced; velocity is only slightly affected in the segment of nerve that has been under the center of the cuff,[35] probably because of selective large fiber block at the edge of the lesion.[33] Recovery from conduction block occurs with time, but it generally takes longer as the duration of compression or the length of nerve compressed increases.

With more severe compressive lesions, segmental or internodal demyelination occurs. Ultimately axonal degeneration occurs distal to the lesion.

Chronic Nerve Compression and Entrapment

Ochoa and Marotte found with *chronic* nerve entrapment that in single fibers both proximal and distal to the site of entrapment the internodes were bulbous at one end and tapered at the other.[36] Proximal to the lesion, the proximal ends of the internodes were bulbous, whereas distal to the lesion, the distal ends were bulbous. The underlying sequence of events postulated by these researchers is shown in Figure 7.7. They believe that asymmetry of the myelin sheath led to its retraction from one side of the node, and thus, to paranodal demyelination. Subsequently, myelin loss occurred from the complete internodal segment, and in severe cases there was complete degeneration of the fiber. Such changes have been found in humans in the median nerve fibers at the wrist and the ulnar nerve fibers at the elbow,[37–39] as well as in the lateral cutaneous nerve of the thigh at the anterior end of the inguinal ligament.[40]

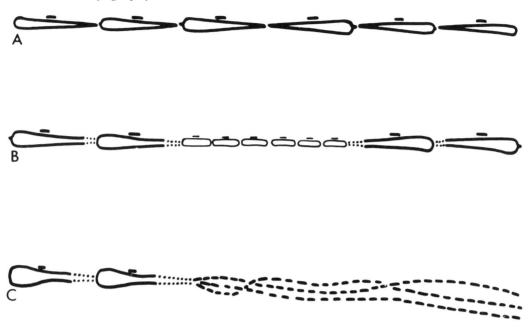

Fig. 7.7 The sequence of changes in chronic compression suggested by Ochoa. (**A**) Distorted internodal segments in a minimal entrapment lesion, with reversal of polarity at the center. (**B**) A more severe lesion with paranodal demyelination affecting the distorted internodes at the edges, and complete demyelination, followed by remyelination, in the center. (**C**) Greater distortion of the internodes on the proximal side of the lesion, with wallerian degeneration distally. (Ochoa J: Nerve fiber pathology in acute and chronic compression. In Omer GE, Spinner M (eds). Management of Peripheral Nerve Problems. W.B. Saunders, Philadelphia, 1980.)

The relative contribution of ischemia and mechanical deformation to the pathologic and electrophysiologic changes that accompany acute or chronic nerve compression awaits more detailed study. However, Gilliatt has reviewed much of the available evidence and concluded that mechanical factors are probably of prime importance in this regard.[33,34] Nevertheless, ischemia may certainly be responsible for some of the clinical or electrophysiologic features of common nerve entrapment syndromes. In patients with carpal tunnel syndrome, for instance, Hongell and Mattsson documented conduction delay or block in sensory fibers with intraoperative recordings.[41] They found that, within a few minutes of decompression, the conduction velocity increased and fibers that had previously been blocked began to respond again to physiologic or electrical stimuli (Fig. 7.8 and 7.9).

The speed of this recovery suggests that ischemia may have been important in causing the conduction block. Also in patients with carpal tunnel syndrome, Fullerton found that the ischemia produced by a cuff around the arm blocked motor conduction at the wrist in a much shorter time than in control subjects, with the block rapidly reversing with release of the cuff.[42] Such an increased sensitivity of motor fibers to ischemia was found to be related to the severity of pain and paresthesias reported in the days preceding the test. It may be relevant, therefore, that the pain of the carpal tunnel syndrome is usually relieved as soon as the nerve is decompressed, as if ischemia had some role in its production, whereas conduction delay in motor fibers takes longer to resolve.

Further experimental evidence of the role of ischemia in patients with nerve entrap-

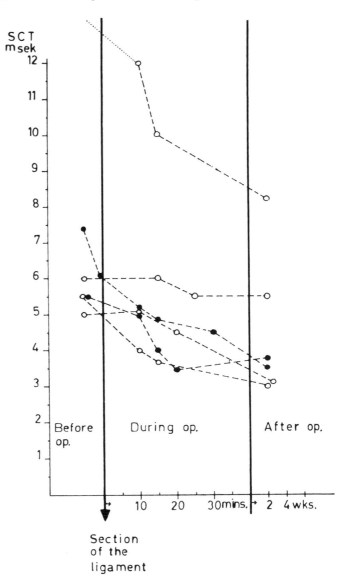

Fig. 7.8 Macroneurographic recording of sensory conduction time immediately before and after sectioning of the anterior carpal ligament, as well as about 2 weeks postoperatively. (Hongell A, Mattsson HS: Neurographic studies before, after, and during operation for median nerve compression in the carpal tunnel. Scand J Plast Reconstr Surg 5:103, 1971.)

ment syndromes comes from the recently published work of Parry and colleagues, who studied the effect of transient focal ischemia on electrophysiologic function of rat sciatic nerves.[43] They found that a reversible conduction block occurred, without associated structural change or significant conduction slowing. Conduction failure was most severe about 45 to 60 minutes after the local blood supply was interrupted. Conduction then returned to normal within 24 hours (Fig. 7.10). Such findings suggest that

metabolic factors may also be important in causing conduction block and so may underlie some of the clinical features of chronic entrapment neuropathies.

Clinical experience suggests that patients with a metabolic disorder, such as diabetes mellitus, are particularly prone to develop a focal entrapment neuropathy. There is also some experimental evidence that the development of an entrapment neuropathy may be influenced by systemic or toxic factors, or by mild, generalized, peripheral

NORMAL

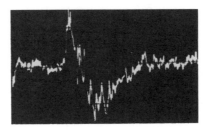

MEDIAN NERVE COMPRESSION

1. <u>Immediately before</u> section of the volar carpal ligament.

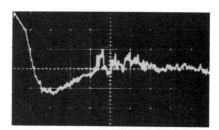

2. <u>4 minutes after</u> section of the ligament.

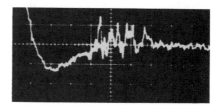

3. <u>30 minutes after</u> section of the ligament.

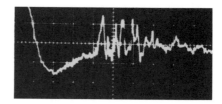

1 msec.

Fig. 7.9 Recording of the potential evoked by electrical stimulation of a finger nerve and recorded with a microelectrode in the corresponding skin nerve fascicle of the median nerve. The normal potential is recorded percutaneously; the potentials recorded from the patient with median nerve compression are recorded from the exposed nerve. Note the improvement in amplitude and complexity of the potential 4 and 30 minutes after sectioning of the anterior carpal ligament. (Hongell A, Mattsson HS: Neurographic studies before, after, and during operation for median nerve compression in the carpal tunnel. Scand J Plast Reconstr Surg 5:103, 1971.)

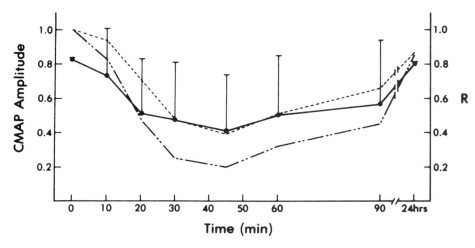

Fig. 7.10 Sequential compound muscle action potentials (CMAPs) elicited by stimulation of 15 rat sciatic-posterior tibial nerves after femoral artery occlusion. Nerves were stimulated proximally in the sciatic notch (sciatic nerve) and distally at the medial malleolus (posterior tibial nerve). Amplitude is expressed as the ratio of postischemic to preischemic values. CMAPs elicited by proximal stimulation (−··−··−) decrease more rapidly and to a greater degree than after distal stimulation (−−−−−−−). The ratio (R) of the proximal-to-distal CMAP amplitudes was calculated, and is shown by a solid line. Responses returned to normal within 24 hours. The larger decrement in the response to proximal stimulation is reflected by R, which is a measure of conduction block. (Parry GJ, Cornblath DR, Brown MJ: Transient conduction block following acute peripheral nerve ischemia. Muscle Nerve 8:409, 1985. Copyright © 1985, John Wiley & Sons, Inc. Reprinted by permission.)

nerve dysfunction. For example, guinea pigs kept for many months in cages with a wire mesh floor develop a focal plantar neuropathy in the hind feet secondary to recurrent compression of the plantar nerves by the cage bars, whereas animals kept in cages with solid floors do not develop this neuropathy.[44] When these animals are given small parenteral doses of diphtheria toxin, they develop this pressure neuropathy much sooner and more easily, and even the animals kept on solid floors develop it. Indeed, plantar nerve damage can only then be prevented if weight-bearing by the hind feet is prevented completely.[45]

Focal entrapment neuropathies are probably much more common than is clinically apparent. Neary and colleagues studied the median and ulnar nerves at routine autopsies of patients without known disease of the peripheral nervous system.[37] They found that the median nerve at the wrist and the ulnar nerve at the elbow commonly showed striking changes in the connective tissue, sometimes in the absence of significant alterations in the nerve fibers. These changes included fascicular enlargement, with or without perineurial thickening. Renaut's bodies were conspicuous at these two sites. Features characteristic of nerve fiber damage included distorted internodes with bulbous swellings at one end, sometimes accompanied by demyelination.

Nerve Transection

The changes of wallerian degeneration are now widely appreciated, although their development over time varies in different animal species. If a nerve is severed or severely compressed in humans, axons and myelin in the distal stump disintegrate rapidly over several days. Neuromuscular transmission rapidly fails, and after about 2 to 3 days, there is a progressive loss of excitability in the distal stump until, within about a week, it becomes completely inexcitable. The maximal conduction velocity in this segment generally remains normal (although the size of the nerve or compound muscle action potential declines progressively) until the nerve is no longer excitable. Proximal to the transection, there may be a variable degree of retrograde axonal degeneration, a reduction in axonal diameter, and some slowing of axonal conduction velocity, and the affected cell bodies show reactive changes. Axonal sprouts appear within 1 to 2 days after nerve transection, growing from the proximal toward the distal end of the stump. However, the rate at which this proceeds and at which axons are able to bridge the gap and reach the distal stump depends upon the type of nerve injury, the distance between the proximal and distal stumps, and a number of other factors.[46] The regenerating axons generally grow at a rate of approximately 2 mm per day. They are thin, unmyelinated, and have a low conduction velocity and a high threshold for electrical stimuli. As remyelination occurs and axons mature, conduction velocity in the regenerating fibers increases and the threshold for excitation diminishes.

Diffuse Peripheral Nerve Pathology

The pathologic basis of diffuse peripheral nerve dysfunction may be either segmental demyelination or axonal degeneration. Axonal degeneration often begins distally, and then spreads more proximally. Schaumburg and Spencer introduced the term *distal axonopathy* to indicate that, in such circumstances, pathologic changes begin multifocally in distal portions of the axons and then spread more proximally, although not in a serial fashion.[47] In many distal axonopathies, the longest and largest fibers are those most susceptible to damage. In focal or diffuse processes characterized by axonal loss, surviving axons to partially denervated muscles may give off terminal and preterminal collateral sprouts that eventually reinnervate muscle fibers that have lost their nerve supply. This may only be evident on needle electromyography (p. 90).

CLINICAL ELECTRODIAGNOSIS OF NERVE LESIONS

Focal Neuropathies

Focal nerve lesions may be identified by demonstrating that axonal degeneration has occurred, that there is a complete or partial conduction block in a particular segment of the nerve, or that there is an abnormal conduction velocity in this segment in comparison to that found in adjacent segments. Needle electromyography may also help to localize a peripheral nerve lesion by indicating which muscles have been affected.

When a nerve is stimulated on one side of a focal lesion and the response (of either nerve or muscle) is recorded after the impulses have traversed the affected segment of nerve, four types of abnormality may be encountered. First, there may be no response whatsoever. Second, there may be a reduction in size of the response. Third, the response may be of abnormal configuration (e.g., dispersed and polyphasic). Fourth, there may be a reduced maximal conduction velocity, as evidenced by an increase in latency of the response. Depending upon the severity of the lesion, however, the response may be normal.

If a nerve is transected, the motor response or nerve action potential obtained by stimulating and recording from nerve fibers distal to the transection remains normal for 2 to 3 days, after which it diminishes in size until it becomes unobtainable over the following 1 to 4 days. From the time the lesion is made, however, stimulation of the nerve above the site of transection fails to elicit any response whatsoever in the nerve below it, or in muscles supplied from the distal stump. In muscles that have lost their nerve supply, needle electromyography fails to reveal any motor units under voluntary control. Electromyographic signs of abnormal spontaneous activity do not appear for a variable interval after nerve transection, depending upon the site of the muscle. They appear earlier in more proximal muscles, and it may take 3 to 5 weeks before abnormal spontaneous activity is found in distally placed denervated muscle. As neuromuscular connections are re-established, the amount of abnormal spontaneous activity in the muscle diminishes, and needle electromyography reveals small motor units under voluntary control. These are typically polyphasic in form, small in amplitude, and short in duration. Single fiber studies show that jitter is markedly increased and frequent impulse blocking occurs. With time, the number of motor unit potentials under voluntary control increases and the parameters of the potentials approach the normal range, although the orderly recruitment of motor units with increasing voluntary activity is lost.[48] Muscles are reinnervated in an orderly proximal-distal sequence, and those that are close to the site of nerve transection are likely to be reinnervated more fully than distal muscles.

Focal compressive lesions may lead to complete axonal degeneration, in which case accurate localization of the site of the lesion may be impossible. The findings are as was described just previously. If only some of the axons degenerate, then the evoked response (motor response or nerve action potential) is reduced in size and area with both proximal and distal stimulation, there may be little change in maximal conduction velocity, and electromyographic signs of partial denervation are found in af-fected muscles after an appropriate interval. As recovery occurs, abnormal spontaneous activity diminishes in these muscles, and large, long-duration, polyphasic motor unit potentials are found, reflecting reinnervation through collateral sprouting from surviving axons.

With complete conduction block, the size and latency of the motor response to stimulation below the level of the lesion remain normal, whereas with more proximal stimulation (i.e., stimulation above the lesion), no response can be obtained. When there is partial conduction block, a response to proximal stimulation can still be obtained, but it is smaller in amplitude and area than the response elicited by stimulation distal to the lesion. Similarly, when conduction block is complete, the nerve action potential is unrecordable if impulses have to traverse the site of the lesion; with partial conduction block, a small potential may be recordable.

In some focal lesions, there is a combination of conduction block in some fibers and axonal degeneration in others, while yet other fibers may remain intact. The electrophysiologic findings in such circumstances show a combination of the features described above. Needle electromyography may help to distinguish conduction block from axonal degeneration. In either context, there is reduced recruitment of motor units, and in severe cases, no units remain under voluntary control. When there is only a conduction block, however, needle electromyography does not reveal any abnormal insertion or spontaneous activity. In contrast, if axonal degeneration has occurred, insertion activity increases and fibrillation potentials are found after a variable time, depending upon the muscle examined.

In mild compressive lesions in which there is neither axonal degeneration nor conduction block, the only electrophysiologic abnormality may be a slowing of conduction across the site of the lesion. The

motor response may be dispersed and reduced in amplitude when elicited by stimulation above rather than below the level of
the lesion, and maximal conduction velocity is reduced. However, unless conduction
block has occurred, the area of the response
is unchanged. Again, the nerve action potential recorded on one side of the lesion
following stimulation on the other is of prolonged latency, and is small and dispersed.
In some cases, a focal nerve lesion leads to
slowing of conduction not only at the site
of the lesion, but also more distally in motor
and sensory fibers. This can be due to selective loss of large axons and to the presence of small, poorly myelinated, regenerating fibers. A failure of the regenerating
fibers to mature and the presence of nar-
rowed distal axons may also be relevant.

It is sometimes possible to localize a
nerve lesion precisely if there is a disproportionate change in latency of the response
to nerve stimulation, with only a slight
change in the site of stimulation. If the
nerve is stimulated sequentially in equal
steps along its course (the "inching" technique), the site of the lesion will be indicated by the point at which the response
latency suddenly increases disproportionately (Fig. 7.11).

Polyneuropathies

Axonal neuropathies are especially common in toxic or metabolic disorders. Conduction velocity usually remains normal or
is only slightly slowed, but there is a decrease in the size of the compound muscle
action potential and of sensory action potentials. Abnormalities are more likely to
be found when the most distal segments of
nerves are studied. Casey and LeQuesne
recorded potentials from the digital nerves
and compared the findings with those from
recordings at the wrist, after stimulating the
tip of the index finger.[49] Among 16 alcoholic
subjects with little or no clinical evidence

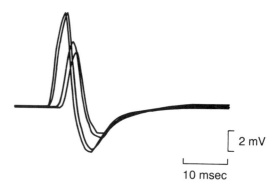

Fig. 7.11 Inching technique to demonstrate the
site of a focal nerve lesion. The muscle responses to four supramaximal stimuli delivered
sequentially at intervals of 2 cm along a motor
nerve are shown. A disproportionate change in
latency and amplitude of the response occurs
between the second and third stimuli, localizing
the lesion to this 2-cm segment of the nerve.

of peripheral neuropathy, they found abnormalities in the distal sensory nerve
trunks in 7, only one of whom had an abnormal sensory potential at the wrist.
Needle electromyography in patients with
axonal neuropathies commonly shows evidence of chronic partial denervation in distal muscles of the extremities.

In certain of the hereditary and inflammatory neuropathies, the predominant
pathologic change is segmental demyelination. The electrophysiologic features of
such *demyelinative neuropathies* are a reduction by more than 40 percent in motor
and sensory conduction velocities[50] and
prolonged terminal motor latencies. In acquired demyelinative neuropathies, superimposed focal changes may be encountered
at common sites of entrapment or at other
sites when the individual nerves are studied, whereas in familial neuropathies, conduction is uniformly slowed and is rarely,
if ever, blocked.[51] Responses typically become increasingly attenuated and dispersed
as conduction distance increases (that is, as
the distance between stimulating and recording electrodes increases). Needle elec-

tromyography fails to reveal any evidence of denervation unless axonal degeneration has also occurred. Further comment in this regard may be found in Chapter 11.

REPORTING THE RESULTS OF NERVE CONDUCTION STUDIES

In reporting the results of nerve conduction studies, specific mention should be made of the individual nerves examined, the sites at which they were stimulated, and the type of electrodes with which recordings were made. The latency and amplitude of the response, the conduction distance, and the calculated conduction velocity should be clearly stated for each segment of nerve that was studied. Since the value obtained for sensory nerve conduction velocity depends, in part, on the method used for measuring and calculating it, this, too, should be indicated. In particular, it should be stated whether measurements were made to the onset or to the peak of the negative potential. If permanent records were obtained during the study, this should also be noted. This factual report, which is best presented in tabular form, should be accompanied by an account of the conclusions reached by the examiner and their clinical relevance.

When the results of nerve conduction studies are being evaluated, comparisons should be made with data obtained in the same laboratory and by the same techniques from normal subjects. This is because there is some variation in the normal values published from different laboratories, partly as a result of methodologic differences.

Care must be taken to avoid reaching diagnostic conclusions on the basis of an inadequate examination. The scope of the examination will have been governed by the clinical findings and the diagnostic problem posed by the patient. A few general points can, however, be made in this regard, and these will indicate the care that must be exercised in interpreting the results obtained with the investigative procedures described above.

In confirming the presence of an isolated peripheral nerve lesion by electrophysiologic means, conduction should be studied not only in the clinically affected nerve but in at least one other nerve so that the possibility of a subclinical polyneuropathy may be excluded. This is emphasized because a generalized neuropathy may present with clinical involvement of only one nerve. The possibility that there is a localized lesion of the affected nerve should also be considered, and conduction should be assessed in the segment of nerve encompassing the likely site of involvement. In order to confirm the existence of a localized lesion on the basis of conduction velocity, however, velocity in the segment of nerve in question must not only be slower than normal, but must be disproportionately slower than that in neighboring segments. Both motor and sensory conduction should be measured so that the functional status of the nerve is evaluated as fully as possible, especially since motor and sensory fibers are not necessarily affected to the same extent by the underlying pathology. Moreover, abnormalities of sensory conduction may be found in patients with normal motor function, and vice versa.

Both motor and sensory conduction should also be assessed in detail in patients with widespread peripheral nerve involvement. In planning the examination of such patients, however, it should be remembered that, in many polyneuropathies, sensory fibers are affected earlier than motor ones, and the legs are affected before the arms. Several nerves in the arms and legs should be examined on both sides of the body to determine whether involvement is symmetric. Some patients with a generalized polyneuropathy may have superimposed entrapment neuropathies, and this must not be taken as evidence of a mononeuritis multiplex. A diagnosis of *demyelinative* neuropathy should not be suggested on the basis of electrophysiologic studies unless conduction velocity is reduced by more than 40 percent, marked prolongation of terminal latencies is noted, compound muscle or sensory action potentials are markedly dispersed, or a conduction block is present. In interpreting the findings, a focal lesion with localized slowing of conduction must be excluded by appropriate studies of different segments of the nerve before it is assumed that conduction velocity is slowed diffusely.

REFERENCES

1. Simpson JA: Fact and fallacy in measurement of conduction velocity in motor nerves. J Neurol Neurosurg Psychiatry 27:381, 1964
2. Gassel MM: Sources of error in motor nerve conduction studies. Neurology 14:825, 1964
3. Henriksen JD: M.S. Thesis, University of Minnesota, 1956
4. LeQuesne PM: Nerve conduction in clinical practice. p. 419. In Licht S (ed): Electrodiagnosis and Electromyography. Elizabeth Licht, New Haven, CT, 1971
5. Lloyd DPC: The interaction of antidromic and orthodromic volleys in a segmental spinal motor nucleus. J Neurophysiol 6:143, 1943
6. Dawson GD, Merton PA: "Recurrent" discharges from motoneurons. p. 221. In Abstracts, 20th International Congress of Physiology. Brussels, 1956
7. McLeod JG, Wray SH: An experimental study of the F wave in the baboon. J Neurol Neurosurg Psychiatry 29:196, 1966
8. Mayer RF, Feldman RG: Observations on the nature of the F wave in man. Neurology 17:147, 1967
9. Fullerton PM, Gilliatt RW: Axon reflexes in human motor nerve fibres. J Neurol Neurosurg Psychiatry 28:1, 1965
10. Guttman L: The intramuscular nerve action potential. J Neurol Neurosurg Psychiatry 32:193, 1969
11. Dawson GD, Scott JW: The recording of nerve action potentials through skin in man. J Neurol Neurosurg Psychiatry 12:259, 1949
12. Dawson GD: The relative excitability and conduction velocity of sensory and motor nerve fibres in man. J Physiol 131:436, 1956
13. Gilliatt RW, Sears TA: Sensory nerve action potentials in patients with peripheral nerve lesions. J Neurol Neurosurg Psychiatry 21:109, 1958
14. Rosenfalck A: Early recognition of nerve disorders by near-nerve recording of sensory action potentials. Muscle Nerve 1:360, 1978
15. Andersen K: Comparison of sensory recording with surface and needle electrodes. Muscle Nerve 8:628, 1985
16. Gilliatt RW, Melville ID, Velate AS, Willison RG: A study of normal nerve action potentials using an averaging technique (barrier grid storage tube). J Neurol Neurosurg Psychiatry 28:191, 1965
17. Bolton CF, Sawa GM, Carter K: The effects of temperature on human compound action potentials. J Neurol Neurosurg Psychiatry 44:407, 1981
18. Bolton CF, Carter KM: Human sensory nerve compound action potential amplitude: Variation with sex and finger circumference. J Neurol Neurosurg Psychiatry 43:925, 1980
19. Checkles NS, Russakov AD, Piero DL: Ulnar nerve conduction velocity—Effect of elbow position on measurement. Arch Phys Med Rehabil 52:362, 1971
20. Harding C, Halar E: Motor and sensory ulnar nerve conduction velocities: Effect of elbow position. Arch Phys Med Rehabil 64:227, 1983
21. Thomas JE, Lambert EH: Ulnar nerve conduction velocity and H-reflex in infants and children. J Appl Physiol 15:1, 1960
22. Gamstorp I: Normal conduction velocity of ulnar, median and peroneal nerves in infancy, childhood and adolescence. Acta Paediatr [Suppl] 146:68, 1963
23. Gamstorp I, Shelburne SA: Peripheral sensory conduction in ulnar and median nerves of normal infants, children and adolescents. Acta Paediatr Scand 54:309, 1965
24. Lang HA, Puusa A, Hynninen P, Kuusela V, Jantti V, Sillanpaa M: Evolution of nerve conduction velocity in later childhood and adolescence. Muscle Nerve 8:38, 1985

25. Cerra D, Johnson EW: Motor nerve conduction velocity in premature infants. Arch Phys Med Rehabil 43:160, 1962
26. Wagman IH, Lesse H: Maximum conduction velocities of motor fibers of ulnar nerve in human subjects of various ages and sizes. J Neurophysiol 15:235, 1952
27. Buchthal F, Rosenfalck A: Evoked action potentials and conduction velocity in human sensory nerves. Brain Res 3:1, 1966
28. Nielsen VK: Sensory and motor nerve conduction in the median nerve in normal subjects. Acta Med Scand 194:435, 1973
29. Andersen K: Surface recording of orthodromic sensory nerve action potentials in median and ulnar nerves in normal subjects. Muscle Nerve 8:402, 1985
30. Hlavova A, Abramson DI, Rickert BL, Talso JF: Temperature effects on duration and amplitude of distal median nerve action potential. J Appl Physiol 28:808, 1970
31. Bolton CF, Carter K, Koval JJ: Temperature effects on conduction studies of normal and abnormal nerve. Muscle Nerve 5:S145, 1982
32. Waxman SG: Pathophysiology of nerve conduction: Relation to diabetic neuropathy. Ann Intern Med 92:297, 1980
33. Gilliatt RW: Acute compression block. p. 287. In Sumner AJ (ed): The Physiology of Peripheral Nerve Disease. W.B. Saunders, Philadelphia, 1980
34. Gilliatt RW: Chronic nerve compression and entrapment. p. 316. In Sumner AJ (ed): The Physiology of Peripheral Nerve Disease. W.B. Saunders, Philadelphia, 1980
35. Gilliatt RW, McDonald WI, Rudge P: The site of conduction block in peripheral nerves compressed by a pneumatic tourniquet. J Physiol 238:31P, 1974
36. Ochoa J, Marotte L: The nature of the nerve lesion caused by chronic entrapment in the guinea-pig. J Neurol Sci 19:491, 1973
37. Neary D, Ochoa J, Gilliatt RW: Sub-clinical entrapment neuropathy in man. J Neurol Sci 24:283, 1975
38. Neary D, Eames RA: The pathology of ulnar nerve compression in man. Neuropathol Appl Neurobiol 1:69, 1975
39. Harriman DGF: Ischaemia of peripheral nerve and muscle. J Clin Pathol, 30: suppl. 11, 94, 1977
40. Jefferson D, Eames RA: Subclinical entrapment of the lateral femoral cutaneous nerve: An autopsy study. Muscle Nerve 2:145, 1979
41. Hongell A, Mattsson HS: Neurographic studies before, after, and during operation for median nerve compression in the carpal tunnel. Scand J Plast Reconstr Surg 5:103, 1971
42. Fullerton PM: The effect of ischaemia on nerve conduction in the carpal tunnel syndrome. J Neurol Neurosurg Psychiatry 26:385, 1963
43. Parry GJ, Cornblath DR, Brown MJ: Transient conduction block following acute peripheral nerve ischemia. Muscle Nerve 8:409, 1985
44. Fullerton PM, Gilliatt RW: Pressure neuropathy in the hind foot of the guinea-pig. J Neurol Neurosurg Psychiatry 30:18, 1967
45. Hopkins AP, Morgan-Hughes JA: The effect of local pressure in diphtheritic neuropathy. J Neurol Neurosurg Psychiatry 32:614, 1969
46. Sunderland S: Nerves and Nerve Injuries. 2nd Ed. Churchill Livingstone, Edinburgh, 1978
47. Schaumburg HH, Spencer PS: Toxic neuropathies. Neurology 29:429, 1979
48. Milner-Brown HS, Stein RB, Lee RG: Pattern of recruiting human motor units in neuropathies and motor neurone disease. J Neurol Neurosurg Psychiatry 37:665, 1974
49. Casey EB, LeQuesne PM: Electrophysiological evidence for a distal lesion in alcoholic neuropathy. J Neurol Neurosurg Psychiatry 35:624, 1972
50. Gilliatt RW: Nerve conduction in human and experimental neuropathies. Proc R Soc Med 59:989, 1966
51. Lewis RA, Sumner AJ: The electrodiagnostic distinctions between chronic familial and acquired demyelinative neuropathies. Neurology 32:592, 1982

8

Other Electrodiagnostic Techniques for the Evaluation of Neuromuscular Disorders

QUANTITATIVE ASPECTS OF ELECTROMYOGRAPHY

In an endeavor to improve the accuracy, reliability, and speed with which electromyography is performed, and to gain further insight into the pathophysiology of neuromuscular disorders, researchers have developed a number of quantitative techniques that merit brief discussion.

Measurement of Motor Unit Parameters

The most commonly used quantitative technique consists of measuring the parameters of individual motor unit potentials. The original technique is described in detail by Buchthal and Pinelli.[1,2] In brief, 20 or more potentials are each recorded photographically five times during slight voluntary activity of the muscle under examination, and their amplitude and duration are measured. The data are then compared with the values obtained from the corresponding muscle in age-matched normal subjects examined in the same laboratory under the same conditions and with the same recording electrode and arrangements. This method has been used in a number of clinical contexts by different workers, but it is time-consuming and provides information concerning primarily the motor unit potentials activated during slight effort.

The accuracy and reliability of this approach have improved with the development of signal delay lines that facilitate recognition of individual potentials and measurement of their various components. Computerized template analysis, in which motor unit identification is based on recurrence and measurement is based on subtraction of superimposed potentials, has permitted study of motor units at higher frequencies, when a larger number of potentials are present.[3] Other computerized approaches have also been used, and these have been reviewed by Daube.[4] These automated methods, in which motor unit potentials are selected for analysis on the basis

129

of amplitude, recurrence of similar forms, or some other predetermined criterion, can distinguish between myopathic and neurogenic disorders, but generally provide little new information.

Motor Unit Territory

The distribution of potentials containing spikes from a single motor unit can be measured by inserting two multielectrodes at right angles to each other across the muscle. Recordings are then made at intervals along the length of each electrode. The motor unit territory in limb muscles is roughly circular in area and normally has a diameter of 5 to 7 mm in the upper extremities and 7 to 10 mm in the lower extremities.[5] The density of active muscle fibers is thought to be reflected by the amplitude of the largest spikes recorded in this way. Motor unit territory is increased by up to about 40 percent in patients with neurogenic weakness, presumably, at least in part, as a result of reinnervation of denervated muscle fibers by collateral sprouting from surviving axons. In contrast, motor unit territory is often reduced in patients with myopathic disorders, such as muscular dystrophy and polymyositis, as a result of the loss of some of the muscle fibers from individual units.[6,7]

Frequency Analysis

Automatic methods of frequency analysis have been used in the diagnosis of muscle disease by several researchers. Richardson described a method of analysis in which the amount of activity at or exceeding 400 Hz in a full interference pattern was compared with that at less than 400 Hz; the results showed a shift to the higher frequencies in myopathies.[8] Walton used an audiofrequency spectrometer for more detailed frequency analysis of the full interference pattern.[9] The apparatus consisted of 27 resonant circuits tuned to different frequencies throughout the range of 40 to 16,000 Hz. Upon contraction of the muscles, the storage condensers in the filter circuits for each of the frequencies were charged in proportion to the amount of activity of the frequency appearing in the waveforms being analyzed. These currents were then fed into a cathode ray oscilloscope for display. Walton found that, in the electromyograms of normal control subjects, activity was confined to the frequency bands below 800 Hz in the major limb muscles, with the peak frequency occurring at 100 to 200 Hz. In contrast, in 98 of 100 patients with muscular dystrophy, there was a shift of the dominant frequency to higher values. In a critical evaluation of this method, Fex and Krakau obtained results similar to those of Walton, but concluded that the method was of limited diagnostic value by itself.[10] The work of Larsson suggests that frequency analysis can distinguish between neuropathic and myopathic disorders and may permit the changes occurring with time to be followed.[11] The development of small computers for spectral analysis should help to advance this approach, but its clinical utility remains to be established.

Estimation of Motor Unit Number

McComas and a number of other workers have attempted to estimate the number of motor units in the extensor digitorum brevis and other limb muscles on the basis of the amplitude of the compound muscle action potentials recorded by surface electrodes following nerve stimulation.[12–14] The technique involves the recruitment of successive motor units singly by grading the intensity of the electrical stimulus to the nerve (Fig. 8.1) so that the mean motor unit potential amplitude may be calculated. The

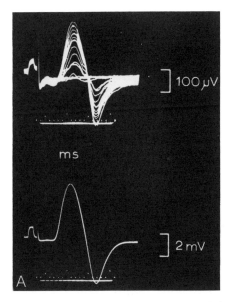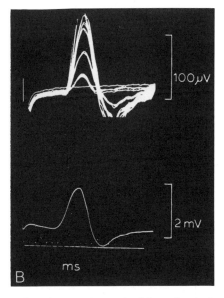

Fig. 8.1 Action potentials in the extensor digitorum brevis muscle evoked by stimulation of the anterior tibial nerve in a control subject (**A**) and a 16-year-old boy with Duchenne type dystrophy (**B**). In both instances, the upper records display superimposed traces of responses as stimulus intensity was gradually increased above threshold; the incremental nature of the potentials is clearly seen. The lower records show the responses to supramaximal stimuli. (McComas AJ, Sica REP, Currie S: Muscular dystrophy: Evidence for a neural factor. Reprinted from Nature, Vol. 226, No. 5252, pp. 1263–1264. Copyright © 1970 Macmillan Journals Limited.)

response of all the motor units in the muscle is then evoked by a maximal nerve stimulus, and the number of units within the muscle is determined by division. The method depends on a number of questionable underlying assumptions[15] and has been criticized on a number of other grounds,[16] in particular, on whether it is sensitive enough to distinguish the small motor units that can occur in myopathic disorders. Despite these objections, McComas and his colleagues concluded that conditions such as the muscular dystrophies, previously regarded as primary degenerative disorders of muscle, are neurogenic in origin because they found an apparent reduction in the number of motor units contained in muscle in these disorders.[17–19]

Ballantyne and Hansen have described a

modification of this method, incorporating on-line computer analysis, which is said to be a more sensitive means of estimating the number of motor units in muscle, especially when the configuration of motor unit potentials is qualitatively altered from normal.[20] They reported normal numbers of motor units in the muscles of patients with Duchenne type, limb-girdle, and facioscapulohumeral muscular dystrophy, but significantly reduced numbers in patients with myotonic dystrophy.[21] The method of McComas and his colleagues has also been modified by Milner-Brown and Brown[22] to correct for fluctuations in the response of motor units to electrical excitation and for any overlap in the firing levels of motor axons. They found that previous estimates of the number of motor units in a muscle were generally too high, and concluded that a number of problems still remained to be solved before electrophysiologic methods could reliably be used to make such estimates.

Computer-assisted motor unit counting, together with determination of the area of individual potentials, has been used to provide a quantitative assessment of reinnervation in various polyneuropathies and neuronopathies.[23] Reinnervation is reflected by an increase in the mean motor unit potential area, whereas a reduction in the number of functioning motor axons reflects the severity of denervation. Ballantyne and Hansen found that, as the number of motor units declines, the degree of reinnervation is greater in neuronopathies (such as motor neuron disease or Alzheimer's disease) than in neuropathies, and is also greater in diabetic neuropathy than in uremic or alcoholic neuropathy.[23] In the Guillain-Barré syndrome, reinnervation was found to continue for periods of up to 7 years from onset of the disorder. Thus, such quantitative studies show that there are marked differences in the capacity for compensatory reinnervation among these various disorders.

Single Fiber Electromyography

Single fiber electromyography is an important technique, the details of which are discussed at length by Ekstedt and Stalberg.[24] In brief, muscle fiber action potentials are recorded from a needle electrode that has a small, active electrode surface mounted in its side. It is inserted into the muscle while the muscle is under slight voluntary activation. The potentials have a constant shape for consecutive discharges, provided that the time resolution of the display is 10 μsec. They are essentially biphasic and often are followed by a small, long-duration, terminal phase. The potentials are usually 5 to 10 mV in amplitude and have a total duration of less than 2

msec; the rise time of the positive-negative deflection is less than 200 μsec when the electrode is appropriately positioned. Activity is usually recorded from only one muscle fiber at a time in an individual motor unit. In a certain number of recording positions, however, activity can be recorded from two or more muscle fibers belonging to the same motor unit. In such circumstances, the time interval between the recorded action potentials depends on differences in conduction time along the nerve and muscle fibers and on the anatomic localization of motor end-plates. This interval between the two action potentials is called the *interpotential interval,* and it has a temporal variability, called the *jitter,* which is attributable mainly to variation in the neuromuscular transmission time in the two motor end-plates involved. The jitter can be expressed numerically as the mean value of consecutive differences (MCD) of 100 interpotential intervals; its value normally lies between 5 and 50 μsec, depending on the muscle examined. The value does not depend on the recording site, suggesting that variability in the conduction velocity of muscle or nerve fibers contributes only a minor portion of the jitter.

Measurement of jitter is a sensitive means of evaluating neuromuscular transmission. When there is uncertain transmission in the terminal nerve twigs or immature motor end-plates, such as occurs following reinnervation, jitter is increased, and there may be an intermittent or constant conduction block. In patients with myasthenia gravis, increased jitter and impulse blocking are the expected findings (Fig. 8.2), especially in muscles that are affected clinically. In patients with myopathy, a slight increase in jitter may be seen in 10 to 15 percent of the recordings, and impulse blocking may be found in 5 to 10 percent.[25] Jitter is normal in myotonia congenita but is increased in myotonic dystrophy. In muscular dystrophy (of the Duchenne, limb-girdle, or facioscapulohumeral varieties), there may be

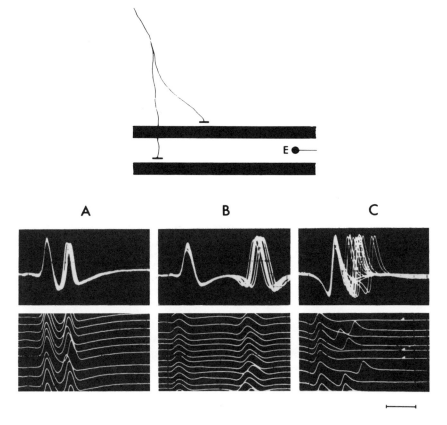

Fig. 8.2 The jitter. Electrode E is recording activity from two muscle fibers belonging to the same motor unit. **(A)** Recording from a normal muscle. **(B,C)** Recording from a myasthenic muscle. The oscilloscope sweep is triggered by the first action potential. Interval variability between the potentials is seen as a variable position of the second potential. In the upper row, 10 to 15 action potentials are superimposed. In the lower row, the oscilloscope sweep is moved downwards. **(A)** shows normal jitter. In **(B)** increased jitter but no impulse blockings is seen. **(C)** shows increased jitter and occasional blockings (*arrows*). Calibration 500 μsec. (Stalberg E: Single Fiber Electromyography. Disa Electronics, 1974.)

an increase in fiber density and abnormally low jitter in some recordings, but more often, there is an increased jitter.[26] In neurogenic disorders, the jitter is markedly increased and blocking is frequently found. When recordings are made from three or more muscle fibers at the same time, it is sometimes apparent that two or more of the components will block only together, and they show a common large jitter in relation to the rest of the action potential complex (Fig. 8.3). This is attributable to impaired

or blocked transmission in the distal axonal branch supplying the muscle fibers whose action potentials are affected in this way.[25]

Single fiber electromyography also can provide an estimate of mean fiber density of motor units. The electrode is positioned so that a muscle fiber action potential is recorded at maximal amplitude. This action potential is then made to trigger the oscilloscope sweep, and the number of synchronous action potentials that are larger than 200 μV and have a rise time of less

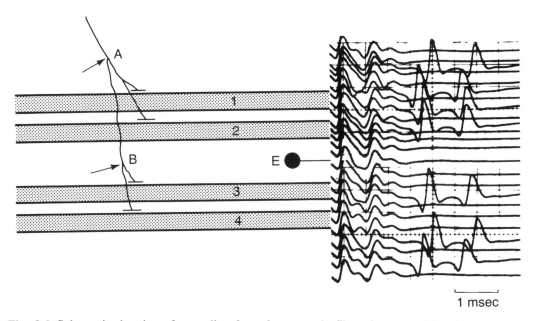

1 msec

Fig. 8.3 Schematic drawing of recording from four muscle fibers innervated by the same nerve axon, two of them (*3* and *4*) by a sprout branching off at *A*. To the right, an original recording from the electrode E of mainly four potentials, two of them blocking together (*3* and *4*). They behave as a unit that also has a large jitter in relation to the rest of the action potential complex. (Stalberg E, Thiele B: Transmission block in terminal nerve twigs: A single fibre electromyographic finding in man. J Neurol Neurosurg Psychiatry 35:52, 1972.)

than 300 μsec is counted for this particular electrode position. To obtain a measure of fiber density in the motor units of the muscle under examination, the process is repeated for at least 20 different positions of the recording electrode, and the mean number of responses is calculated. The number of fiber potentials recorded with random electrode placements in this way depends on the muscle examined and on the age of the patient. It is normally less than 1.5 for extensor digitorum communis in young adults. Seldom is it possible to record from three or more muscle fibers belonging to the same normal motor unit in any one electrode position. After reinnervation, however, fiber density is increased as a result of collateral sprouting, and it may be possible to record potentials from up to about 10 fibers of the same motor unit with the

electrode in one position. The increased fiber density occurring in muscular dystrophy has been attributed to a localized increase in the number of muscle action potential generators; it is believed that there is a remodeling of the motor unit due to fiber loss, and to regeneration and reinnervation.[26]

Macroelectromyography

Conventional electromyography yields no information about the size of motor units (i.e., the total number and size of the component fibers). Macroelectromyography is a recently developed technique that may provide such information.[27,28] A modified single fiber electrode is used. Electrical activity obtained by the electrode shaft during voluntary muscle activity is averaged after triggering from a single muscle fiber action potential, so that the contribution from one motor unit is extracted (Fig. 8.4).

Macro motor unit potentials reflect activity in the entire motor unit, and their shape varies according to the number and size of muscle fibers, to motor end-plate scatter, and to the recording site.[28] Macro motor

unit potentials are generally of low amplitude in primary myopathies, and they may have a more fractionated appearance than normal. However, macro motor unit potentials may have normal or only slightly reduced amplitudes in muscular dystrophy, even in severely weak muscles, despite other electrophysiologic abnormalities, such as abnormal configuration of the po-

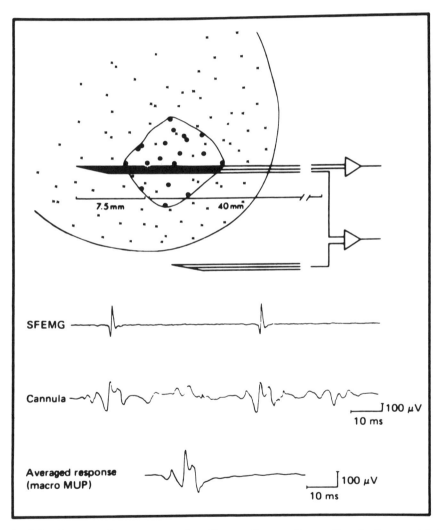

Fig. 8.4 Principle of macro electromyography. The small recording surface in the special electrode is positioned to record action potentials from one muscle fiber. This is used to trigger the averager to which the activity recorded with the cannula is fed. (Stalberg E, Antoni L: Computer-aided EMG analysis. p. 186. In Desmedt JE (ed): Progress in Clinical Neurophysiology. Vol. 10. S. Karger AG, Basel, 1983.)

tentials. The amplitude and area of the potentials are typically increased when reinnervation has occurred, such as in polyneuropathies or mononeuropathies.[28] By combining the technique with conventional and single fiber electromyography, new insights about the anatomy and physiology of both healthy and disordered motor units can be gained.

Scanning Electromyography

Scanning electromyography, a new technique, was developed to study motor units in order to obtain a better understanding of their topography. It indicates both the spatial and temporal distribution of activity in individual units.[29] A single fiber electrode is inserted into the slightly contracted muscle and positioned so that a low-threshold motor unit potential is recorded. A concentric needle electrode is then inserted into the fiber at a distance of more than 2 cm away. The single fiber electrode is made to trigger the oscilloscope, and the concentric needle is moved until it records a potential time locked to the sweep (that is, activity from the triggering motor unit). It is pushed through the motor unit territory until its electrical activity is no longer recorded. It is then connected to a step motor able to pull it in steps of 50 μm, or multiples thereof, after each sweep, or after some preset number of sweeps. The technique relies heavily on the use of a computer in all stages of processing. The graphics produced are interpreted visually to assess motor unit fractions, distribution, and overall complexity (Fig. 8.5).

The shape of the motor unit potentials within one motor unit shows considerable variation. The electrical activity usually has one or two sites of maximal amplitude within the territory of an individual unit in the biceps muscle, and up to four such sites in the tibialis anterior muscle. These distinct portions are called motor unit fractions. Each fraction, which usually corresponds to the motor unit potential recorded in conventional electromyography, probably reflects activity from fibers innervated by a single major branch of the axon. In myopathies, each motor unit fraction is typically smaller and shorter than normal, whereas in neurogenic disorders the amplitude of the signals is typically increased, the number of motor unit fractions is unchanged, and, because of volume conduction, electrical activity is recorded over a larger area.

Analysis of the Pattern of Electrical Activity of Muscle

Quantitative analysis of the pattern of electrical activity of muscle during contraction against a standard load (usually 2 kg, as shown in Fig. 8.6) has been used to distinguish between patients with myopathy and normal subjects. Fitch and Willison measured the features of an interference pattern, which are usually evaluated subjectively, by converting the signal into two serial pulse trains.[30] A turn pulse was generated each time the signal changed its direction from positive to negative or vice versa, provided that the deflection exceeded a certain level of significance (usually 100 μV). An amplitude pulse was generated whenever the potential between each turn in the signal reached 100 μV, irrespective of the direction of potential change (Fig. 8.7). The two pulse trains were counted over specified intervals to determine the number of spikes (turns) for each 5-second period, the amplitude of the potential changes between spikes, and the distribution of time intervals between spikes. A small computer was used for more detailed analysis.[31]

This method has been applied to the diagnosis of myopathic disorders.[32] The characteristic finding is an increase in the mean turns count, as might be expected from the

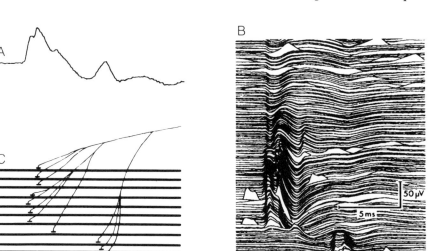

Fig. 8.5 Scanning electromyography. Recording from the tibialis anterior muscle showing motor unit fractions. **(A)** Macro electromyography. **(B)** Scanning electromyography. **(C)** Schematic interpretation. (Stalberg E, Antoni L: Computer-aided EMG analysis. p. 186. In Desmedt JE (ed): Progress in Clinical Neurophysiology. Vol. 10. S. Karger AG, Basel, 1983.)

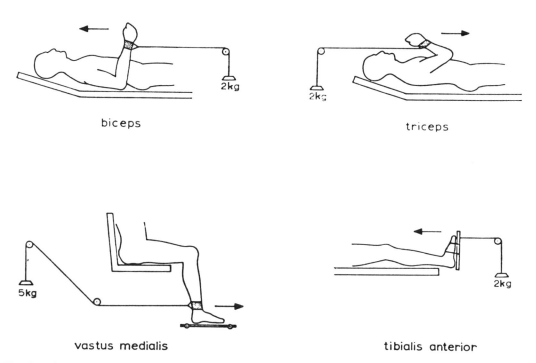

Fig. 8.6 Arrangement of the patient for quantitative analysis of the pattern of electrical activity of muscle, as performed by Willison and colleagues. (Hayward M, Willison RG: The recognition of myogenic and neurogenic lesions by quantitative EMG. p. 448. In Desmedt JE (ed): New Developments in Electromyography and Clinical Neurophysiology. Vol. 2. S. Karger AG, Basel, 1973.)

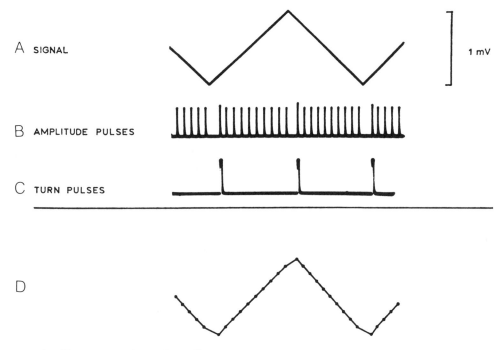

Fig. 8.7 Oscilloscope tracings of a calibration signal (**A**) and outputs of pulse generators (**B,C**). A reconstruction of the signal (**D**) was obtained by plotting the information given by the pulse trains. (Hayward M, Willison RG: The recognition of myogenic and neurogenic lesions by quantitative EMG. p. 448. In Desmedt JE (ed): New Developments in Electromyography and Clinical Neurophysiology. Vol. 2. S. Karger AG, Basel, 1973.)

shortened duration of motor unit potentials. In patients with chronic partial denervation, Hayward and Willison found that a change in mean amplitude between turns was characteristic, whereas there was no significant change in the mean spike count.[33,34] This was attributed to an increase in the density of muscle fibers in individual motor units secondary to reinnervation.

The requirement of a constant load has limited the utility of this approach. However, Fuglsang-Frederiksen and Mansson analyzed by a similar technique the electrical activity of muscle at different degrees of voluntary activity.[35] They measured the activity during contractions against a load related to the subject's maximal voluntary effort, rather than against a fixed load, and found that a force of 2 kg resulted in a fewer number of turns when subjects were capa-

ble of high maximal force than when the maximal force they could generate was low. If subjects exerted the same relative force, however, the number of turns was not dependent on maximal force. They concluded, therefore, that a fixed relative force (e.g., 30 percent of maximum) was less likely to yield false positive data or to obscure abnormalities than was a fixed absolute load.

When the pattern of electrical activity was analyzed during a force that was a fixed fraction (30 percent) of maximum in 41 patients with myopathy, the ratio of the number of turns in 5 seconds to mean amplitude between turns provided a diagnostic yield of 70 percent. The yield was increased to 87 percent when abnormalities in the number of turns per 5 seconds, the incidence of short time intervals between turns, and mean amplitude were included. In the same muscles, measurement of the mean duration of motor unit potentials during weak effort enabled a diagnosis of myopathy to be made in 60 percent of the patients, and if attention was also directed toward the number of polyphasic potentials, a diagnosis could be established in 89 percent of patients. The two methods supplemented each other, as in some instances the myopathy could only be identified by one of the two procedures.[36]

Patients with neurogenic weakness were investigated in a later study by the same authors.[37] They again found that the best diagnostic yield from the pattern of electrical activity was obtained when the force was 30 percent of maximum. The number of spikes (turns) per 5 seconds was diminished in 70 percent of their patients, a fact which they attributed mainly to a prolonged duration of motor unit potentials. They also found an increased incidence of long-duration intervals between turns and an increased amplitude between turns.

It may be difficult to assess the force of a muscle if it works in conjunction with others. Attempts have been made to avoid measurement of force, and modifications of techniques using a specified percentage of maximal force have been suggested. With this in mind, Fuglsang-Frederiksen and colleagues quantified the electrical activity of the brachial biceps muscle during a gradual increase in force from zero to maximum within 10 seconds in patients with neuromuscular disorders.[38] In patients with myopathy, the ratio of turns per 100 msec to mean amplitude at 10 percent and 20 percent of maximal force was increased more often (82 percent and 76 percent of patients, respectively) than it was at greater force. In many (64 percent) patients with neurogenic disorders, the number of turns was decreased at a force of 20 percent and 30 percent of maximum. Thus, it has been suggested that, in muscles in which force is easily determined, electrical activity should

be analyzed at both 10 percent and 30 percent of maximum. In other muscles, the ratio of turns to mean amplitude should be analyzed at "moderate force" (estimated on the oscilloscope at the onset of overlap of individual motor unit potentials). In patients with neurogenic disorders, the analysis of turns at a given force of, for example, 30 percent of maximum is required.

Using a modification of Willison's method, Stalberg and associates plotted mean amplitude against the number of turns at different force levels and found that most data points from normal muscle were within an area of this plot that they called a "cloud."[39] The interference pattern was measured several times at each recording site while the force was varied from minimum to maximum. Normal values differed with age, muscle, sex, and type of recording electrode. They found that, in neuropathic disorders, data points occurred above the normal cloud, whereas in myopathies some data points fell below it. Whether this approach will have any major clinical application remains to be established.

Recently, Stalberg and associates developed a different method for analyzing the interference pattern which was based more on the way that a clinical electromyographer assesses it, using three new parameters.[40] In particular, they developed an *activity parameter* to quantitate the "fullness" of the interference pattern and to represent the time (msec) within a 1-second period during which it is inferred that motor unit potentials are present. The so-called *upper centile amplitude,* developed to quantitate the amplitude of the largest spikes of the interference pattern, was defined as the amplitude that is exceeded by only 1 percent of segments in the measured epoch. The third parameter, the *number of small segments*, measures the low-amplitude (less than 2 mV), high-frequency components of the interference pattern. They found that the activity and the logarithm of the upper centile amplitude correlated strongly with the force of muscle contraction at which the interference pattern was measured. The number of small segments initially increased with the force of contraction, but became relatively constant at higher force levels.

In a subsequent study, these researchers measured the interference pattern in the biceps muscle and defined normal values in men and women for these parameters from 500-msec epochs of the interference pattern.[41] They plotted the upper centile amplitude and number of small segment values against activity for each epoch, and defined an area on these plots, called a "cloud," that contained more than 90 percent of the data points from each study. In patients with neuropathy, the characteristic pattern was increased upper centile amplitude with a normal or decreased number of small segments. In patients with myopathy, the number of small segments was increased and the upper centile amplitude was normal or diminished. In all studies, they found that the interpretation of the interference pattern from the plots accorded well with the qualitative assessments made independently by an electromyographer. They therefore suggested that the technique might be useful in detecting mild abnormalities that are equivocal on conventional electromyographic studies, and in quantitating the severity and progression of nerve and muscle disease. Their technique has the advantage of not requiring any measurement of force, and further studies of the technique are, therefore, awaited with interest.

CONDUCTION STUDIES IN DIFFERENT POPULATIONS OF NERVE FIBERS

Conduction slowing or block in some nerve fibers, despite normal maximal nerve conduction velocity, may be evident in conventional nerve conduction studies by changes in the configuration or amplitude of the compound nerve or muscle action potential when the nerve is stimulated at different sites along its course. However, much more information would be obtained about the functional status of an individual nerve if conduction could be measured in different populations of fibers that constitute that nerve. A number of methods have been developed for estimating the distribution of nerve fiber conduction velocities in the hope that such studies would increase the sensitivity of conventional nerve conduction measurements for detecting peripheral nerve disease, and help to characterize the underlying pathology.[42] Unfortunately, such approaches generally involve much mathematical manipulation and, because of the limitations of stimulating and recording from small or unmyelinated fibers, are concerned primarily with conduction only in relatively large, myelinated nerve fibers.[43]

One method of measuring the difference in velocity between different fibers in a single nerve trunk has been used for many years, and is based on a "collision" technique. Thomas and associates attempted to determine the range of motor conduction velocity via collision of orthodromic and antidromic impulses in the same nerve fibers,[44] and their approach has been refined by others.[45,46]

The technique described by Hopf is the most widely used and involves the use of paired supramaximal stimuli at different interstimulus intervals.[45] It is best described by reference to a particular nerve. If a supramaximal stimulus is delivered to the median nerve at the wrist, it not only elicits a compound muscle action potential of the abductor pollicis brevis muscle, but also gives rise to an antidromically conducted compound nerve action potential. This latter potential may prevent the generation of a compound muscle action potential by a second supramaximal stimulus delivered to the median nerve at the elbow. This is because (depending on the interstimulus intervals) the orthodromically conducted impulses generated by this second stimulus are extinguished by collision with the antidromically conducted impulses from the first stimulus. As the interval between the stimuli is increased, the antidromic action potentials conducted along fast-conducting fibers will come to have passed the elbow by the time that the second stimulus is delivered and, if these fibers are no longer refractory, they will then be activated by the second stimulus, propagating impulses orthodromically to the muscle and producing a second compound muscle action potential. The size of this second response will be proportional to the number of unblocked motor nerve fibers. As the interstimulus interval is increased further, more of the slow-conducting fibers will be activated by the second stimulus until the size of the compound muscle action potential elicited by the second stimulus is the same as that of the first stimulus. The relationship of interstimulus interval to the amplitude or area of the second compound muscle action potential (or to certain other parameters of this muscle response relative to the response to the first stimulus) can provide a measure of the distribution in conduction velocities of motor fibers in the nerve.[47]

Another approach involves studying the distribution of conduction velocities in sensory and mixed nerves by reconstructing the compound nerve action potential from the known characteristics of single fiber action potentials. The form and dimensions of the compound potential will depend on the delays (which reflect conduction velocities) of the single fiber action potentials. However, it is necessary to take into account the various factors relating to conduction velocity that influence the dimensions of single fiber action potentials. Unfortunately, the relative importance of these individual factors is not always clear, and the parameters of single fiber action potentials for a specific clinical recording situation are rarely known.[43]

The distribution of conduction velocities in motor nerves or in the motor fibers of mixed nerves can similarly be determined by reconstructing the compound muscle action potential. Although motor unit potentials are readily observed, the variation in parameters of normal potentials and the alterations that occur with neuromuscular disease lead to difficulties when the distribution of conduction velocities is to be estimated, because the contribution of each motor unit potential to the compound muscle action potential is not necessarily constant or linearly related to conduction velocity. Some authors have attempted to surmount this problem by calculating a "mean" motor unit potential from which an "expected" muscle compound action potential is reconstructed using histologic data.[48] By varying the conduction velocity distributions systematically, the effect on the simulated compound muscle action potential is then observed.

Attempts have also been made to determine in sensory or mixed nerves the distribution of conduction velocities, without knowledge of the parameters of single fiber action potentials, by analyzing two compound nerve action potentials from the same nerve. The nerve can either be stimulated at one point and the resulting compound nerve action potentials recorded at two sites separated by a known distance from each other and from the site of stimulation,[49] or one recording site and two stimulation sites may be used.[50,51] The distribution of conduction velocities is estimated by analyzing the differences between the two compound nerve action potentials with regard to the difference in their conduction distances from the site of stimulation. This approach involves several major assumptions, including the assumption that there is uniform or specifiable conduction in all nerve fibers in the segment studied, so the technique cannot be used in the presence of focal nerve disease.[43] In addition, the compound nerve action potentials have to be of optimal quality, with minimal stimulus artifact, and are best recorded using a referential derivation. The distribution of conduction velocities obtained by such means extends to a low of about 30 m/sec.

If a motor nerve is stimulated at two separate points along its course, the shapes of the compound muscle action potentials differ because of the different rates at which the constituent nerve fibers conduct impulses. Analysis of the compound muscle action potentials obtained by such stimulation may permit the distribution of conduction velocities in the motor nerve fibers to be determined in a manner similar to that outlined previously for sensory fibers. Again, this type of analysis requires that certain assumptions be made that are not entirely in accord with the available experimental evidence. Nevertheless, using this technique, a relatively narrow range of conduction velocities (12 to 24 m/sec) has been obtained, which is similar to that obtained by the collision technique.

Clinical Applications

At present, such approaches have greater research value than clinical relevance. Nevertheless, Cummins and Dorfman have studied the reliability of the methods, their sensitivities to controllable variables, and the range of normal distribution of conduction velocities.[52] They have also compared the distribution of conduction velocities in normal persons with those obtained from diabetic patients having various degrees of peripheral nerve involvement. They found that diabetic patients with minimal or no clinical evidence of polyneuropathy showed varying degrees of shift in the distribution of conduction velocities toward slower conduction values, sometimes even when conventional nerve conduction studies were normal. Few reports are available on the findings in other contexts, but approaches of this sort may well enable subtle differences in conduction properties of normal and diseased human nerves to be distinguished.

BLINK REFLEX

The blink reflex has been studied in some detail since its clinical description by Overend in 1896[53] and its initial electrophysiologic characterization by Kugelberg in 1952.[54] The blink reflex may be recorded in the laboratory, permitting its accurate quantitative analysis. The afferent arc of the reflex is subserved by the trigeminal nerve, a branch of which can be stimulated mechanically or electrically. The facial nerve mediates the efferent arc.

The blink reflex has been useful in the evaluation of patients with suspected involvement of the trigeminal or facial nerve, patients with multiple sclerosis or other brain stem lesions, and patients with a variety of polyneuropathies.

Method

The reflex is best recorded with the patient lying quietly on a couch, with eyes closed, in a warm, darkened room. The response can be elicited most conveniently by electrical stimulation of the supraorbital nerve using surface electrodes. The cathode is placed over the supraorbital foramen on one side, and the anode is positioned on the forehead. Alternatively, the infraorbital nerve may be stimulated unilaterally, with the cathode being placed over the infraorbital foramen and the anode being placed below it. However, components of the reflex may not be obtained with this method (p. 144). Stimulation of the mental nerve is usually even less satisfactory for clinical purposes. For supraorbital stimulation, the stimulus intensity is adjusted so that the reflex response is maximal and stable on repeated trials, and the interval between successive stimuli is set to be at least 30 seconds in order to minimize interactions between them. Responses are recorded from both sides of the face by surface electrodes placed laterally over the orbicularis oculi muscles, with a reference electrode placed on the side of the nose. A ground electrode can be placed submentally, on the neck, or around the arm (Fig. 8.8). A frequency response of 20 Hz to 32 kHz for the amplifiers is satisfactory.

Responses may be measured directly from the screen of the oscilloscope or recorded photographically for later analysis. They may be obscured in part by stimulus artifact, which can be difficult to control, especially with stimulation of the supraorbital nerve, because the active recording electrode is then so close to the stimulating cathode. Kimura and his group have overcome this problem by designing a special amplifier with a short blocking time (1 msec) and low noise.[55]

In blink reflex studies, conduction along the facial nerve itself is generally tested also by stimulating the nerve percutaneously at the stylomastoid foramen, with the cathode just in front of the mastoid process, and recording the compound muscle action potential from the ipsilateral ocularis oculi muscle. The latency of this direct response is then measured from stimulus artifact to onset of response.

The reflex response consists of two distinct components (Fig. 8.9). The initial component, designated R1, is elicited only on the side that is stimulated, whereas the later component, R2, is normally present on both sides following unilateral stimulation. Although R1 is relatively stable with repeated trials, R2 is more variable. The R2 component is generally more long-lasting and of higher amplitude than R1. The pathways subserving the responses are not known with certainty, but the arc subserving R1 seems to have a pontine course, whereas R2 is dependent upon pontine and lateral medullary pathways.[56–58]

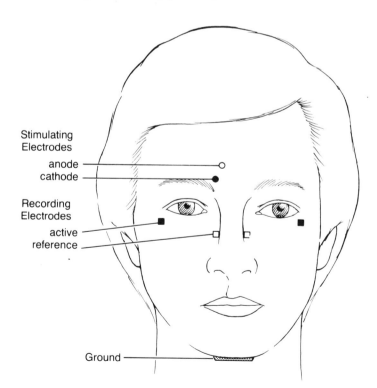

Fig. 8.8 Arrangements for eliciting the blink reflex.

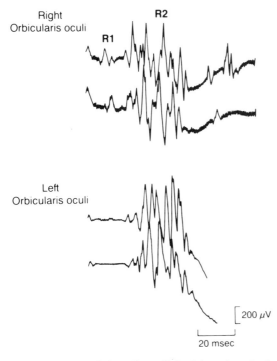

Fig. 8.9 The blink reflex elicited by electrical stimulation of the right supraorbital nerve in a normal adult. Two separate responses are shown. The R1 component of the response is present only on the side that is stimulated, whereas R2 is present bilaterally.

If the R1 component cannot be recorded easily, it is often helpful to deliver paired stimuli with an interstimulus interval of 5 msec. The facilitation resulting from the first stimulus may then permit R1 to be elicited by the second.[59] The R1 component is not consistently present when the reflex is elicited by stimulation of the infraorbital nerve; for this reason, supraorbital stimulation is preferred for clinical purposes.

For clinical purposes, the latencies of the direct response and of R1 and R2 are measured. For R1 and R2, the shortest value of 8 to 10 separate trials is taken as the latency. The ratio of the latency of R1 to that of the direct response can be calculated in order to compare conduction through the distal portion of the facial nerve to conduction in the reflex arc as a whole. There is normally no difference in the responses obtained on the two sides. Kimura regards R1 as abnormally delayed if its latency is greater than 13 msec, and considers R2 to be delayed if its latency exceeds 41 msec when recorded ipsilaterally and 44 msec when recorded contralaterally.[60] He found the interside difference in latency of R1 to be less than 1.2 msec. For R2, the latency difference between the ipsilateral and contralateral response recorded simultaneously following unilateral stimulation is normally less than 5 msec; the latency difference between R2 evoked by stimulation on each side in turn should be less than 7 msec.

Delay or absence of the R1 component of the reflex response indicates a disturbance of the trigeminal or facial nerve, or both, on that side. The manner in which R2 is involved should indicate the site of the lesion when R1 is abnormal. Trigeminal nerve lesions produce an afferent defect of the blink reflex, characterized by bilateral delay or attenuation of R2 when the affected side of the face is stimulated. With facial nerve lesions, R2 is abnormal on the affected side, whichever side is stimulated.

Clinical Applications of Blink Reflex Studies

The blink reflex has been used to evaluate the function of the trigeminal nerve in patients with facial pain. The response is generally normal in patients with idiopathic trigeminal neuralgia, whereas in patients with a paratrigeminal syndrome, abnormalities may be encountered.[61,62] Thus, the blink reflex can be helpful in distinguishing between these two disorders when clinical differentiation is difficult. Similarly, blink reflex abnormalities may be encountered in patients with structural lesions producing subclinical trigeminal nerve involvement, as occurs with certain aneurysms or acoustic neuromas (discussed below).

Abnormalities in the blink reflex may be

found in patients with Bell's palsy; these sometimes progress over the course of several days or even longer, providing electrophysiologic evidence that the condition may advance with time. Indeed, the response may initially be nearly normal, becoming much more abnormal after a few days.[63] The R1 response is generally delayed or absent during the first few weeks, suggesting that there has been demyelination or other pathologic change of the involved nerve segment. The findings do not, however, permit the early identification of patients with a bad prognosis, and therefore cannot be used to select patients for treatment with steroids. They do, nevertheless, provide a guide to prognosis. In patients in whom the distal segment of the facial nerve remains excitable until the reflex responses return, good clinical recovery generally occurs within a few months. However, recovery is much slower in those who lose distal excitability without recovery of the reflex, due to distal degeneration of the nerve.[63]

In patients with hemifacial spasm or facial synkinesis following aberrant reinnervation after a facial nerve palsy, supraorbital nerve stimulation may lead to a response in one or several facial muscles, in addition to the response elicited in the orbicularis oculi, provided that additional recording electrodes are placed.[64,65]

In certain polyneuropathies, there may be a delay in the direct response and in the R1 component, providing objective evidence of facial nerve involvement. Abnormalities may be found even when clinical evidence of facial nerve involvement is equivocal or absent. Abnormalities have been reported in Guillain-Barré syndrome, as well as in diabetic and hereditary motor and sensory neuropathy.[66,67]

In patients with acoustic neuroma, the blink reflex may be abnormal. Lyon and Van Allen reported blink reflex abnormalities in five patients with verified acoustic neuromas.[68] In addition to loss of the R1 on the affected side in every case, the R2 component on the involved side was delayed regardless of which supraorbital nerve was stimulated. They concluded that there was trigeminal and facial nerve involvement on the affected side, although only two patients had facial weakness clinically. In another study, an abnormality of the early (R1) component of the blink reflex was found in each of 11 patients with cerebellopontine angle tumors who were studied electrophysiologically, indicating trigeminal or facial nerve dysfunction, or both.[69] In eight patients, the R2 findings on the uninvolved side, in response to supraorbital stimulation on the affected side, indicated trigeminal nerve dysfunction which, in two patients, was subclinical. However, studies of the brain stem auditory evoked potential and radiologic imaging procedures (computed tomography or magnetic resonance imaging) are more useful for screening purposes.

Kimura reported on the findings obtained during blink reflex studies in 260 patients with suspected multiple sclerosis.[60] The R1 component was delayed on one or both sides in 96 of 145 patients (66 percent) in whom the diagnosis was definite, in 32 of 57 patients (56 percent) with probable multiple sclerosis, and in 17 of 58 patients (29 percent) with possible multiple sclerosis. The incidence of abnormal R1 increased as the duration of illness increased in each diagnostic category. The R1 was abnormal in 78 percent of patients with pontine signs, in 57 percent of those with other brain stem signs, and in 40 percent of patients who had no clinical evidence of brain stem dysfunction. Alterations in the R2 component were less specific, but when they occurred in association with a normal R1, they were usually accompanied by clinical signs suggesting a lateral medullary lesion.

In patients with Wallenberg's syndrome, the R1 component of the response is generally normal on the affected side. R2 is commonly delayed, absent, or markedly attenuated bilaterally with stimulation of the affected side of the face, but is normal bilaterally when the unaffected side is stimulated.[58] The R2 component of the blink reflex may also be disturbed by lesions that indirectly influence the excitability of polysynaptic connections. For example, the response is commonly absent or markedly attenuated in comatose patients, regardless of the cause of coma or the site of the underlying pathology.[70] Blink reflex abnormalities are common in patients during the acute phase of hemispheric cerebrovascular accidents, and there is no consistent correlation between the localization of the hemispheric lesion and the type of reflex abnormality.[71]

F RESPONSE

The F response may be recorded easily from most skeletal muscles. If the sweep speed of the oscilloscope is changed so that the traces can be seen for 40 msec or more after the stimulus during routine motor conduction studies, an F response will be found to follow the direct (M) response or compound muscle action potential (Fig. 8.10). The electrical stimulus that generates the direct motor response leads also to antidromic volleys in motor axons and thereby to the activation of a certain number of anterior horn cells. This may result in reactivation of the membrane of the initial segment or first node (provided that the absolute refractory period is over), and thereby to orthodromic impulses along a few of the motor axons, so that a small, late response follows the direct response. The F response represents only a small percentage of the motor neuron pool invaded antidromically and is elicited from neurons regardless of their peripheral excitability or conduction characteristics.[72]

The F response is variable in size, configuration, and latency—and even in its very presence—from trial to trial, and usually is very small (less than 5 percent) compared to the compound muscle action po-

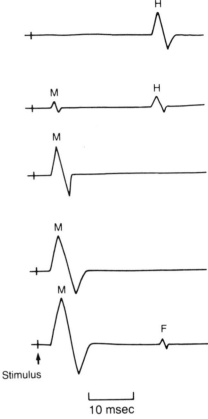

Fig. 8.10 Diagrammatic representation of the relationship between the direct (M) response, F response, and H reflex, and the intensity of the eliciting stimulus. With low-intensity stimulation of the tibial nerve, an H reflex is elicited from the soleus muscle. As the intensity of stimulation increases, the H reflex declines and a small M wave is seen. With a higher stimulus intensity, the H reflex disappears and the M wave increases in size until it is maximal. Following the maximal M wave, a small F response is sometimes seen.

tential. This variation in latency and configuration presumably relates to the activation of different anterior horn cells—with axons having different conduction velocities—in different trials. The *extent of scatter* in a series of F responses has been taken as a measure of temporal dispersion among different motor fibers with different conduction characteristics.[72-74] There is very little variation in latency of successive F responses recorded from any single motor unit.[75] The F response latency also varies with height or limb length, and depends on the sites of stimulation and recording. The greater the conduction distance (that is, the distance between the stimulation site and the cord plus the distance between the cord and the recording site), the longer is the F response latency.

Studies of the F response provide information about the rate of conduction in alpha motor fibers, but not about the function of sensory fibers. When recorded for clinical purposes, a supramaximal stimulus with a duration of 100 μsec is applied to the motor nerve, and the response is recorded from the resting muscle with surface electrodes. For clinical studies, 10 or more F responses are generally recorded from an individual muscle following motor nerve stimulation at 2 Hz or less. This is most conveniently undertaken by displaying the 10 (or more) F responses on a storage oscilloscope that automatically moves successive sweeps in the vertical axis. The *latency of the shortest response* is then determined, with the assumption that this represents conduction in one of the largest-diameter motor fibers in the nerve that is stimulated. Certainly, there does appear to be a correlation between the earliest or minimal F response latency and the maximal motor conduction velocity in the distal segment of the same nerve, as measured by conventional techniques.[76] However, it is not clear that this relationship applies to different pathologic states, especially if the pathologic process is patchy in distribution and severity, and selectively affects some fiber populations more than others. Fisher undertook a detailed analysis of F response latency and found that, based on a series of 10 responses, mean latency values were more reproducible than minimal latency values and provided a statistically consistent measure of F response conduction.[77] Other au-

thors have examined the question of the optimal number of F waves that should be recorded when the minimal latency is to be determined.[78] They found that the minimum value of 20 had only a 59 percent probability of being within 0.5 msec and a 76 percent probability of being within 1 msec of the minimum value obtained from at least 100 responses. However, because of the time required to collect a large sample of responses, they considered a total of 20 to be a satisfactory compromise.

Some authors have used formulas to convert F response latency to conduction velocity or conduction time, but such an approach is both inaccurate and unnecessary. It is not possible to measure accurately the conduction distance, and the precise time required for retrograde activation of anterior horn cells is unknown, although a value of 1 msec is generally assumed for the purposes of such formulas.

When F responses are to be recorded using a relatively proximal site of stimulation, the response may be distorted by the preceding direct (M) response. Accordingly, a collision technique involving stimulation of the nerve at two separate sites may have to be employed, as advocated by Kimura.[79] The principles of this technique are illustrated in Figure 8.11.

In patients with polyneuropathies and entrapment neuropathies, F response latency studies may reveal a delay in conduction when slowing in the distal segment (as monitored by the direct or M response) is normal or equivocal. Eisen and associates evaluated conduction in the proximal segments of the median and ulnar nerves using F responses.[80] The results of these and conventional motor and sensory studies in patients with a variety of proximal and distal entrapment syndromes were compared to the findings in 60 control subjects. They found that 67 percent of patients with proximal lesions had abnormalities in their F response studies, whereas conventional motor studies were normal. They also found that 23 percent

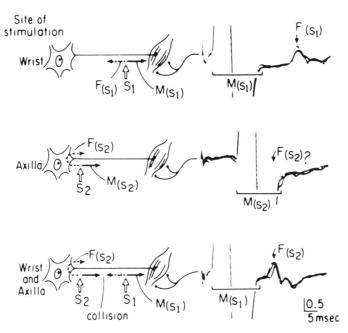

Fig. 8.11 Normal M wave (*horizontal brackets*) and F response (*small arrows*) recorded from the abductor digiti minimi muscle with surface electrodes. From top to bottom, supramaximal stimulus to the ulnar nerve at the wrist (S_1) and at the axilla (S_2), and simultaneous paired stimuli at the wrist and axilla (S_1 and S_2). Three consecutive traces are superimposed for each tracing. The M wave and the F response elicited by wrist stimulation were widely separate. With stimulation at the axilla, however, only the M wave was recorded; the F response was apparently absent because it occurred before the completion of the M wave. With paired stimuli, the orthodromic impulse from the axilla and the antidromic impulse from the wrist were extinguished by collision, leaving intact the M wave, M (S_1), from the wrist and the F response, F (S_2), from the axilla. The figures on the left are schematic diagrams showing the orthodromic (*solid arrows*) and antidromic (*dotted arrows*) impulses carrying the M wave and the F response, respectively. In the bottom figure, the collision between F (S_1) and M (S_2) leaves M (S_1) and F (S_2) intact. (Kimura J: F-wave velocity in the central segment of the median and ulnar nerves. A study in normal subjects and in patients with Charcot-Marie-Tooth disease. Neurology 24:539, 1974).

of patients with carpal tunnel syndrome also had abnormal F response studies, suggesting an additional element of proximal entrapment since the F response latencies were abnormally prolonged in relation to the corresponding M latency.

In patients with polyneuropathies, the minimal F response latency may be delayed to an extent corresponding to the slowing of peripheral motor conduction velocity. However, when pathologic involvement is greater proximally than distally, or when there is proximal conduction block in the fastest-conducting fibers, there may be disproportionate prolongation of the minimal F response latency, as in the Guillain-Barré syndrome.[81–83] Occasionally, this latency may be prolonged significantly in patients with peripheral neuropathies in whom conventional motor and sensory conduction studies show no abnormality, presumably because proximal involvement is more severe or because the cumulative delay over this extended course permits recognition when delay over a shorter segment is insufficient to be identified.[83,84] Lachman and co-workers, for example, found abnormalities of late responses in 18 percent of patients with either axonal or demyelinative neuropathies in whom conventional nerve conduction studies were normal.[83]

F response studies have had a disappointing yield in patients with suspected root lesions. This may be because only motor fibers are evaluated by the method, and because a slowing of conduction along a restricted segment of the lengthy course mediating the F response may well be masked by the normal conduction velocity along the greater part of this course. Moreover, it does not seem surprising that normal values are obtained on stimulation of a polysegmental peripheral nerve in patients with isolated root lesions. However, in patients with neoplastic lesions of the eighth cervical and first thoracic nerve roots secondary to epidural metastases, F response studies may be helpful in documenting pathology.[85]

The determination of minimal F response latency has been of greater help in the evaluation of patients with plexopathies. In patients with wasting of the hand caused by a cervical rib and band, for example, there may be an increase in F response latency, as recorded from the hypothenar muscles following stimulation of the ulnar nerve at the wrist on the affected side, compared with the findings on the asymptomatic side.[86]

The peak-to-peak *amplitude* of the F response has also been studied for clinical purposes. It is influenced by the character of the recording electrodes and their relationship to the end-plate zone, the skin impedance and depth of the motor unit within the muscle, and the size and number of the motor units contributing to the response that is recorded. To minimize variation caused by such factors, F response amplitude is best expressed as a percentage of the maximal M wave recorded simultaneously.

In a study of single motor units, Yates and Brown were unable to find any relationship between the absolute amplitude and latency of the F response.[87] The F response amplitude is increased in spasticity except when this condition is of recent onset, when the response may be reduced on the affected side.[88] Further discussion of this topic is provided in Chapter 15.

The F response *persistence*—that is, the number of responses elicited by a specific number of stimuli—may be another useful measure, as may the *duration* of the F response complex,[74] but these parameters await detailed appraisal. The measurement of *minimal-maximal* F response *latency difference* was referred to earlier (p. 146).

H REFLEX

The H reflex represents a monosynaptic reflex in which the afferent arc consists of group Ia fibers from muscle spindles and the efferent arc consists of alpha motor fibers (Figs. 7.3 and 8.10). The reflex response is elicited by stimuli that are lower in intensity than those required to elicit a direct M response. Indeed, with the supramaximal stimuli generally used in conventional motor conduction studies to elicit the direct response, the H reflex is blocked. The H reflex is elicited with ease from the soleus muscle and certain other muscles, such as the forearm flexor muscles.[89,90] In contrast to the F response, however, the H reflex is generally not easily elicited from most other skeletal muscles in adults, except when there is an upper motor neuron lesion. When elicited at low rates of stimulation (for example, one stimulus every 2 to 30 seconds), the response is relatively consistent in configuration and amplitude, unlike the F response, but there may be some variation in its latency. Its amplitude depends on stimulus intensity and is reduced during sleep and with vibration of the muscle, but when maximal, it is about half the size of the maximal M response in normal subjects.

Since the H reflex is routinely recordable only from the calf muscles, it is of limited clinical utility. It is best elicited using long-duration (1 msec) stimuli delivered by bipolar surface electrodes that have been placed over the tibial nerve in the popliteal fossa, with the cathode proximal to the anode. The stimuli should be of such an intensity that they produce either a small M wave or no visible motor response at all. The surface recording electrodes are placed over the medial part of the soleus muscle (active electrode) and over the Achilles tendon (reference electrode). The response can be recorded most easily if the subject is asked to make a *small* isometric contraction during the period of stimulation. This unmasking or facilitation of the H reflex by muscular contraction was initially reported by Upton and associates.[91] By this means, H reflexes (or responses that have been regarded as H reflex responses) can be recorded from the thenar and hypothenar muscles of normal adults.[92]

The H reflex latency depends on several factors including the time required for activation of the group 1a spindle afferent fibers, the conduction time along these fibers to the cord and along the alpha motor axons to the neuromuscular junctions from the cord, the central delay in the cord (involving conduction, synaptic transmission, and activation of anterior horn cells) and delay at the neuromuscular junction, and the time required for conduction of action potentials along muscle fibers to the recording site. There may be considerable differences in latencies of individual motor unit potentials activated by the H reflex, reflecting differences in either peripheral conduction velocity, central activation time, or both. The latency will vary with limb length and height in different subjects; this factor must therefore be considered when normal values are obtained. Latency (as recorded from the soleus muscle) is usually approximately 30 msec in adults, but its mean value increases by about 1 msec for each decade of age.[93] An interside difference in latency of 2 msec is abnormal.

H reflexes have been used to study central excitability of motor neurons, as discussed in Chapter 15, but their major clinical use has been in the evaluation of patients with lesions of the peripheral nervous system. Because they are usually only recordable from the calf muscles, the use of H reflexes for this purpose is much more limited than that of the F response. Nevertheless, abnormalities (loss or delay) of the H reflex have been reported in patients with various types of polyneuropathy[83] and also in patients with S1 root lesions.[93]

Traditionally, the Achilles tendon reflex and the electrically elicited H reflex have been thought to be monosynaptic spinal reflexes that differ only in the fact that the H reflex bypasses receptor mechanisms and is generated by a more synchronous afferent volley. Physiologic studies show that the afferent volleys responsible for both of these reflex responses are contaminated by activity in a wide variety of afferents rather than consisting of a homogeneous volley in group Ia afferent fibers. Burke and associates have demonstrated that the afferent populations activated by the two stimuli differ, as does the pattern of activity in each afferent.[94] Because of this and other differences they describe, it is clear that to regard the H reflex as the electrophysiologic equivalent of the ankle jerk is both facile and incorrect.

SOMATOSENSORY EVOKED POTENTIALS

In the last few years, somatosensory evoked potentials have been recorded with increasing frequency to evaluate the functional status of the peripheral and central somatosensory pathways. For clinical purposes, these potentials are elicited most conveniently by electrical stimulation that activates mainly the large-diameter, fast-conducting group Ia muscle and group II cutaneous afferent fibers. Both mixed and cutaneous nerves can be stimulated, and the skin in the region of a particular nerve or nerve root can be stimulated directly.

Electrical stimuli give rise to a relatively synchronous volley and thus are generally preferred to natural stimuli. However, although natural stimuli are harder to localize and result in a more asynchronous volley, they have the advantage of testing the functional integrity of the sensory receptors or the terminal portions of the sensory fibers. Electrical stimuli of short duration (200 μsec) that are repeated at 3 or 5 Hz are convenient; they are usually of an intensity that is just above motor threshold so that a small muscle twitch is produced when a mixed nerve is stimulated. For clinical purposes, the median or ulnar nerve can be stimulated with ease at the wrist, as can the peroneal nerve at the knee and the posterior tibial nerve at the ankle. If cutaneous nerves are to be stimulated, then any accessible specific nerve can be used, including the lateral femoral cutaneous nerve or sural nerve in the legs, the digital nerves in the hands, the superficial radial nerve at the wrist, and the trigeminal nerve in the face.

Surface electrodes are convenient for recording. When responses to stimulation of a nerve in the limbs are to be recorded over the head, both a cephalic bipolar and a referential recording montage should be used. Responses are usually also recorded over the spine. They should always be recorded peripherally in the limbs to determine whether there is a postganglionic lesion of the afferent pathways. With stimulation of a nerve in the arm, a convenient recording montage, using a four-channel recording system, is to record from the contralateral C3'/C4' electrode placement referenced to Fz (channel 1), as well as to contralateral Erb's point (channel 2). Recordings are also made from over the second cervical spine referenced to Fz (channel 3), and from ipsilateral to contralateral Erb's point (channel 4). When recording the responses to stimulation of a nerve in the legs, one channel is commonly used to record over the spine between L3 and L1, and another to record between Cz' and Fpz' or Fz.

Responses are best recorded using a relatively broad bandpass, such as 10 to 3,000 Hz. Between 500 and 2,000 trials are usually averaged when responses are elicited from nerves in the arms, but up to about 4,000 trials may be required when a nerve in the legs is stimulated. At least two averages are obtained to ensure that the findings are reproducible.

The responses are examined with regard to the latency and interpeak latency of the various components, the presence or absence of individual components, and the amplitude of the potentials. In most laboratories, latency or interpeak latency is not considered abnormal unless it exceeds the normal mean by three standard deviations. It is more difficult to attribute any significance to amplitude asymmetry because there is such variation between individuals and even between the two sides in the same individual. More sophisticated methods of analysis, to obtain some measure of configuration and dispersion, are not used routinely but would probably enhance the sensitivity of the technique.

Latency varies with limb length and height, and also increases in the elderly. Furthermore, immaturity of the peripheral and central nervous systems may lead to differences in the responses recorded in infants and adults, and it may not be until children are 7 or 8 years old that conduction velocity along the entire somatosensory pathway reaches the adult range.[95]

It has been suggested that the various components of the somatosensory evoked potential reflect the sequential activation of different neural generators as the volley ascends the nervous system. Such a concept has the merit of simplicity, but is probably incorrect. In particular, physical changes that occur in the surrounding volume conductor may lead to the generation of distinct peaks or waves.[96–98] The individual components of the potential are generally labeled by their polarity and normal mean latency. Typical responses, as obtained in my laboratory, are illustrated in Figures 8.12 and 8.13, where their probable origin or significance is also indicated.

Clinical Applications

Somatosensory evoked potentials have been used to evaluate both the peripheral and central nervous systems. The presence of an abnormal response does not, however, indicate the nature of the underlying disease. With regard to the peripheral nervous system, it was hoped that the recording of somatosensory evoked potentials would be useful when conventional techniques proved inadequate because the lesion was so proximal that it was inaccessible. Thus, attention has been focused on the role of somatosensory evoked potentials in evaluating patients with lesions involving the peripheral nerves proximally, the limb plexuses, and the spinal nerve roots. F response studies have similarly been used in such contexts, but these evaluate conduction in motor rather than sensory fibers.

In patients with injuries to the brachial plexus, somatosensory evoked potentials have been used to determine whether the likely site of injury is preganglionic or postganglionic, since this determination has prognostic relevance. The degree of any attenuation of the N9 peak recorded at Erb's point reflects the proportion of fibers damaged postganglionically, whereas attenua-

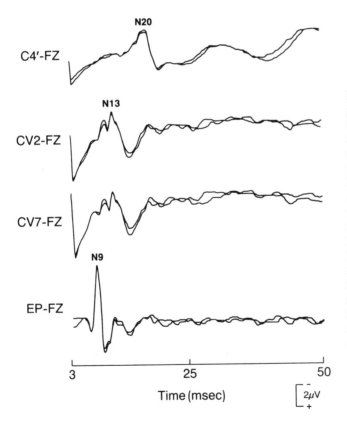

Fig. 8.12 Somatosensory evoked potentials elicited in response to stimulation of the left median nerve at the wrist in a normal adult and recorded over Erb's point (EP), the C7 and C2 spinous processes at the back of the neck (CV7 and CV2), and the contralateral "hand" area of the scalp (C4') using a midfrontal (FZ) reference. Two trials, each of 512 responses, are superimposed to illustrate the reproducibility of the response. The Erb's point potential is generated peripherally, the N13 response is probably generated, at least in part, in the dorsal column nuclei, and the N20 response is generated in the cerebral cortex.

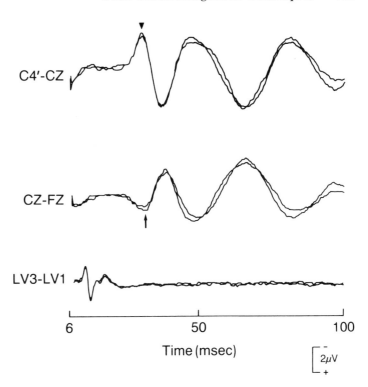

Fig. 8.13 Normal somatosensory evoked potentials elicited by stimulation of the left peroneal nerve at the knee and recorded between the third and first lumbar spines (LV3-LV1), and between the vertex (CZ) and the contralateral centroparietal (C4′) and midfrontal (FZ) reference points. Two trials, each of 1,024 responses, are superimposed. There is a well-formed, reproducible cauda equina potential over the lumbar spine, an initial positivity over the scalp in the CZ-FZ derivation (*arrow*) that is generated cortically, and a corresponding negativity in the C4′-CZ derivation (*arrowhead*).

tion of N13 relates to the total proportion of damaged fibers. Jones and associates compared the electrophysiologic findings obtained preoperatively with the surgical findings in 16 patients with unilateral traction lesions of the branchial plexus.[99] An attenuation of the N13 component by more than 40 percent on the affected side, as compared with the normal side, was taken to indicate damage of the C6 and C7 nerve roots when the median nerve was stimulated, and of C8 and/or T1 when found in the ulnar-derived somatosensory evoked potential. Attenuation of the N9 peak to the same extent or more than that of N13 was taken to indicate a postganglionic lesion. When the N9 peak was less attenuated than the N13, the extent of postganglionic involvement was reflected by the reduction of this peak, and the extent of preganglionic damage was indicated by the additional amount by which the N13 component was attenuated. Using this approach, however, Jones and associates correctly localized the lesion in only 8 of their 16 patients, and in three instances a serious discrepancy was found in the site of the lesion as determined electrophysiologically and that determined at operation. Occasionally, there was an apparent conflict between the findings obtained by somatosensory evoked potentials and those deduced by recording of sensory nerve action potentials, perhaps due to recoil of an avulsed root for some distance from the spinal cord with its ganglion still attached so that the N9 potential recorded from the Erb's point region was affected, whereas the sensory nerve action potential recorded more distally remained intact.

Others have also used somatosensory evoked potentials to investigate injuries of the brachial plexus. In general, it is necessary to stimulate a number of nerves, arising from different cord segments, if useful information is to be obtained. The median, ulnar, and radial nerves can easily be stimulated at the wrist, and the musculocutaneous nerve can be stimulated more proximally. In one study, median nerve stimulation yielded somewhat variable results in patients with C5 and C6 root lesions, but somatosensory evoked potentials recorded over the cervical spine and scalp in response to musculocutaneous nerve stimulation were sometimes markedly attenuated or absent.[100]

When somatosensory evoked potentials are used to evaluate patients with lesions of the plexus, the findings may be misleading if lesions are present at more than one site. Thus, postganglionic damage may obscure the electrophysiologic sequelae of a preganglionic lesion involving the same nerve fibers. However, intraoperative stimulation of specific nerve roots (while responses are recorded from the scalp) may help to determine whether there is functional continuity when clinical findings are inconclusive, especially if torn roots are to be treated by grafting.[101]

Somatosensory evoked potentials have also been used to evaluate patients with suspected thoracic outlet syndrome. As indicated in Chapter 13, electrophysiologic evaluation may reveal typical findings in patients with neurogenic thoracic outlet syndrome. In other patients with suspected thoracic outlet syndrome, however, clinical examination is normal, and neither needle electromyography nor nerve conduction studies reveals any abnormality. In such circumstances, it was hoped that the somatosensory evoked potential findings might provide objective evidence of the lesion, especially if these findings were abnormal with stimulation of the ulnar nerve at the wrist, but normal with median nerve stimulation. In my experience, however, abnormalities of somatosensory evoked potentials are not found in patients with suspected thoracic outlet syndrome who have neither clinical nor other electrophysiologic abnormalities to support the diagnosis.[102] The other published evidence on this point is conflicting. In one study, evoked potential abnormalities were found in 13 of 19

patients with suspected thoracic outlet syndrome who were studied by median and ulnar nerve stimulation; these abnormalities usually resolved following surgical treatment.[103] However, a detailed account of the findings and the criteria for abnormality were not provided. In another study, abnormalities in median- and ulnar-derived somatosensory evoked potentials were not encountered in seven patients who had no objective neurologic signs and in whom conventional nerve conduction studies and needle electromyography were normal.[104] In five patients with objective clinical signs, the somatosensory evoked potentials elicited in response to ulnar nerve stimulation at the wrist were abnormal, with either an absent or markedly attenuated N13 but a relatively normal N9 peak, or with a small delayed N9 peak and prolonged N9-N13 interpeak interval.[104]

In patients with cervical spondylotic radiculopathy or myelopathy, somatosensory evoked potentials elicited by stimulation of nerves in the arms may be abnormal. Components of the response may be delayed or absent in patients with objective neurologic signs of spondylotic radiculopathy, regardless of whether there is also a myelopathy.[105,106] However, the electrophysiologic findings provide no clue as to the nature, severity, or long-term prognosis of the neurologic disorder.

Eisen and associates have attempted to improve the yield of evoked potential studies in patients with root lesions by stimulating cutaneous nerves, in which there is greater segmental specificity, rather than mixed nerve trunks in the extremities.[107] They stimulated the musculocutaneous nerve for evaluation of the C5 segment, the median nerve fibers in the thumb for assessment of C6, the median nerve fibers along the adjoining surfaces of the second and third fingers for C7 evaluation, and the ulnar nerve in the little finger for assessment of C8. Using a similar approach, they also evaluated patients with lumbosacral

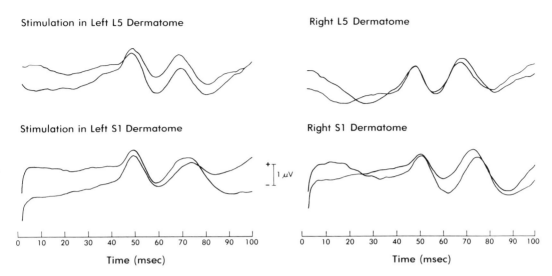

Fig. 8.14 Responses recorded over the scalp of a normal subject between vertex (CZ) and contralateral C3′ or C4′ electrodes to dermatomal stimulation in the L5 and S1 territories on either side. In each case, the average of 512 responses is shown for each trial, and two trials have been superimposed to demonstrate the reproducibility of the findings. An upward deflection indicates positivity at the CZ electrode. (Aminoff MJ, Goodin DS, Barbaro NM, Weinstein PR, Rosenblum ML: Dermatomal somatosensory evoked potentials in unilateral lumbosacral radiculopathy. Ann Neurol 17:171, 1985.)

radiculopathies, stimulating the saphenous nerve at the knee or at the ankle to assess function in the L3 or L4 segments, respectively; the superficial peroneal nerve above the ankle to evaluate L5; and the sural nerve at the ankle to evaluate S1. They found that, in 16 of 28 patients, the somatosensory evoked potentials elicited by such cutaneous nerve stimulation were abnormal, usually because of amplitude reduction and abnormal morphology, but occasionally because of a prolonged latency.

Another approach to improve the diagnostic yield of somatosensory evoked potentials in patients with root lesions was evaluated by Aminoff and associates, who used dermatomal stimulation in the L5 or S1 region in patients with verified lumbosacral root lesions.[108] The typical response consisted of a positive-negative-positive complex recorded at the vertex with reference to either the midfrontal region or the contralateral C3′/C4′ position, with the in-

itial positive peak having a latency of about 50 msec (Fig. 8.14). Using this technique, some authors—without published normative data—reported a yield as high as 92 percent in patients with surgically verified L5 or S1 root lesions,[109] but Aminoff and co-workers[108] found that the yield was less than 30 percent in their study, and certainly was far less than that of needle electromyography.[110] The most common abnormality is a grossly attenuated or absent response, but occasionally a prolonged latency occurs (Fig. 8.15).

Somatosensory evoked potential studies have been used to evaluate patients with peripheral nerve lesions when sensory nerve action potentials cannot be recorded by conventional techniques. Somatosensory evoked potentials may be recorded over the scalp in patients with polyneuropathies or mononeuropathies in whom no response can be recorded peripherally, and the difference in latency of the scalp-

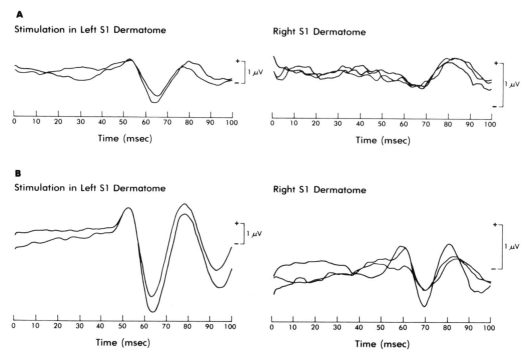

Fig. 8.15 Dermatomal somatosensory evoked potentials recorded between vertex (CZ) and contralateral C3' or C4' electrodes in response to stimulation in the S1 dermatome on either side in two patients. Two or three trials, each the average of 512 responses, have been superimposed. An upward deflection indicates positivity at the CZ electrode. In **A** there is loss of the first positive component of the response to stimulation in the right S1 dermatome; in **B** a prolonged response latency is evident with right S1 stimulation. These findings suggest a right S1 radiculopathy in each case. (Aminoff MJ, Goodin, DS, Barbaro NM, Weinstein PR, Rosenblum ML: Dermatomal somatosensory evoked potentials in unilateral lumbosacral radiculopathy. Ann Neurol 17:171, 1985.)

recorded response elicited by stimulation of the nerve at two separate sites can then be used to determine conduction velocity in the intervening segment of peripheral nerve. Parry and Aminoff investigated eight patients with acquired demyelinating peripheral neuropathies in whom sensory conduction velocity could not be determined using conventional techniques.[111] In every case, satisfactory responses were always present over the scalp (Fig. 8.16). In 11 of 15 nerves studied, afferent conduction velocity was slowed, and in 10, the slowing was similar to the degree of slowing in motor fibers, as determined by conventional motor conduction studies. In four

other nerves, however, afferent conduction velocity was within the normal range despite slowing of motor conduction. The reason that somatosensory evoked cerebral potentials can be recorded despite an absence of peripheral sensory nerve action potentials[112,113] is not clear. It is possible that the peripheral sensory nerve action potentials are not recorded because of dispersion of peripheral impulse traffic by the underlying pathology and that central reorganization leads to synchronization at different synaptic levels so that the volleys are amplified. However, if this is indeed the explanation, misleading information about the functional status of the nerve may be

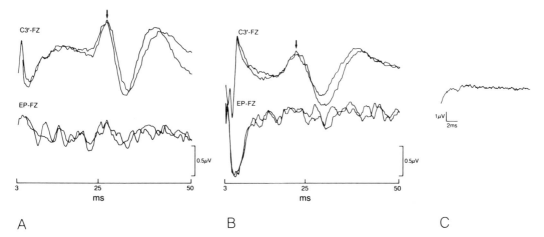

Fig. 8.16 Somatosensory evoked potentials recorded over Erb's point (EP-FZ) and contralateral scalp (C3'-FZ) with stimulation of the right ulnar nerve at the wrist (**A**) and elbow (**B**). Two separate trials are superimposed. A well-formed, reproducible N20 response (*arrow*) is seen over the scalp, but no reproducible response is present over Erb's point. Afferent conduction velocity in the forearm, as determined by the difference in latency of the N20 peak, was 50 m/sec. (**C**) The sensory nerve action potential (SNAP), recorded at the wrist in response to stimulation of the ulnar digital fibers in the little finger. Sixty-four responses have been averaged to reveal a small, poorly formed potential having an onset latency of 4.1 msec and an amplitude of 0.7 μv. (Parry GJ, Aminoff MJ: Somatosensory evoked potentials in chronic acquired demyelinating peripheral neuropathy. Neurology 37:313, 1987.)

obtained if central amplification of a very attenuated response arising from a few normally conducting axons leads to an apparently normal sensory conduction velocity.

The same principle—central amplification of a small or unrecordable peripheral response—has been used to follow recovery in patients with peripheral nerve injuries. It may be possible to record over the scalp a response to stimulation of the regenerating nerve when a potential cannot be recorded peripherally from the nerve itself.

In patients with the Guillain-Barré syndrome, somatosensory evoked potential studies sometimes permit electrophysiologic demonstration of pathology affecting proximal, inaccessible segments of peripheral nerves when conventional nerve conduction studies are normal. Brown and Feasby found predominantly proximal con-

duction slowing in a number of patients[114]—for example, by an increase in the interval between the response recorded at Erb's point and the N13 component or by the presence of a small, dispersed N13. Similarly, Synek found somatosensory evoked potentials to be useful in evaluating conduction along inaccessible proximal segments of nerves in the lower limbs of patients with disorders as diverse as meralgia paresthetica, nerve tumors, and trauma.[115]

In patients with distal axonopathies, animal studies suggest that abnormalities in somatosensory evoked potentials may precede any abnormality of peripheral nerve conduction. This has been attributed to early pathologic changes in the terminal and preterminal portions of the long axons in the posterior columns of the spinal cord.[116] However, in studies of a number of patients with suspected toxic neuropathies, I have never encountered a patient with an abnormal somatosensory evoked potential but normal findings on conventional nerve conduction studies.

Somatosensory evoked potentials have also been widely used to evaluate the function of the central nervous system, but such applications are of lesser interest to clinical electromyographers. In this regard, they have been used most widely to detect subclinical lesions in patients with suspected multiple sclerosis. Indeed, the diagnostic yield with this technique probably exceeds that of any other single electrophysiologic approach. Abnormalities may consist of delayed or absent components of the response, or responses with an abnormal configuration. Similar abnormalities, however, may be encountered in patients with vitamin B_{12} deficiency, hereditary ataxias, or familial spastic paraplegia, and such disorders may sometimes be labeled erroneously as multiple sclerosis.

Somatosensory evoked potential studies have been used to evaluate patients with spinal cord injuries, as well as for intraoperative monitoring of patients undergoing spinal surgery. With regard to the former, the presence of a normal response over the scalp to stimulation of a nerve below the level of cord injury implies a good prognosis. Early return of a previously absent response is similarly helpful in suggesting that the cord is in continuity. However, in patients with either complete or incomplete cord lesions, somatosensory evoked potential studies may initially be abnormal, with loss of the response to stimulation of a nerve below the level of the lesion; this finding, therefore, cannot be taken to predict the totality of the lesion. The role of somatosensory evoked potential studies in monitoring cord function during surgery requires further definition,[117] and a detailed discussion of this aspect here is unnecessary and premature.

Somatosensory evoked potentials have been recorded in patients with brain stem and hemispheric lesions, and have been used to evaluate comatose patients or patients who are thought to be brain-dead. Its role in this regard and the findings in patients with other disorders of the central nervous system are beyond the scope of the present work, but the reader is referred to a recent review by Eisen and Aminoff[117] for further details.

One further point may be made. Somatosensory evoked potentials have sometimes been recorded in patients with sensory disturbances of an uncertain origin in an attempt to determine whether these disturbances are organic or nonorganic. Normal responses have been elicited from nerves in the apparently anesthetic limbs of patients with nonorganic sensory disturbances, and the responses obtained in patients with hypnotically induced anesthesia are similarly normal.[118] However, responses to weak or strong stimuli applied to anesthetic regions of the skin are said to be smaller than those elicited by comparable stimuli to unaffected regions in patients with hysterical anesthesia, although there are no differences in the responses to strong stimuli applied to the nerves of affected and unaffected limbs.[119,120] Accordingly, the findings derived from peripheral nerve conduction studies and somatosensory evoked potentials should not be relied upon to determine whether sensory loss is organic or nonorganic in origin, although they are one factor to consider in making this determination.

REFERENCES

1. Buchthal F, Pinelli P: Muscle action potentials in polymyositis. Neurology 3:424, 1953
2. Buchthal F, Pinelli P: Action potentials in muscular atrophy of neurogenic origin. Neurology 3:591, 1953
3. Prochazka VJ, Conrad B, Sindermann F:

Computerized single-unit interval analysis and its clinical application. p. 462. In Desmedt JE (ed): New Developments in Electromyography and Clinical Neurophysiology. Vol. 2. S. Karger AG, Basel, 1973

4. Daube JR: Quantitative EMG in nerve-muscle disorders. p. 33. In Stalberg E, Young RR (eds): Clinical Neurophysiology. Butterworths, London, 1981

5. Buchthal F, Erminio F, Rosenfalck P: Motor unit territory in different human muscles. Acta Physiol Scand 45:72, 1959

6. Erminio F, Buchthal F, Rosenfalck P: Motor unit territory and muscle fiber concentration in paresis due to peripheral nerve injury and anterior horn cell involvement. Neurology 9:657, 1959

7. Buchthal F, Rosenfalck P, Erminio F: Motor unit territory and fiber density in myopathies. Neurology 10:398, 1960

8. Richardson AT: Newer concepts in electrodiagnosis. St. Thomas Hosp Rep 7:164, 1951

9. Walton JN: The electromyogram in myopathy: Analysis with the audiofrequency spectrometer. J Neurol Neurosurg Psychiatry 15:219, 1952

10. Fex J, Krakau CET: Some experiences with Walton's frequency analysis of the electromyogram. J Neurol Neurosurg Psychiatry 20:178, 1957

11. Larsson LE: On the relation between the EMG frequency spectrum and the duration of symptoms in lesions of the peripheral motor neuron. Electroencephalogr Clin Neurophysiol 38:69, 1975

12. McComas AJ, Fawcett PRW, Campbell MJ, Sica REP: Electrophysiological estimation of the number of motor units within a human muscle. J Neurol Neurosurg Psychiatry 34:121, 1971

13. Brown WF: A method for estimating the number of motor units in thenar muscles and the changes in motor unit count with ageing. J Neurol Neurosurg Psychiatry 35:845, 1972

14. Sica REP, McComas AJ, Upton ARM, Longmire D: Motor unit estimations in small muscles of the hand. J Neurol Neurosurg Psychiatry 37:55, 1974

15. Brown WF, Milner-Brown HS: Some electrical properties of motor units and their effects on the methods of estimating motor unit numbers. J Neurol Neurosurg Psychiatry 39:249, 1976

16. Panayiotopoulos CP, Scarpalezos S, Papapetropoulos T: Electrophysiological estimation of motor units in Duchenne muscular dystrophy. J Neurol Sci 23:89, 1974

17. McComas AJ, Campbell MJ, Sica REP: Electrophysiological study of dystrophia myotonica. J Neurol Neurosurg Psychiatry 34:132, 1971

18. McComas AJ, Sica REP, Currie S: An electrophysiological study of Duchenne dystrophy. J Neurol Neurosurg Psychiatry 34:461, 1971

19. Sica REP, McComas AJ: An electrophysiological investigation of limb-girdle and facioscapulohumeral dystrophy. J Neurol Neurosurg Psychiatry 34:469, 1971

20. Ballantyne JP, Hansen S: A new method for the estimation of the number of motor units in a muscle. I. Control subjects and patients with myasthenia gravis. J Neurol Neurosurg Psychiatry 37:907, 1974

21. Ballantyne JP, Hansen S: New method for the estimation of the number of motor units in a muscle. 2. Duchenne, limb-girdle and facioscapulohumeral, and myotonic muscular dystrophies. J Neurol Neurosurg Psychiatry 37:1195, 1974

22. Milner-Brown HS, Brown WF: New methods of estimating the number of motor units in a muscle. J Neurol Neurosurg Psychiatry 39:258, 1976

23. Ballantyne JP, Hansen S: A quantitative assessment of reinnervation in the polyneuropathies. Muscle Nerve 5:S127, 1982

24. Ekstedt J, Stalberg E: Single fibre electromyography for the study of microphysiology of the human muscle. p. 89. In Desmedt JE (ed): New Developments in Electromyography and Clinical Neurophysiology. Vol. 1. S. Karger AG, Basel, 1973

25. Stalberg E, Ekstedt J: Single fibre EMG and microphysiology of the motor unit in normal and diseased human muscle. p. 113. In Desmedt JE (ed): New Developments in Electromyography and Clinical Neurophysiology. Vol. 1. S. Karger AG, Basel, 1973

26. Hilton-Brown P, Stalberg E: The motor

unit in muscular dystrophy, a single fibre EMG and scanning EMG study. J Neurol Neurosurg Psychiatry 46:981, 1983

27. Stalberg E: Macro EMG, a new recording technique. J Neurol Neurosurg Psychiatry 43:475, 1980

28. Stalberg EV: Macro EMG. Minimonograph No. 20. American Association of Electromyography and Electrodiagnosis, 1983

29. Stalberg E, Antoni L: Computer-aided EMG analysis. p. 186. In Desmedt JE (ed): Progress in Clinical Neurophysiology. Vol. 10. S. Karger AG, Basel, 1983

30. Fitch P, Willison RG: Automatic measurement of the human electromyogram. J Physiol 178:28P, 1965

31. Dowling MH, Fitch P, Willison RG: A special purpose digital computer (Biomac 500) used in the analysis of the human electromyogram. Electroencephalogr Clin Neurophysiol 25:570, 1968

32. Rose AL, Willison RG: Quantitative electromyography using automatic analysis: Studies in healthy subjects and patients with primary muscle disease. J Neurol Neurosurg Psychiatry 30:403, 1967

33. Hayward M, Willison RG: The recognition of myogenic and neurogenic lesions by quantitative EMG. p. 448. In Desmedt JE (ed): New Developments in Electromyography and Clinical Neurophysiology. Vol. 2. S. Karger AG, Basel, 1973

34. Hayward M, Willison RG: Automatic analysis of the electromyogram in patients with chronic partial denervation. J Neurol Sci 33:415, 1977

35. Fuglsang-Frederiksen A, Mansson A: Analysis of electrical activity of normal muscle in man at different degrees of voluntary effort. J Neurol Neurosurg Psychiatry 38:683, 1975

36. Fuglsang-Frederiksen A, Scheel U, Buchthal F: Diagnostic yield of analysis of the pattern of electrical activity and of individual motor unit potentials in myopathy. J Neurol Neurosurg Psychiatry 39:742, 1976

37. Fuglsang-Frederiksen A, Scheel U, Buchthal F: Diagnostic yield of the analysis of the pattern of electrical activity of muscle and of individual motor unit potentials in neurogenic involvement. J Neurol Neurosurg Psychiatry 40:544, 1977

38. Fuglsang-Frederiksen A, Dahl K, Monaco ML: Electrical muscle activity during a gradual increase in force in patients with neuromuscular diseases. Electroencephalogr Clin Neurophysiol 57:320, 1984

39. Stalberg E, Chu J, Bril V, Nandedkar S, Stalberg S, Ericsson M: Automatic analysis of the EMG interference pattern. Electroencephalogr Clin Neurophysiol 56:672, 1983

40. Nandedkar SD, Sanders DB, Stalberg EV: Automatic analysis of the electromyographic interference pattern. Part I. Development of quantitative features. Muscle Nerve 9:431, 1986

41. Nandedkar SD, Sanders DB, Stalberg EV: Automatic analysis of the electromyographic interference pattern. Part II. Findings in control subjects and in some neuromuscular diseases. Muscle Nerve 9:491, 1986

42. Dorfman LJ, Cummins KL, Leifer LJ (eds): Conduction Velocity Distributions: A Population Approach to Electrophysiology of Nerve. Alan R Liss, Inc., New York, 1981

43. Dorfman LJ: The distribution of conduction velocities in peripheral nerves: A review. Muscle Nerve 7:2, 1984

44. Thomas PK, Sears TA, Gilliatt RW: The range of conduction velocity in normal motor nerve fibres to the small muscles of the hand and foot. J Neurol Neurosurg Psychiatry 22:175, 1959

45. Hopf HC: Electromyographic study on so-called mononeuritis. Arch Neurol 9:307, 1963

46. Gilliatt RW, Hopf HC, Rudge P, Baraitser M: Axonal velocities of motor units in the hand and foot muscles of the baboon. J Neurol Sci 29:249, 1976

47. Leifer LJ: Nerve-fiber conduction velocity distributions: Motor nerve studies using collision neurography. p. 233. In Dorfman LJ, Cummins KL, Leifer LJ (eds): Conduction Velocity Distributions: A Population Approach to Electrophysiology of Nerve. Alan R Liss, Inc., New York, 1981

48. Lee RG, Ashby P, White DG, Aguayo AJ: Analysis of motor conduction velocity in the human median nerve by computer simulation of compound muscle action potentials. Electroencephalogr Clin Neurophysiol 39:225, 1975

49. Cummins KL, Dorfman LJ, Perkel DH: Nerve fiber conduction-velocity distributions. II. Estimation based on two compound action potentials. Electroencephalogr Clin Neurophysiol 46:647, 1979

50. Barker AT, Brown BH, Freeston IL: Modeling of an active nerve fiber in a finite volume conductor and its application to the calculation of surface action potentials. IEEE Trans Biomed Eng 26:53, 1979

51. Barker AT, Brown BH, Freeston IL: Determination of the distribution of conduction velocities in human nerve trunks. IEEE Trans Biomed Eng 26:76, 1979

52. Cummins KL, Dorfman LJ: Nerve fiber conduction velocity distributions: Studies of normal and diabetic human nerves. Ann Neurol 9:67, 1981

53. Overend W: Preliminary note on a new cranial reflex. Lancet 1:619, 1896

54. Kugelberg E: Facial reflexes. Brain 75:385, 1952

55. Walker DD, Kimura J: A fast-recovery electrode amplifier for electrophysiology. Electroencephalogr Clin Neurophysiol 45:789, 1978

56. Kimura J: Alteration of the orbicularis oculi reflex by pontine lesions. Study in multiple sclerosis. Arch Neurol 22:156, 1970

57. Kimura J, Lyon LW: Orbicularis oculi reflex in the Wallenberg syndrome: Alteration of the late reflex by lesions of the spinal tract and nucleus of the trigeminal nerve. J Neurol Neurosurg Psychiatry 35:228, 1972

58. Ongerboer de Visser BW, Kuypers HGJM: Late blink reflex changes in lateral medullary lesions. An electrophysiological and neuro-anatomical study of Wallenberg's syndrome. Brain 101:285, 1978

59. Penders CA, Delwaide PJ: Physiologic approach to the human blink reflex. p. 649. In Desmedt JE (ed): New Developments in Electromyography and Clinical Neurophysiology. Vol. 3. S. Karger AG, Basel, 1973

60. Kimura J: Electrically elicited blink reflex in diagnosis of multiple sclerosis. Review of 260 patients over a seven-year period. Brain 98:413, 1975

61. Kimura J, Rodnitzky RL, Van Allen MW: Electrodiagnostic study of trigeminal nerve. Orbicularis oculi reflex and masseter reflex in trigeminal neuralgia, paratrigeminal syndrome, and other lesions of the trigeminal nerve. Neurology 20:574, 1970

62. Ongerboer de Visser BW, Goor C: Electromyographic and reflex study in idiopathic and symptomatic trigeminal neuralgias: Latency of the jaw and blink reflexes. J Neurol Neurosurg Psychiatry 37:1225, 1974

63. Kimura J, Giron LT, Young SM: Electrophysiological study of Bell palsy: Electrically elicited blink reflex in assessment of prognosis. Arch Otolaryngol 102:140, 1976

64. Auger RG: Hemifacial spasm: Clinical and electrophysiologic observations. Neurology 29:1261, 1979

65. Kimura J, Rodnitzky RL, Okawara S-H: Electrophysiologic analysis of aberrant regeneration after facial nerve paralysis. Neurology 25:989, 1975

66. Kimura J: An evaluation of the facial and trigeminal nerves in polyneuropathy: Electrodiagnostic study in Charcot-Marie-Tooth disease, Guillain-Barré syndrome, and diabetic neuropathy. Neurology 21:745, 1971

67. Kimura J: The blink reflex as a clinical test. p. 347. In Aminoff MJ (ed): Electrodiagnosis in Clinical Neurology. 2nd Ed. Churchill Livingstone, New York, 1986

68. Lyon LW, Van Allen MW: Alteration of the orbicularis oculi reflex by acoustic neuroma. Arch Otolaryngol 95:100, 1972

69. Eisen A, Danon J: The orbicularis oculi reflex in acoustic neuromas: A clinical and electrodiagnostic evaluation. Neurology 24:306, 1974

70. Lyon LW, Kimura J, McCormick WF: Orbicularis oculi reflex in coma: Clinical, electrophysiological, and pathological correlations. J Neurol Neurosurg Psychiatry 35:582, 1972

71. Kimura J, Wilkinson JT, Damasio H, Adams HR, Shivapour E, Yamada T: Blink reflex in patients with hemispheric cerebrovascular accident (CVA). Blink reflex in CVA. J Neurol Sci 67:15, 1985

72. Kimura J, Yanagisawa H, Yamada T, Mitsudome A, Sasaki H, Kimura A: Is the F wave elicited in a select group of motoneurons? Muscle Nerve 7:392, 1984

73. Panayiotopoulos CP: F chronodispersion:

A new electrophysiologic method. Muscle Nerve 2:68, 1979

74. Shahani BT: Application of newer F response parameters in the diagnosis of peripheral neuropathies. Muscle Nerve 5:S163, 1982

75. Trontelj JV: A study of the F response by single fibre electromyography. p. 318. In Desmedt JE (ed): New Developments in Electromyography and Clinical Neurophysiology. Vol. 3. S. Karger AG, Basel, 1973

76. Young RR, Shahani BT: Clinical value and limitations of F-wave determination. Muscle Nerve 1:248, 1978

77. Fisher MA: F response latency determination. Muscle Nerve 5:730, 1982

78. Peioglou-Harmoussi S, Howel D, Fawcett PRW, Barwick DD: F-response behaviour in a control population. J Neurol Neurosurg Psychiatry 48:1152, 1985

79. Kimura J: F-wave velocity in the central segment of the median and ulnar nerves. A study in normal subjects and in patients with Charcot-Marie-Tooth disease. Neurology 24:539, 1974

80. Eisen A, Schomer D, Melmed C: The application of F-wave measurements in the differentiation of proximal and distal upper limb entrapments. Neurology 27:662, 1977

81. Kimura J: Proximal versus distal slowing of motor nerve conduction velocity in the Guillain-Barré syndrome. Arch Neurol 3:344, 1978

82. King D, Ashby P: Conduction velocity in the proximal segments of a motor nerve in the Guillain-Barré syndrome. J Neurol Neurosurg Psychiatry 39:538, 1976

83. Lachman T, Shahani BT, Young RR: Late responses as aids to diagnosis in peripheral neuropathy. J Neurol Neurosurg Psychiatry 43:156, 1980

84. Walsh JC, Yiannikas C, McLeod JG: Abnormalities of proximal conduction in acute idiopathic polyneuritis: Comparison of short latency evoked potentials and F-waves. J Neurol Neurosurg Psychiatry 47:197, 1984

85. Ongerboer de Visser BW, van der Sande JJ, Kemp B: Ulnar F-wave conduction velocity in epidural metastatic root lesions. Ann Neurol 11:142, 1982

86. Wulff CH, Gilliatt RW: F waves in patients with hand wasting caused by a cervical rib and band. Muscle Nerve 2:452, 1979

87. Yates SK, Brown WF: Characteristics of the F response: A single motor unit study. J Neurol Neurosurg Psychiatry 42:161, 1979

88. Fisher MA, Shahani BT, Young RR: Assessing segmental excitability after acute rostral lesions. I. The F response. Neurology 28:1265, 1978

89. Jabre JF: Surface recording of the H-reflex of the flexor carpi radialis. Muscle Nerve 4:435, 1981

90. Deschuytere J, Rosselle N, De Keyser C: Monosynaptic reflexes in the superficial forearm flexors in man and their clinical significance. J Neurol Neurosurg Psychiatry 39:555, 1976

91. Upton ARM, McComas AJ, Sica REP: Potentiation of "late" responses evoked in muscles during effort. J Neurol Neurosurg Psychiatry 34:699, 1971

92. Eisen A, Hoirch M, White J, Calne D: Sensory group 1a proximal conduction velocity. Muscle Nerve 7:636, 1984

93. Braddom RI, Johnson EW: Standardization of H reflex and diagnostic use in S1 radiculopathy. Arch Phys Med Rehabil 55:161, 1974

94. Burke D, Gandevia SC, McKeon B: The afferent volleys responsible for spinal proprioceptive reflexes in man. J Physiol 339:535, 1983

95. Desmedt JE: Somatosensory evoked potentials in man: Maturation, cognitive parameters, and clinical uses in neurological disorders. p. 83. In Lehmann D, Callaway E (eds): Human Evoked Potentials. Plenum Press, New York, 1979

96. Kimura J, Mitsudome A, Yamada T, Dickins QS: Stationary peaks from a moving source in far-field recording. Electroencephalogr Clin Neurophysiol 58:351, 1984

97. Kimura J, Mitsudome A, Beck DO, Yamada T, Dickins QS: Field distribution of antidromically activated digital nerve potentials: Model for far-field recording. Neurology 33:1164, 1983

98. Lueders H, Lesser R, Hahn J, Little J, Klem G: Subcortical somatosensory evoked potentials to median nerve stimulation. Brain 106:341, 1983

99. Jones SJ, Wynn Parry CB, Landi A: Diagnosis of brachial plexus traction lesions by sensory nerve action potentials and somatosensory evoked potentials. Injury 12:376, 1981

100. Synek V: Somatosensory evoked potentials from musculocutaneous nerve in the diagnosis of brachial plexus injuries. J Neurol Sci 61:443, 1983

101. Landi A, Copeland SA, Wynn Parry CB, Jones SJ: The role of somatosensory evoked potentials and nerve conduction studies in the surgical management of brachial plexus injuries. J Bone Joint Surg 62B:492, 1980

102. Aminoff MJ, Olney RK, Parry GJ, Raskin NH: Relative utility of different electrophysiologic techniques in the evaluation of brachial plexopathies. (Submitted for publication).

103. Glover JL, Worth RM, Bendick PJ, Hall PV, Markand OM: Evoked responses in the diagnosis of thoracic outlet syndrome. Surgery 89:86, 1981

104. Yiannikas C, Walsh JC: Somatosensory evoked responses in the diagnosis of thoracic outlet syndrome. J Neurol Neurosurg Psychiatry 46:234, 1983

105. Ganes T: Somatosensory conduction times and peripheral, cervical and cortical evoked potentials in patients with cervical spondylosis. J Neurol Neurosurg Psychiatry 43:683, 1980

106. El Negamy E, Sedgwick EM: Delayed cervical somatosensory potentials in cervical spondylosis. J Neurol Neurosurg Psychiatry 42:238, 1979

107. Eisen A, Hoirch M, Moll A: Evaluation of radiculopathies by segmental stimulation and somatosensory evoked potentials. Can J Neurol Sci 10:178, 1983

108. Aminoff MJ, Goodin DS, Barbaro NM, Weinstein PR, Rosenblum ML: Dermatomal somatosensory evoked potentials in unilateral lumbosacral radiculopathy. Ann Neurol 17:171, 1985

109. Scarff TB, Dallmann DE, Toleikis JR, Bunch WH: Dermatomal somatosensory evoked potentials in the diagnosis of lumbar root entrapment. Surg Forum 32:489, 1981

110. Aminoff MJ, Goodin DS, Parry GJ, Barbaro NM, Weinstein PR, Rosenblum ML: Electrophysiologic evaluation of lumbosacral radiculopathies: Electromyography, late responses and somatosensory evoked potentials. Neurology 35:1514, 1985

111. Parry GJ, Aminoff MJ: Somatosensory evoked potentials in chronic acquired demyelinating peripheral neuropathy. Neurology 37:313, 1987

112. Desmedt JE, Noel P: Averaged cerebral evoked potentials in the evaluation of lesions of the sensory nerves and of the central somatosensory pathway. p. 352. In Desmedt JE (ed): New Developments in Electromyography and Clinical Neurophysiology. Vol. 2. S. Karger AG, Basel, 1973

113. Eisen A, Purves S, Hoirch M: Central nervous system amplification: Its potential in the diagnosis of early multiple sclerosis. Neurology 32:359, 1982

114. Brown WF, Feasby TE: Sensory evoked potentials in Guillain-Barré polyneuropathy. J Neurol Neurosurg Psychiatry 47:288, 1984

115. Synek VM: Assessing sensory involvement in lower limb nerve lesions using somatosensory evoked potential techniques. Muscle Nerve 8:511, 1985

116. Arezzo JC, Schaumburg HH, Vaughan HG, Spencer PS, Barna J: Hind limb somatosensory evoked potentials in the monkey: The effects of distal axonopathy. Ann Neurol 12:24, 1982

117. Eisen A, Aminoff MJ: Somatosensory evoked potentials. p. 535. In Aminoff MJ (ed): Electrodiagnosis in Clinical Neurology. 2nd Ed. Churchill Livingstone, New York, 1986

118. Halliday AM, Mason AA: The effect of hypnotic anaesthesia on cortical responses. J Neurol Neurosurg Psychiatry 27:300, 1964

119. Levy R, Behrman J: Cortical evoked responses in hysterical hemianaesthesia. Electroencephalogr Clin Neurophysiol 29:400, 1970

120. Levy R, Mushin J: The somatosensory evoked response in patients with hysterical anaesthesia. J Psychosom Res 17:81, 1973

9

Nerves in the Upper Limb

The principles and basic technical aspects of nerve conduction studies were considered in Chapter 7. Details of the electrode placements used for studying the individual peripheral nerves of the upper limb are provided in this chapter, together with an account of the clinical and electrophysiologic features of the various lesions that affect these nerves. It must be emphasized, however, that when patients with mononeuropathies are being investigated, the function of at least one other nerve should also be examined to exclude more generalized peripheral nerve involvement. Furthermore, in patients with an entrapment neuropathy on one side, the other side should also be examined electrophysiologically, despite the absence of symptoms, because the common entrapment neuropathies often occur bilaterally.

Before considering the individual peripheral nerves, certain general comments must be made regarding anomalies in the normal pattern of innervation.

ANOMALOUS INNERVATION OF THE HAND MUSCLES

Anomalies in the innervation of the hand muscles are common, and can be a source of confusion and error when nerve conduc-

tion studies are performed. The size of the problem is indicated by Rowntree, who found that the intrinsic hand muscles were anomalously innervated in 20 percent of 226 patients with lesions of the median or ulnar nerves.[1]

As a consequence of such anomalies, patients with complete lesions of one of these nerves may either fail to exhibit the expected motor deficit or develop a more widespread impairment of muscle function than might have been anticipated. The entire course of the aberrant fibers is sometimes anomalous, but in other cases, fibers pass via branches linking the median and ulnar nerves so that only the proximal or distal part of their course is abnormal. As for the affected muscles, their nerve supply may be either entirely anomalous, or partly anomalous and partly normal.

Using electrophysiologic techniques, Wilbourn and Lambert found that 31 percent of subjects had an anomalous crossover of fibers from the median to the ulnar nerve in the forearm,[2] and the incidence of this communication may be considerably higher in the family members of propositi with this anatomic variant.[3] Such an anomaly is sometimes referred to as the Martin-Gruber anastomosis. Its presence is often suggested by the findings during routine motor nerve conduction studies. In normal subjects, the compound muscle action potential elicited by supramaximal stimulation of the median nerve at the wrist is about the same size as, or slightly greater than, the response to stimulation of the nerve at the elbow. When there is an anomalous communication between median and ulnar nerves in the forearm, however, the response to wrist stimulation may be significantly smaller than that to elbow stimulation (Fig. 9.1). This is because some of the axons present in the median nerve at the elbow leave it in the forearm to travel with the ulnar nerve, and so are not excited by stimulation of the median nerve at the wrist. Before the presence of such an anomaly is assumed, however, technical factors that might lead to similar findings must be excluded. In particular, the intensity of the stimulating current must be adjusted to ensure that it is indeed supramaximal at the wrist, and not so excessive that the current spreads to other nerves at the elbow.

The presence of a Martin-Gruber anastomosis may complicate the evaluation of patients with median nerve entrapment at the wrist, and can lead to erroneous calculation of motor conduction velocity in the forearm segment of the median nerve (p. 186).

Some of the fibers crossing from the median to the ulnar nerve may supply muscles normally innervated by the ulnar nerve. Stimulation of the median nerve at the elbow will then elicit a response from ulnar-innervated hand muscles, whereas median nerve stimulation at the wrist will elicit no response in these muscles. In these circum-

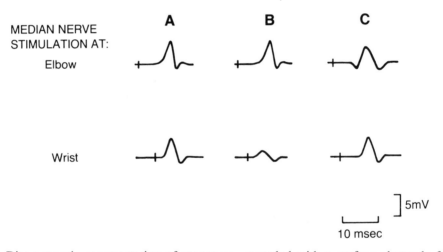

MEDIAN NERVE STIMULATION AT:

Elbow

Wrist

A   B   C

5mV

10 msec

Fig. 9.1 Diagrammatic representation of responses, recorded with a surface electrode from the abductor pollicis brevis muscle, to supramaximal stimulation of the median nerve at the elbow and wrist. **(A)** Normal responses. **(B)** Responses obtained in a normal subject with an anomalous communication between the median and ulnar nerves in the forearm. The response elicited by stimulation at the elbow is significantly larger than the response obtained by stimulation at the wrist. **(C)** Response obtained in a patient with carpal tunnel syndrome and a coexisting anomalous communication between the median and ulnar nerves in the forearm. The response to stimulation at the wrist has a prolonged latency. With stimulation at the elbow, the response has an initial positivity secondary to volume conduction of a response generated in ulnar-innervated muscles by fibers crossing from the median to the ulnar nerve in the forearm. Moreover, the latency of the response to stimulation at the elbow is relatively normal because fibers bypass the segment with slowed conduction velocity; this may lead to spuriously fast forearm conduction velocity as determined by the difference in latency with proximal and distal stimulation.

stances, the response of the hypothenar muscles or the first dorsal interosseous muscle to ulnar nerve stimulation at the wrist may be considerably greater than that which occurs with ulnar nerve stimulation at the elbow, thereby resembling the findings in patients with ulnar nerve lesions causing conduction block at the elbow. The significance of such findings should, therefore, be determined during the course of ulnar nerve conduction studies by confirming that the stimulus is indeed supramaximal at both sites, by stimulating the ulnar nerve just below the elbow to determine whether the response size is altered as compared to the response to more proximal stimulation, and also by examining the responses to median nerve stimulation.

It is important to remember the possibility of such anomalies when patients with peripheral nerve lesions are being evaluated, particularly when the clinical findings do not conform with those that might have been anticipated. The nature and size of the individual muscle responses evoked by proximal and distal stimulation of the median and ulnar nerves should then be examined in the hope of clarifying the issue.

ULNAR NERVE

Clinical Aspects

The ulnar nerve is derived from the medial cord of the brachial plexus and contains fibers from the C7, C8, and T1 segments. It supplies various muscles in the forearm and hand, as shown in Table 9.1, and sends cutaneous branches to part of the hand and to the medial one and a half digits.

The nerve descends the arm and then traverses the ulnar groove between the olecranon and the medial epicondyle, where it lies superficially and is easily palpated. After passing through the cubital tunnel, the nerve passes down the forearm under the belly of the flexor carpi ulnaris. The nerve

Table 9.1. Muscles Innervated by the Ulnar Nerve

Ulnar nerve	Flexor carpi ulnaris Flexor digitorum profundus to fourth and fifth digits
Superficial terminal branch	Palmaris brevis
Deep terminal branch	Abductor digiti minimi Opponens digiti minimi Flexor digiti minimi Third and fourth lumbricals Adductor pollicis The interossei Flexor pollicis brevis

lies superficial to and is between the tendons of flexor digitorum sublimis and flexor carpi ulnaris at the wrist and, having entered the canal of Guyon at the level of the wrist crease, divides into two branches. The deep branch supplies the abductor digiti minimi, and then passes across the palm, supplying the ulnar-innervated intrinsic hand muscles. The superficial branch supplies the skin on the palmar aspect of the little finger and the medial half of the ring finger. Another branch of the ulnar nerve— the dorsal cutaneous sensory branch— comes off the parent nerve about 2 to 3 inches above the ulnar styloid process, supplying the dorsal aspect of these same fingers, as well as the ulnar part of the back of the hand and wrist (Fig. 9.2).

LESIONS IN THE ELBOW REGION

Lesions are especially liable to occur in the region of the elbow joint as the nerve runs in the groove behind the medial epicondyle and descends in the cubital tunnel. In the condylar groove, the ulnar nerve is particularly susceptible to pressure or trauma. An increase in the carrying angle of the elbow—whether congenital in origin or secondary to trauma or degenerative changes—may cause it to be stretched excessively when the elbow is flexed. The term *tardy ulnar palsy* refers to the devel-

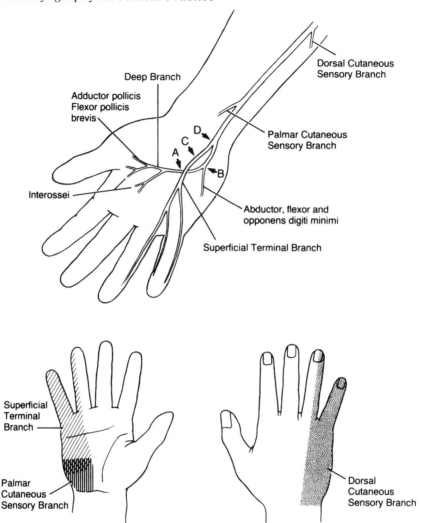

Fig. 9.2 Anatomy of the ulnar nerve in the lower part of the forearm and hand. The cutaneous regions supplied by different sensory branches of the ulnar nerve are indicated in the lower part of the figure. The ulnar nerve may be injured at several different sites in the hand. Injury to the deep terminal branch (at *A*) leads to weakness of the ulnar-innervated hand muscles except for the hypothenar group. With more proximal involvement of this branch (*B*), there is weakness of all the ulnar-innervated hand muscles, but no sensory loss. In some instances, there may be sensory loss secondary to a lesion of the superficial sensory branch (at *C*), whereas a combined motor and sensory deficit occurs in the hand with involvement of the ulnar nerve itself, or both its deep and superficial terminal branches (as at *D*).

opment of an ulnar neuropathy as a late complication of injury, usually in association with residual bony deformity of the elbow. Constriction of the nerve in the cubital tunnel has received less attention until comparatively recently. The roof of this tunnel is formed by the aponeurosis of the flexor carpi ulnaris between the olecranon and the medial epicondyle, and its floor is the medial ligament of the elbow.[4] Thickening or distortion of either of these structures constricts the nerve, and the resulting symptoms may be aggravated by flexion of the elbow, which causes the tunnel to narrow as a result of tightening of its roof or bulging of its floor inward.

Differentiating between lesions at these two sites can be exceedingly difficult, but is of paramount importance because their surgical treatment differs. A severe lesion at either site causes appropriate sensory changes and weakness of ulnar-innervated muscles in the forearm and hand. In the cubital tunnel syndrome, however, there is no evidence of previous injury to the elbow or of joint deformity, and the ulnar nerve may be palpably taut and enlarged in the ulnar groove. Moreover, there may be relative sparing of the flexor carpi ulnaris because its motor axons are in a separate fascicle, with branches that are given off from the parent nerve either before, or very soon after, the parent nerve enters the tunnel.[4] Nerve stimulation techniques may permit more accurate determination of the site of the lesion.

Pathologic studies suggest that subclinical ulnar nerve lesions at the elbow occur fairly commonly. Neary and co-workers, for example, found pathologic evidence of compressive ulnar nerve lesions at the elbow in 5 of 12 nerves examined at autopsy in patients who had no clinical evidence of the lesion.[5]

LESIONS IN THE HAND

Lesions may develop at the wrist or in the palm of the hand, and are usually related to trauma, which is often repetitive, or to compression from ganglia or benign tumors. These lesions may be divided into different patterns of clinical presentation, depending on their presumed sites (Fig. 9.2).[6] First, the deep terminal (palmar) branch of the nerve can be involved after it has supplied the hypothenar muscles and rounded the

hook of the hamate. All of the ulnar-innervated hand muscles are weak except the hypothenar group, and there are no sensory changes. Second, the deep terminal branch can be involved more proximally so that, although there is no sensory loss, all of the hand muscles supplied by the nerve, including the hypothenar ones, are affected. Third, an even more proximal lesion can involve either the ulnar nerve itself, or both its deep and superficial terminal branches, so that both sensory and motor changes occur in the hand, the latter involving the hypothenar muscles as well as the interossei, adductor pollicis, and two medial lumbricals. Function of the dorsal cutaneous sensory branch is normal. Less commonly, there may be sensory loss secondary to involvement of the superficial sensory branch, but with preserved motor function and normal sensation in the territory of the dorsal cutaneous branch. Finally, although rare, there may be weakness limited to the interossei or the hypothenar muscles, with impaired sensation in the region of the superficial cutaneous branch of the ulnar nerve, but preserved sensation in the territory of the dorsal sensory branch of the nerve.[7] The deep palmar branch seems especially vulnerable as it rounds the hook of the hamate, presumably because it is compressed as it runs between the pisohamate ligament and the overlying tendinous arch.[8]

Electrophysiologic Aspects

It is sometimes impossible to localize a lesion of the ulnar nerve on clinical grounds, and electrophysiologic techniques therefore have an important role in this regard. In addition to electromyographic sampling of the muscles supplied by the ulnar nerve, motor and sensory conduction can conveniently be studied in this nerve, thereby determining with precision the site of a local lesion. Some of the available data relating

Table 9.2. Ulnar Nerve Conduction Studies—Normal Mean Values

Motor Conduction Studies

	Distal Latency (msec)	Conduction Velocity (m/sec)			Source
		Forearm	Upper Arm	Across Elbow	
Recording from abductor digiti minimi	2.9 (SD 0.4)				Ebeling et al.[6]
	2.7[a] (SD 0.3)	58.9[a] (SD 2.2)	64.4[a] (SD 2.6)		Mayer[9]
		56.2 (SD 4.6)			Thomas et al.[10]
		56.4 (SD 4.8)	63.4 (SD 5.3)		Trojaborg[11]
	3.0 (SD 0.4)	54.6 (SD 6.7)	59.2 (SD 8.2)	53.2 (Ext) (SD 7.8)	Eisen[12]
		62.5 (SD 4.5)		49.9 (Ext) (SD 7.9)	Checkles et al.[13]
		61.8 (SD 5.0)		62.7 (Flex) (SD 5.5)	Checkles et al.[13]
	2.4 (SD 0.3)	69.0 (SD 5.5)		52.0 (Ext) (SD 4.0)	Payan[14]
Recording from first dorsal interosseous	3.8 (SD 0.5)				Ebeling et al.[6]
		55.0 (SD 4.9)			Thomas et al.[10]

Nerve Action Potentials

Finger to Wrist			Wrist to Above Elbow		Elbow to Axilla		Source
Velocity (m/sec)	Latency to Peak (msec)	Amplitude (μV)	Velocity (m/sec)	Amplitude (μV)	Velocity (m/sec)	Amplitude (μV)	
	2.2–3.4	8–28					Gilliatt & Sears[15]
64.7 (SD 3.9)			64.8[a] (SD 3.8)		69.1[a] (SD 4.3)		Mayer[9]
				33–117		33–100	Gilliatt & Thomas[16]
55.0 (SD 4.50)		14.5 (SD 7.0)	66.0 (SD 3.0)				Payan[14]

[a] Data for subjects between 10 and 35 years of age.
Ext, extended; Flex, flexed; SD, standard deviation.

to the normal ulnar nerve are summarized in Table 9.2.

MOTOR CONDUCTION STUDIES

In performing motor conduction studies, bipolar surface electrodes may be used for stimulation, with the cathode being placed distal to the anode and positioned over the ulnar nerve (Fig. 9.3) at any of the following sites:

1. The proximal wrist crease
2. About 5 cm below the medial epicondyle ("below elbow")
3. 1 to 5 cm above the tip of the medial epicondyle ("above elbow")
4. About 10 cm or more above the tip of the medial epicondyle, in the axilla

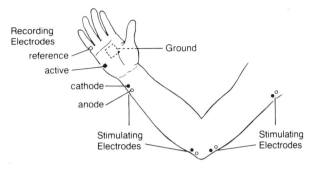

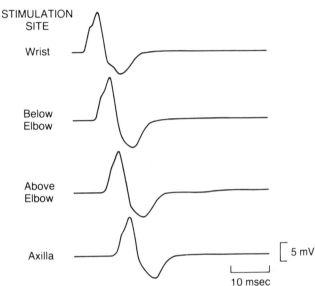

Fig. 9.3 Arrangement for motor conduction studies of the ulnar nerve. The responses recorded with a surface electrode from the abductor digiti minimi muscle to supramaximal stimulation of the nerve at different sites are indicated in the lower part of the figure.

5. Erb's point (i.e., the angle between the clavicle and the posterior border of the sternomastoid).

Muscles from which motor responses can conveniently be recorded with surface or needle electrodes are the abductor digiti minimi, the first dorsal interosseous, and the adductor pollicis. The ground lead is placed on the back of the hand. Depending on the sites selected for stimulation, motor conduction velocity in the forearm, across the elbow, in the upper arm, and more proximally can be calculated by subtraction. If surface electrodes are used for recording, the amplitude of the compound muscle action potential evoked by stimulating the

nerve at different sites can also be compared.

When conduction velocity is being determined across the elbow segment of the nerve, the elbow must be maintained in exactly the same position while the nerve is stimulated above and below it, and while the distances involved are measured.[17] Conduction across the elbow is sometimes found to be slower than in the forearm in normal subjects, but this seems to depend, at least in part, on the manner in which the distances are measured. Eisen found that, in 15 percent of normal ulnar nerves, the conduction velocity across the elbow was at least 10 m/sec less than in adjacent portions of the nerve, when studied with the elbow extended.[12] Checkles and co-workers found motor conduction velocity to be markedly reduced when determined with the elbow extended rather than flexed to 70 degrees,[13] and others have found a somewhat similar effect of elbow position on motor and sensory conduction velocity across the elbow.[18] In general, however, comparable values for maximal motor conduction velocity across the elbow and in the forearm are obtained when the elbow is in the flexed position.[13,17]

NERVE ACTION POTENTIALS

Sensory conduction is evaluated orthodromically by stimulating the ulnar digital fibers in the little finger and recording the action potential of the afferent volley at the wrist (Fig. 9.4). Ring electrodes are convenient for stimulation, a cathode being placed near the metacarpophalangeal joint at the base of the finger and an anode at the terminal interphalangeal joint, the stimulated finger being separated from its neighbors by hydrophobic cotton to prevent current spread. The recording electrodes at the wrist are placed over the nerve trunk, the position of which is defined by observing the motor response to stimulation. When no motor response can be evoked, the electrodes are placed over the tendon of the flexor carpi ulnaris, adjacent to which the nerve normally runs, and their position is then altered very slightly to yield the largest responses to stimulation of the finger. Either needle or surface electrodes are suitable for recording purposes, but the latter are easier to apply, less distressing for the patient, and perfectly satisfactory for most clinical purposes. The saddle electrode described by Dawson and Scott is particularly convenient for this purpose.[19] The ground lead is attached to the back of the hand.

The recording of nerve action potentials in successive portions of the limb may be important when attempting to localize a lesion of the nerve. A small or absent sensory action potential may be found at the wrist when sensory fibers are involved at any point distal to the posterior root ganglia, and so is not of more specific localizing value.

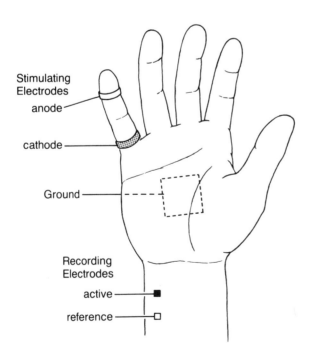

Stimulating Electrodes

anode

cathode

Ground

Recording Electrodes

active

reference

Fig. 9.4 Arrangement for recording orthodromic sensory nerve action potentials from the ulnar nerve at the wrist.

Nerve action potentials can be recorded just above the elbow after stimulation at the wrist, and in the axilla after stimulation above the elbow, the ground being placed between the stimulating and recording electrodes. If nerve action potentials are to be recorded across the elbow segment of the nerve, the elbow should be in the flexed position.[18] The afferent volleys are composed of antidromically conducted impulses in motor fibers, as well as orthodromic impulses in sensory ones.

The dorsal sensory branch of the ulnar nerve comes off the main trunk of the nerve some 2 to 3 inches above the ulnar styloid process, and accordingly, is spared in lesions in the wrist or hand. By contrast, with ulnar lesions at the elbow, conduction in this branch is likely to be affected. A technique for recording conduction in this branch has recently been described.[20,21] The nerve is stimulated about 8 to 10 cm above the ulnar styloid process, between the flexor carpi ulnaris tendon and the ulna. The response is recorded along the fifth metacarpal bone, with a reference electrode placed over the fifth metacarpophalangeal joint about 3 cm more distally (Fig. 9.5).

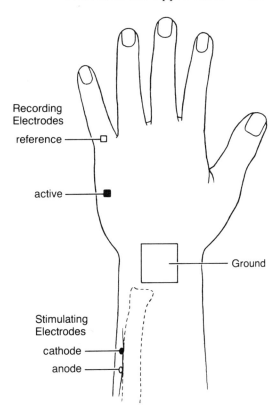

Fig. 9.5 Arrangement for studying conduction in the dorsal sensory branch of the ulnar nerve.

ELECTROPHYSIOLOGIC FINDINGS WITH LESIONS AT THE ELBOW

Sensory fibers are usually the first to be affected. The finding of absent or markedly attenuated ulnar sensory action potentials at the wrist with stimulation of the digital fibers in the little finger is of little localizing value, but does suggest that the lesion is distal to the dorsal root ganglia. Moreover, it provides some indication of the extent of any axonal degeneration that has occurred. In some instances, nerve action potentials are unrecordable at the wrist or immediately above the elbow; in others, these potentials have a diminished amplitude and/or prolonged conduction time, and conduction velocity is often slowed to a greater degree across the elbow than in the forearm or hand.[14]

In their study of patients with the cubital tunnel syndrome, Odusote and Eisen found that, on the affected side, the sensory nerve action potential recorded above the elbow was dispersed in 85 percent of patients who had either no clinical signs or just a mild sensory deficit.[22] The increased dispersion could be localized to the elbow region in most patients, which underscores the value of recording nerve action potentials in the various segments of the ulnar nerve.

Slowing of motor conduction velocity may be restricted to the elbow segment,[23] especially if there is no clinical motor deficit.[14] However, the finding of slowed motor conduction velocity across this segment of the nerve may be hard to interpret for the reasons outlined earlier—namely, the critical influence of elbow position on apparent conduction velocity, and the fact that, in normal subjects with the elbow extended, conduction velocity across the elbow segment is commonly more than 10 m/sec slower than in neighboring segments of the nerve.[12] In some patients with ulnar nerve lesions at the elbow, motor conduction velocity is also slowed in the forearm, and it may be mildly reduced in the upper arm as well.[16] When performing motor conduction studies in patients with suspected lesions at the elbow, it should be remembered that motor fibers to the first dorsal interosseous muscle are sometimes affected to a greater extent than those to the abductor digiti minimi, or vice versa, so that slowing is more apparent in one group than in the other.[14]

Recording the muscle response by surface electrodes and measuring its amplitude (Fig. 9.6) may be helpful in establishing the diagnosis. A decrement of 20 percent or more in the size of the response evoked by stimulation of the nerve above the elbow, compared with the response to stimulation at the wrist, supports the possibility of an ulnar nerve lesion at the elbow, and may be the only motor abnormality that is found. In all cases, however, the possibility of a Martin-Gruber anastomosis must be excluded by stimulating the ulnar nerve just below the elbow and stimulating the median nerve before any definite conclusions are reached (p. 166). If the response obtained in ulnar-innervated muscle has a negative onset with stimulation of the median nerve at the elbow but not with stimulation at the wrist, then at least a part of the nerve supply to these muscles must travel anomalously in the median nerve until reaching the forearm.

Any decrement in size of the compound muscle action potential obtained by stimulation of the ulnar nerve above a lesion at the elbow is often accompanied by increased duration and dispersion of the response. This reflects segmental demyelination with conduction delay; a reduction in the area of the response relates to conduction block.

When a significant decrement in size of the compound muscle action potential is found with ulnar nerve stimulation above the elbow, when compared to the response obtained with stimulation below the elbow or at the wrist, an attempt should be made to localize the lesion more precisely. To accomplish this, the ulnar nerve in the elbow region is stimulated in sequential steps approximately 2 cm apart so as to determine the site at which the amplitude and configuration of the muscle response shows an abrupt change,[24] as shown in Figure 7.11.

Electromyographic sampling of ulnar-innervated muscles may also help to establish the diagnosis of an ulnar nerve lesion, localize the site of pathology, and determine its severity. The findings provide a guide to the relative duration of the lesion, the speed of its evolution, the extent of axonal damage, and the rapidity with which recovery is likely to occur. With lesions at the elbow, the incidence of abnormalities is equal in the abductor digiti minimi and first dorsal interosseous muscles. Examination of other muscles in the hand—i.e., those supplied by the median nerve (such as the abductor pollicis brevis)—helps to exclude the possibility of a C8 or T1 radiculopathy, or a lesion of the lower trunk of the brachial plexus. The presence of abnormalities in the flexor carpi ulnaris indicates that the lesion must be at the level of the elbow or more rostrally, although the absence of abnormalities in this muscle does not exclude a rostral lesion (with sparing of the branch to the muscle). The flexor digitorum profundus to the fourth and fifth digits is affected by lesions at the elbow, but these muscles are hard to examine electrophysiologically.

In some patients with a complete ulnar

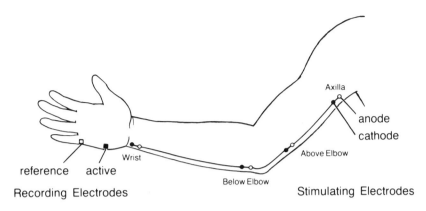

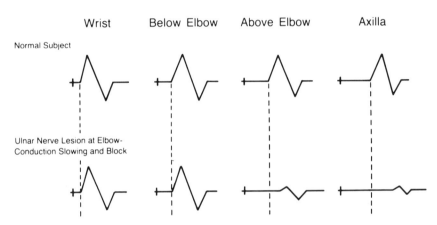

Fig. 9.6 Diagrammatic representation of the findings in a patient with an ulnar nerve lesion at the elbow. With stimulation above the elbow or in the axilla, the response elicited from the abductor digiti minimi by a supramaximal stimulus is markedly reduced in amplitude and area compared to the response elicited by distal stimulation.

neuropathy due to severe injury about the elbow, there is only mild weakness in the hands and, at electromyography, only partial denervation of ulnar-innervated muscles. This is because an anomalous course with subsequent communication between the median and ulnar nerves has permitted many fibers destined for the ulnar nerve in the forearm to bypass the lesion. This possibility must always be considered if a correct prognosis is to be made and if patients are to be managed appropriately.

In order for it to have any localizing value, the motor or sensory conduction velocity across the elbow must not only be slower than normal, but also relatively slower than that in the forearm. Payan found in his comprehensive study that the lesion could be localized to the elbow region by motor studies in 35 of 50 cases and by sensory studies in 34 cases; in 23 cases, the lesion could have been localized by either means.[14] Since there may be electrical evidence of motor involvement in patients with only sensory symptoms and signs, as well as evidence of sensory abnormalities in patients with purely motor involvement clinically, a fully comprehensive study should always be performed in patients suspected of having a lesion at the elbow.

During spontaneous improvement or postoperative recovery after transposition of the ulnar nerve, Payan found that motor and sensory conduction velocity increased across the elbow segment.[25] This increase was followed by restoration of the sensory potential recorded at the wrist, at which time clinical improvement also became noticeable. In patients with the cubital tunnel syndrome, decompressive surgery is followed by a similar increase in motor conduction velocity across the elbow, an increase in the size of the compound muscle action potential elicited by stimulation above the elbow, and an increased interference pattern on the needle examination.[26]

ELECTROPHYSIOLOGIC FINDINGS WITH LESIONS IN THE HAND

When the deep branch of the ulnar nerve is affected distal to the point at which it gives off its branches to the abductor digiti minimi, stimulation of the ulnar nerve at the wrist evokes a response of normal latency in this muscle, but the latency of the response of the first dorsal interosseous muscle is increased. The sensory action potentials recorded at the wrist after stimulation of the little finger are normal in latency and amplitude. In addition, there may be mild slowing of motor conduction velocity in the forearm, especially in fibers to the first dorsal interosseous muscle.[6] With more proximal lesions, the latency of the compound muscle action potential of the abductor digiti minimi may also be prolonged, and abnormalities of sensory conduction in the superficial cutaneous (palmar) branch may be found.[6]

Table 9.3. Muscles Innervated by the Median Nerve

Median nerve	Pronator teres
	Flexor carpi radialis
	Palmaris longus
	Flexor digitorum sublimis
	Abductor pollicis brevis
	Flexor pollicis brevis
	Opponens pollicis
	First and second lumbricals
Anterior interosseous branch	Flexor digitorum profundus to second and third digits
	Flexor pollicis longus
	Pronator quadratus

MEDIAN NERVE

Clinical Aspects

The median nerve originates from the lateral and medial cords of the brachial plexus, and contains fibers from the C6, C7, C8, and T1 segments of the cord. It supplies various muscles in the forearm and hand, as shown in Table 9.3, and innervates the skin of part of the hand and lateral three and a half digits. The skin of the third digit is supplied from fibers arising in the C7 nerve root and traversing the middle trunk of the brachial plexus, whereas the sensory fibers to the thumb and index finger are derived predominantly from C6 (and, to a lesser extent, C7), traversing the upper or middle trunk to reach the lateral cord of the plexus.

The median nerve enters the forearm between the two heads of the pronator teres muscle, which it supplies. As it descends, it supplies various mucles in the forearm, either directly or through the anterior interosseous nerve (see Table 9.3). The median nerve then passes beneath the anterior carpal ligament in the carpal tunnel to enter the hand. A motor branch is given off to supply certain muscles of the thenar eminence (see Table 9.3), and terminal branches supply the first and second lumbrical muscles. Cutaneous branches supply the skin of the lateral part of the palm, as well as the palmar surface (and dorsal surface of the terminal phalanges) of the lateral three-and-a-half digits.

The nerve is particularly prone to damage immediately above the elbow, where it may be compressed by the ligament of Struthers, in the forearm itself (pronator teres syndrome), at the wrist (carpal tunnel syndrome), and in the intermetacarpal tunnel.

ENTRAPMENT BY THE LIGAMENT OF STRUTHERS

Before it has supplied the pronator teres muscle, the median nerve may be compressed by the ligament of Struthers. This ligament is attached to the medial epicondyle of the humerus and to an anomalous supracondylar process about 5 cm above the epicondyle.[27] The nerve and, often, the brachial artery pass beneath it (Fig. 9.7). The disorder that occurs as a result of nerve compression at this site resembles the pronator syndrome, but clinical and needle examination of the pronator teres may show

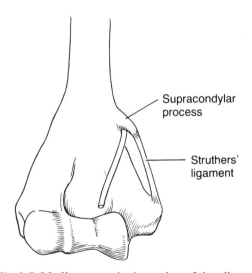

Supracondylar process

Struthers' ligament

Fig.9.7 Median nerve in the region of the elbow. The ligament of Struthers can be seen attached to the medial epicondyle of the humerus and an anomalous supracondylar process.

abnormalities that are usually not present in the latter disorder. Obliteration of the radial pulse (because of compression of the brachial artery) when the elbow is extended should suggest the diagnosis, whereas the presence of a supracondylar process on radiographs[28] supports the diagnosis but may be present in asymptomatic subjects as well. Surgical release of the ligament of Struthers is curative.

PRONATOR TERES SYNDROME

The median nerve gives off a purely motor branch, the anterior interosseous nerve, below the elbow as it descends between the two heads of the pronator teres, and then descends under the arch of the flexor digitorum sublimis. A lesion of either the parent nerve itself or the anterior interosseous nerve may develop in this region, sometimes following trauma or muscle hypertrophy, or as a result of an anomalous band between the pronator teres and the arch of the flexor digitorum sublimis.[29–31] When the anterior interosseous nerve is involved, there is no sensory loss, and weakness is confined to the pronator quadratus, flexor pollicis longus, and the flexor digitorum profundus to the second and third digits. When the main trunk of the median nerve is affected, however, weakness is more widespread, and sensory changes occur in an appropriate distribution. In either case, the presenting symptoms are often pain and tenderness about the upper forearm and the elbow.

Symptoms develop acutely when they follow trauma, but often develop more insidiously in relation to, for example, repetitive elbow flexion and pronation as may occur in butchers, leather cutters, and in certain other occupations. Weakness is often mild, and may not be detected clinically. There may be conspicuous enlargement of the pronator teres muscle on the affected side.[30] Symptoms and signs may erroneously be attributed to a cervical radiculopathy at the C6 or C7 level.

Treatment depends on the cause of the disorder. Precipitating factors, including those that are occupationally related, should be avoided, and a treatment regimen of rest and anti-inflammtory analgesics may be helpful. Local injection of steroids is recommended by some. Surgical exploration may be necessary if conservative measures do not lead to improvement within about 3 months, and may need to be undertaken immediately if nerve dysfunction follows a penetrating injury.

Weakness in the distribution of the anterior interosseous nerve may occur as the presenting feature of neuralgic amyotrophy[32] or of a partial median nerve lesion in the antecubital region.[33] This presumably occurs because the fibers destined to form the anterior interosseous nerve are organized into discrete fiber bundles relatively early in their course, but it can lead to diagnostic difficulty unless there are other clinical or electrophysiologic signs that enable the lesion to be localized correctly.

CARPAL TUNNEL SYNDROME

Compression of the median nerve occurs much more commonly in the carpal tunnel at the wrist than in the forearm. Predisposing factors to the development of this disorder include a reduction in the normal size of the carpal tunnel (e.g., occurring congenitally or as a result of trauma or degenerative or inflammatory arthritis) and an increase in the volume of its content (e.g., as occurs with tenosynovitis or in the presence of a ganglion). The carpal tunnel syndrome may also be related to pregnancy, acromegaly, myxedema, or amyloidosis, and it may have an occupational basis. In some instances, it is the presenting feature of a subclinical polyneuropathy, and this possibility must always be excluded by appropriate electrophysiologic studies. In many cases, no specific etiologic factors are apparent.

Pain and paresthesias are early symptoms and may be confined to the hand in a median nerve distribution, but in some cases they appear to involve the little finger as well. They may spread to the forearm, and occasionally to the upper arm, and are often particularly troublesome at night. Movement of the hand and arm usually helps to relieve these symptoms. Examination reveals impaired cutaneous sensation in a median nerve distribution in the hand. If motor involvement has occurred, weakness and wasting of the abductor pollicis brevis muscle and, usually, the opponens pollicis muscles, may be found as well. However, if motor involvement is mild, it may not be possible to detect any weakness unless the findings on the symptomatic and asymptomatic sides are compared. In early cases, there may be no clinical evidence whatsoever of motor involvement. Passive flexion or extension at the wrist for about a minute may aggravate or produce symptoms.[34]

The development of clinical dysfunction probably relates, at least in part, to mechanical factors, but ischemia may also play a role in symptom production. In carpal tunnel syndrome, there is some evidence that the median nerve is abnormally susceptible to ischemia.[35,36] Nerve decompression usually leads to immediate or rapid relief of pain, as if the pain related to ischemia, whereas other motor and sensory symptoms take longer to resolve.

Mild carpal tunnel syndrome is treated by the avoidance of precipitating activities (which are often occupational) and by nocturnal splinting of the wrist in a neutral position. Some authorities also recommend local injections of steroids into the carpal tunnel. A failure of conservative measures, or the development of neurogenic atrophy of the thenar eminence, is an indication for surgical decompression of the carpal tunnel. This generally leads to complete relief of pain and resolution of mild sensory or motor deficits. More severe and long-standing deficits require longer to recover, and may never resolve completely.

Electrophysiologic Aspects

MOTOR CONDUCTION STUDIES

The median nerve can be stimulated with bipolar surface electrodes, the cathode being placed distal to the anode and positioned at the following sites:

1. The palm of the hand at the most distal point from which a response can be elicited in appropriate (median-innervated) muscles. Kimura stressed that the anode should be placed distal rather than proximal to the stimulating cathode because the thenar nerve can sometimes be activated near the anode, leading to an erroneous determination of conduction velocity.[37]

2. The proximal crease of the wrist between the tendons of flexor carpi radialis and palmaris longus, or just proximal to this level

3. The elbow, next to the brachial artery

4. The upper arm or axilla, next to the brachial artery

5. Erb's point

The motor response is usually recorded from the abductor pollicis brevis muscle with surface or needle electrodes, the ground being placed on the back of the hand. When surface electrodes are used, the active one (G1) is placed over the motor point of the muscle, and the reference one (G2) is positioned over its tendon (Fig. 9.8). The distal motor latency is determined and, depending on the sites selected for stimulation, the motor conduction velocity in the

Table 9.4. Median Nerve Conduction Studies—Normal Mean Values

Motor Conduction Studies

	Distal Latency (msec)		Conduction Velocity (m/sec)		
	Wrist Stimulation	Palmar Stimulation	Forearm	Upper Arm	Source
Recording from abductor pollicis brevis	3.2[a] (SD 0.3)		59.3[a] (SD 3.5)	65.9[a] (SD 5.0)	Mayer[9]
			56.1 (SD 5.3)	67.9 (SD 7.7)	Trojaborg[11]
	3.6 (SD 0.4)	2.1 (SD 0.3)	59.0 (SD 5.0)		Kimura[37]

Nerve Action Potentials

Finger-Palm Segment		Finger-Wrist Segment		Wrist to Elbow		Elbow to Axilla		
Latency (msec)	Amplitude (μV)	Latency (msec)	Amplitude (μV)	Velocity (m/sec)	Amplitude (μV)	Velocity (m/sec)	Amplitude (μV)	Source
		2.5–4.0[d]	9–45					Gilliatt & Sears[15]
				67.7[d] (SD 4.4)		70.4[a] (SD 4.8)		Mayer[9]
1.41[c] (SD 0.2)	44.8[b] (SD 22.0)	2.82[c] (SD 0.3)	41.3[b] (SD 19.3)	63.2 (SD 6.3)	30.9[b] (SD 14.8)			Kimura[37]

[a] Data for subjects between 10 and 35 years of age.
[b] Amplitude measured from baseline to negative peak.
[c] Latency to onset of initial negative response.
[d] Latency to peak of negative response.
SD, standard deviation.

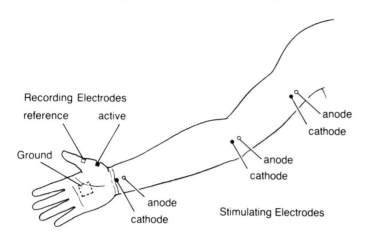

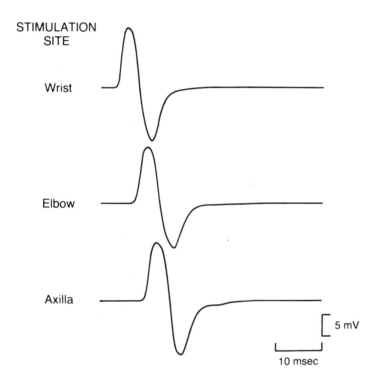

Fig. 9.8 Arrangement for performing motor conduction studies of the median nerve. The responses recorded from the thenar muscles by supramaximal stimulation of the median nerve at different sites are shown in the lower part of the figure.

forearm, upper arm, and more proximal segment of the nerve can be calculated. Normal values are given in Table 9.4.

NERVE ACTION POTENTIALS

Sensory action potentials can be recorded either orthodromically or antidromically. When an orthodromic technique is preferred, the digital fibers of the median nerve can be stimulated by a ring cathode placed at the base of one of the first three digits (usually the index finger), while another ring electrode, placed at the terminal interphalangeal joint, serves as the anode (Fig. 9.9). The finger to be stimulated is isolated from the adjacent digits by hydrophobic cotton to prevent current spread, and the ground electrode is attached to the

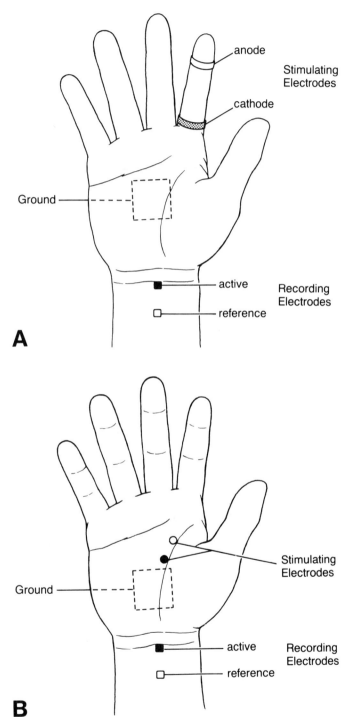

Fig. 9.9 Arrangement for recording orthodromic sensory nerve action potentials from the median nerve at the wrist with digital (**A**) and palmar (**B**) stimulation.

back of the hand. The recording electrode is placed over the median nerve trunk at the wrist, and the reference one is positioned more proximally. Surface electrodes, such as the saddle type described by Dawson and Scott,[19] are satisfactory for clinical purposes. Sensory action potentials can also be obtained antidromically by stimulating the nerve trunk at the wrist while the response is recorded from one of the digits. The position of the nerve trunk should be defined by motor stimulation techniques, but it is normally between the tendons of flexor carpi radialis and palmaris longus.

Sensory action potentials can also be elicited by palmar stimulation while recording from the digit and also from the wrist (Figs. 9.9 and 9.10). This permits evaluation of sensory conduction in the segment between digit and palm, and between palm and wrist. The stimulation site in the palm is about 5 cm distal to the wrist.

Nerve action potentials can be recorded in the forearm by stimulating the nerve at the wrist and recording over it at the elbow. They may also be recorded in the upper arm by stimulating at the elbow and recording in the axilla, with the ground being placed between the stimulating and recording electrodes.

Abnormalities of the sensory action potential amplitude in the distal segment of the median nerve are not necessarily of localizing value. The potential may, for example, be unrecordable due to involvement of sensory fibers at any point distal to the posterior root ganglia.

ELECTROPHYSIOLOGIC FINDINGS IN PRONATOR TERES SYNDROME

When the *anterior interosseous nerve* is involved, the only electromyographic signs are of chronic partial denervation in the pronator quadratus and the flexor pollicis longus; similar changes may also be found in the flexor digitorum profundus to the second and third digits, but are not always present.[38] Motor and sensory conduction studies of the median nerve are normal, but conduction velocity in the anterior interosseous nerve itself may be slow, as determined by recording the response of the pronator quadratus muscle to nerve stimulation at the elbow.[38]

If the *median nerve* itself is involved, electromyographic abnormalities are more extensive, being found in the superficial as well as the deep flexors, and in the abductor pollicis brevis. The distribution of affected muscles clearly conforms, however, to the territory of the median nerve rather than to that of the C6 or C7 nerve root. Thus, the needle examination of the biceps (C6), triceps (C7), and wrist and finger extensors (C7) yields normal findings, thereby helping to exclude a cervical radiculopathy. Buchthal and co-workers reported that the latencies of the potentials evoked in one or another of the flexor muscles by stimulating the nerve at the elbow may be prolonged, and abnormalities of sensory conduction sometimes occur.[39] Morris and Peters found slowing of motor conduction velocity in the forearm in the majority of their cases, but the distal motor latency and sensory action potential recorded at the wrist were normal,[29] in contrast to the findings in the carpal tunnel syndrome.

Compression of the median nerve by the ligament of Struthers may result in electrophysiologic abnormalities similar to those occurring in the pronator syndrome. However, needle examination of the pronator teres muscle sometimes reveals abnormalities in the former but not usually in the pronator syndrome.

ELECTROPHYSIOLOGIC FINDINGS IN CARPAL TUNNEL SYNDROME

Since the report by Simpson in 1956 that conduction is delayed in the motor fibers of the median nerve distal to the wrist,[23] there

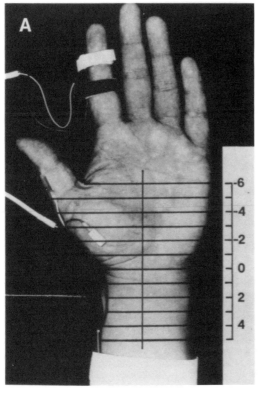

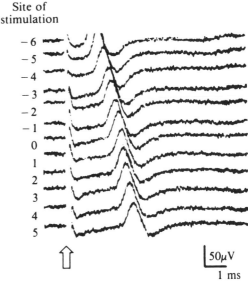

Fig. 9.10 (A) Twelve sites of stimulation in 1-cm increments along the median nerve. The 0 level is at the distal crease of the wrist, corresponding to the origin of the transverse carpal ligament. Sensory nerve and muscle action potentials are recorded from the second digit and the abductor pollicis brevis muscle, respectively. (B) Sensory nerve action potentials in a normal subject recorded after stimulation at the multiple points across the wrist that are shown in A. The site of each stimulus is indicated on the left. The latency increases linearly as the stimulus site is moved proximally in 1-cm increments. (Kimura J: The carpal tunnel syndrome. Localization of conduction abnormalities within the distal segment of the median nerve. Brain 102:619, 1979, Oxford University Press.)

have been a host of other papers describing the electrophysiologic abnormalities that may occur in this syndrome. Although the distal motor latency is characteristically prolonged, it is within the normal range in about 25 percent of patients with clinical and other electrophysiologic evidence of carpal tunnel syndrome. In such circumstances, an abnormality of conduction may still be suggested if the distal latency differs by more than 1 msec in the affected and unaffected hands.[40] However, comparison of the distal latency on the two sides may

be misleading if the patient has a symptomatic carpal tunnel syndrome on one side and an asymptomatic or subclinical lesion on the other, and is of very limited value in patients with bilateral symptoms. Increased distal latency may be accompanied by slowing of motor conduction velocity in the forearm, but this is less pronounced than the terminal slowing. In advanced cases, the size of the thenar compound muscle action potential may also be reduced.

In many patients, sensory action potentials are either unrecordable at the wrist or are of low amplitude and prolonged latency, sensory conduction in the forearm being normal (Fig. 9.11). In about 10 percent of cases, however, sensory conduction may be normal from one digit, but abnormal when another is stimulated;[39] examination of sensory conduction from the different digits innervated by the median nerve may, therefore, permit the diagnosis to be established when the findings obtained by a less detailed examination are normal. A change in the configuration or amplitude of the sensory action potential when the nerve is stimulated at different sites along the palm may also help to localize the lesion.

Electromyographic sampling of the abductor pollicis brevis or opponens pollicis muscles may reveal spontaneous fibrillation potentials and positive sharp waves; an increased incidence of long-duration, poly-

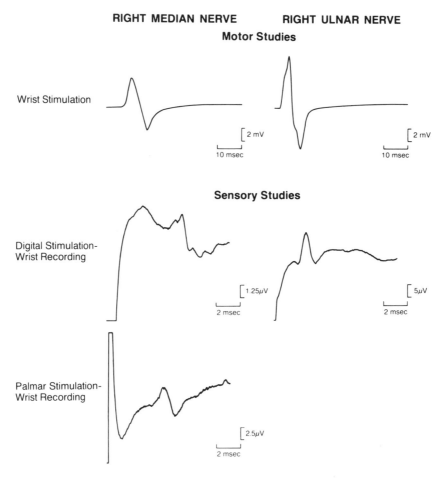

Fig. 9.11 Electrophysiologic findings in patient with right carpal tunnel syndrome. With supramaximal stimulation of the median nerve at the wrist, the response elicited from the thenar muscles is mildly delayed in latency and reduced in amplitude, especially when compared to the corresponding findings in the abductor digiti minimi muscle elicited by wrist stimulation of the ulnar nerve. Sensory conduction studies show that the median sensory action potential recorded at the wrist with digital or palmar stimulation is prolonged in latency, with particular prolongation in the response recorded with palmar stimulation.

phasic motor unit potentials; and a reduced interference pattern during maximal volitional activity. These signs of chronic partial denervation are sometimes found even when the distal motor latency in the median nerve is normal; for this reason, electromyographic sampling should never be omitted. The carpal tunnel syndrome cannot be diagnosed on electrophysiologic grounds, however, unless some focal abnormality of motor or sensory conduction is found in the distal portion of the median nerve.

Abnormalities of sensory conduction may be found in patients with normal motor latencies. Conversely, but less commonly, prolonged motor latencies are occasionally found in patients without sensory abnormalities, perhaps because the thenar branch of the median nerve courses in a separate tunnel through the transverse carpal ligament.[41] Both motor and sensory studies should, therefore, be undertaken when patients with a suspected carpal tunnel syndrome are being assessed. Motor conduction studies may be the only way of localizing the lesion when the sensory action potential is lost.

There remains a group of patients in whom a diagnosis of carpal tunnel syndrome seems inescapable on clinical grounds, but in whom the above electrophysiologic studies reveal no significant abnormality. Several additional neurophysiologic techniques have, therefore, been used to improve the diagnostic yield, with varying success.

Schwartz and associates found that Phalen's wrist flexion maneuver not only reproduced sensory symptoms of carpal tunnel syndrome, but also caused an increase in motor or sensory latency in many patients.[42] In two of their patients, latencies were abnormal only after wrist flexion, suggesting that the maneuver may be useful in the electrodiagnosis of borderline cases. If only because of its simplicity, such an approach would seem worthy of trial.

Another approach has been to compare the terminal motor latency of the median nerve to that of the ulnar nerve in the same hand; the diagnosis of carpal tunnel syndrome is supported if it exceeds the ulnar distal latency by 1.8 msec or more.[40] Alternatively, the latency of the median sensory action potential may be compared to that of the ulnar or radial nerve, provided that the length of nerve under study is kept constant. Johnson and colleagues recorded medial and ulnar sensory nerve action potentials antidromically in the fourth digit (i.e., the ring finger) after stimulation of each nerve 14 cm proximal to the recording electrodes.[43] They found that their latency differed by 0.3 msec or less in 93 percent of 74 normal hands, whereas in 18 cases of carpal tunnel syndrome, the difference ranged from 1 to 2.1 msec.

Shahani and co-workers have used the terminal latency index to provide a monitor of function in distal nerve segments as compared to more proximal portions of the same nerve.[44] The index is calculated by dividing the terminal distance (expressed in millimeters) by the product of proximal conduction velocity (in meters per second) and terminal latency (in milliseconds). In patients with carpal tunnel syndrome this index was below the lower limit of the normal range (0.356 to 0.550), as it was in patients with dying-back axonal neuropathies. In the latter context, however, the change was diffuse, affecting a number of different nerves rather than just the median nerve.

These various approaches have not met with general acceptance. By contrast, methods for determining motor or sensory conduction time in the segment across the carpal tunnel have proved to be very useful. Motor axons may be stimulated in the palm, as well as at the wrist, while the response of the median-innervated thenar muscles is recorded. Similarly, sensory action potentials can be recorded orthodromically at the palm and the wrist after digital stimulation,[45] and digital potentials may be recorded antidromically in response to stimulation of fibers in the wrist and palm.[46] In patients with the carpal tunnel syndrome who are evaluated with an orthodromic technique, sensory conduction abnormalities may be limited to the palm-to-wrist segment of the median nerve.[39,47] With palmar stimulation, both sensory and motor axons may show focal slowing under the transverse carpal ligament.[46] In a more detailed study, Kimura[37] found that, with serial stimulation of sensory fibers from midpalm to distal forearm, there was a predictable change in latency of 0.16 to 0.21 msec/cm as the stimulus site was moved proximally in steps of 1 cm, whereas in many patients with carpal tunnel syndrome, there was a sharply localized increase in latency across a 1-cm segment, most often 2 to 4 cm distal to the origin of the transverse carpal ligament (Fig. 9.12). The wrist-to-palm latency was significantly greater in patients with carpal tunnel syndrome than in controls for both sensory or motor axons.

The Martin-Gruber anastomosis (i.e., median-to-ulnar communication in the forearm) was referred to earlier (p. 165). Changes in configuration of the motor response elicited by stimulation of the median nerve at the elbow and wrist, or a response that is smaller when elicited by wrist rather than elbow stimulation, should suggest the possibility of this anomaly. Its presence can be confirmed by recording a response from hand muscles normally supplied by the ulnar nerve when the median nerve is stimulated at the elbow. In most patients with the carpal tunnel syndrome and a coexisting anomaly of this sort, the compound muscle action potential recorded over the thenar eminence with median nerve stimulation at the elbow is characterized by an initial positive deflection that is not seen when the

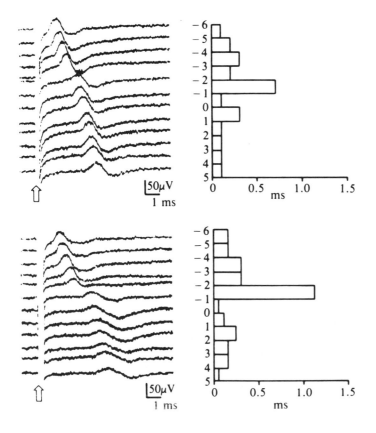

Fig. 9.12 Sensory nerve action potentials elicited by median nerve stimulation at multiple sites, as shown in Figure 9.10, in a patient with carpal tunnel syndrome. The histogram on the right shows the conduction time over successive 1-cm segments. A sharply localized slowing is seen from −2 to −1 in both hands, representing a maximal conduction velocity of 14 m/sec on the left (*top set of tracings*) and 9 m/sec on the right (*bottom set of tracings*). There is a distinct change in the waveform of the sensory action potential at the point of localized conduction delay. (Kimura J: The carpal tunnel syndrome. Localization of conduction abnormalities within the distal segment of the median nerve. Brain 102:619, 1979, Oxford University Press.)

median nerve is stimulated at the wrist (Fig. 9.1). This initial positivity is due to volume conduction of a response generated in ulnar-innervated muscles, such as the first dorsal interosseous and adductor pollicis, by fibers crossing from the median to the ulnar nerve in the forearm. In one study, this positivity was encountered in 16 of 63 patients (25 percent), and so was found to be a useful additional criterion in the diagnosis of carpal tunnel syndrome.[48] Others have reported on patients with carpal tunnel syndrome in whom the latency of the motor response elicited by median nerve stimulation at the elbow was relatively normal because the median-to-ulnar communication in the forearm resulted in bypassing of the affected segment in which conduction velocity was slowed.[49,50]

Surgical decompression of the carpal tunnel is frequently followed by improvement in motor and sensory conduction as recovery progresses,[51,52] but in other instances, conduction slowing persists in the distal portion of the median nerve.[53] Electrophysiologic findings at operation have shown that decompression causes an improvement in median sensory function within 30 minutes, as referred to in Chapter 7.

RADIAL NERVE

Clinical Aspects

The radial nerve, which is a continuation of the posterior cord of the brachial plexus, contains fibers originating from the C5, C6, C7, and C8 segments of the cord. Either directly or through the posterior interosseous nerve, which is a purely motor branch that it gives off in the elbow region, the radial nerve supplies a number of muscles, mainly extensors, in the arm and forearm (Table 9.5). It also supplies the skin of the lower, lateral aspect of the arm, the back of the forearm, the lateral part of the dor-

Table 9.5. Muscles Innervated by the Radial Nerve

Radial nerve	Triceps
	Anconeus
	Brachioradialis
	Extensor carpi radialis longus
Posterior interosseous branch	Extensor carpi radialis brevis
	Supinator
	Extensors digitorum and digiti minimi
	Extensor carpi ulnaris
	Abductor pollicis longus
	Extensors pollicis longus and brevis
	Extensor indicis

sum of the hand, and the back of the proximal phalanges of the first two or three digits. Although it can be damaged anywhere along its course, it is particularly liable to injury in the axilla, in the arm as it descends in the spiral groove of the humerus, and in the region of the elbow. The designation "Saturday night palsy" refers to a compression injury of the radial nerve, either in the axillary region or in the arm, that usually occurs while the patient is intoxicated and deeply asleep. Treatment of such lesions is generally conservative, and includes a cock-up splint for the wrist joint if paralysis lasts for longer than 7 to 10 days.

Pressure, angulation, or stretch of the nerve by neighboring anatomic structures may also occur. The radial nerve may be compressed in the spiral groove by the lateral head of the triceps muscle, especially when it contains a fibrous arch,[54] and the posterior interosseous nerve may be compressed by the supinator muscle, or a fibrous band, especially in response to repetitive motor activity involving the muscle.

AXILLARY LESIONS

Lesions in the axilla are usually due to compression (e.g., from improperly fitted crutches) or trauma, and lead to weakness or paralysis of all the muscles supplied by the radial nerve, including the triceps. Sensory changes may also occur, but they are often surprisingly inconspicuous despite the extensive cutaneous branches of the parent nerve. These changes may be prominent only in a small region on the back of the hand between the thumb and index finger.[55]

LESIONS IN THE ARM

Post-traumatic lesions of the radial nerve in the spiral groove are not uncommon, especially if the humerus has been fractured. The neurologic disturbance generally spares the triceps muscle, which is supplied by a more proximal portion of the nerve. Pressure palsies commonly occur below the insertion of the deltoid, where the nerve pierces the lateral intermuscular septum to lie superficially.

LESIONS IN THE ELBOW REGION

Radial nerve lesions may be related to trauma at or above the elbow, and the posterior interosseous nerve, which innervates the extensors of the wrist and fingers, may similarly be involved immediately below the elbow. In the latter case, however, the extensor carpi radialis longus is spared, so that the ability to extend the wrist is retained.

The posterior interosseous nerve may be compressed by the arcade of Frohse, sometimes following apparently trivial trauma. Vascular leashes crossing the nerve may also compress it.[56] There is weakness or paralysis of the extensors carpi ulnaris, digitorum, digiti minimi, indicis, and pollicis longus and brevis, and of the abductor pollicis longus. The extensor carpi radialis longus is spared because it is innervated by the

radial nerve itself, and the extensor carpi radialis brevis and supinator are spared because they are supplied by the posterior interosseous nerve before it is compressed.[56]

LESIONS AT THE WRIST

The superficial radial nerve may be compressed at the wrist, for example, by a watchband or handcuffs. Numbness and dysesthesias occur in the distribution of this nerve, and there may be pain at the wrist. Removal of the compressive article is generally rewarding. The nerve may also be damaged by intravenous lines, or lacerated by injury, leading to sensory changes in the territory it supplies.

Electrophysiologic Aspects

Electromyographic sampling may help to clarify the pattern of muscle involvement following a radial nerve lesion, and thus may help to localize the site of the lesion. It may also provide a guide to prognosis. Additional information may also be obtained by nerve conduction studies.

MOTOR CONDUCTION STUDIES

Bipolar surface electrodes can be used to stimulate the radial nerve, with the cathode being placed distal to the anode and over the nerve at the following sites:

1. In the region of the elbow, about 5 cm proximal to the lateral epicondyle of the humerus, or between the biceps tendon and brachioradialis muscle in the cubital fossa
2. In the arm, either in the spiral groove about 4 cm posterior to the insertion of the deltoid muscle, or after the nerve has pierced the intermuscular septum at a point approximately one-third of the distance from the rostral end of the line drawn be-

tween the insertion of the deltoid and the lateral epicondyle[57]

3. At Erb's point.

Responses can conveniently be recorded from the brachioradialis and extensor digitorum muscles using concentric needle or surface disc electrodes. The ground is placed between the stimulating and recording electrodes.

Motor conduction velocity can also be studied in more distal fibers of the radial nerve. While the response of the extensor indicis muscle is recorded by a needle inserted into it about 4 cm above the ulnar styloid process, the branch to this muscle is stimulated some 4 cm more proximally as it lies between extensor digiti minimi and extensor carpi ulnaris in the forearm.[58] The radial nerve is then stimulated at the elbow to permit conduction velocity in the forearm to be determined by subtraction.

Normal values for maximal conduction velocity in radial motor fibers are given in Table 9.6.

NERVE ACTION POTENTIALS

A convenient technique for recording evoked sensory potentials in the radial nerve was described by Downie and Scott.[59] The recording electrodes were mounted 2.5 cm apart on a plastic base and placed so that the active one was situated over the largest palpable branch of the radial nerve as it crosses the tendon of extensor pollicis longus, whereas the distal reference electrode was positioned over the first dorsal interosseous muscle. For stimulation, surface electrodes were placed over the nerve in the middle of the forearm next to the cephalic vein (Fig. 9.13) and then systematically moved about from this point until an evoked potential was obtained by antidromic conduction. If the position of the stimulating and recording electrodes was reversed, orthodromically conducted po-

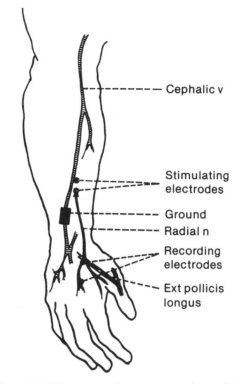

Fig. 9.13 Diagrammatic representation of the electrode placements for recording evoked sensory potentials from the radial nerve. (Downie AW, Scott TR: An improved technique for radial nerve conduction studies. J Neurol Neurosurg Psychiatry 30:332, 1967. Reproduced by permission of the Authors and Editors of the Journal of Neurology, Neurosurgery and Psychiatry.)

tentials could be recorded (Fig. 9.14). Latency to peak, rather than to onset, of the nerve action potential was measured, and this was correlated with the distance from the stimulating cathode to the midpoint between the recording electrodes (rather than to the active recording electrode). Using this technique, Downie and Scott found that the amplitude of the nerve action potential ranged between 5 and 20 μV (with a mean of 11.4 μV) in 50 control subjects, and that conduction velocity varied between 47 and 64 m/sec (with a mean of 53.7 m/sec).[59]

A number of other techniques for eval-

Table 9.6. Motor Conduction Velocity in Fibers of the Radial Nerve—Normal Mean Values

	Conduction Velocity (m/sec)		
Fibers to	Forearm	Upper Arm	Source
Brachioradialis		74 (SD 6.7)	Gassel & Diamantopoulos[57]
Extensor digitorum		72 (SD 6.1)	Gassel & Diamantopoulos[57]
Extensor indicis	61.6 (SD 5.9)	72 (SD 6.3)	Jebsen[58]

SD, standard deviation

uating sensory conduction in the radial nerve have been described, some of which were compared by Critchlow and co-workers in a study aimed at developing a method that would be simple, reliable, and relatively painless.[60] They found that the method of Downie and Scott[59] was most satisfactory, but the antidromic technique was preferred to the orthodromic arrangement because it was more comfortable, yielded larger responses, and resulted in less variation within and between subjects. Moreover, a few subjects were found to have recordable antidromic responses but absent orthodromic ones.

Radial sensory action potentials may be

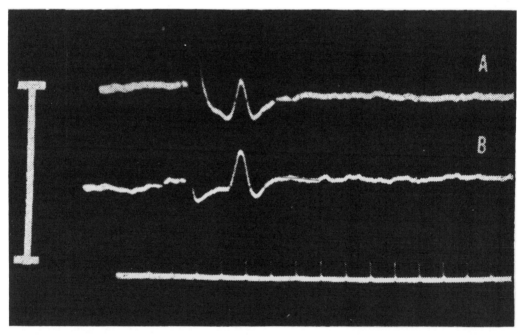

Fig. 9.14 Sensory action potentials recorded from the radial nerve. (**A**) Single sweep, orthodromic conduction. (**B**) Single sweep, antidromic conduction; vertical bar, 50 µV; time marker at 1-msec intervals. (Downie AW, Scott TR: An improved technique for radial nerve conduction studies. J Neurol Neurosurg Psychiatry 30:332, 1967. Reproduced by permission of the Authors and Editors of the Journal of Neurology, Neurosurgery and Psychiatry.)

attenuated or absent with a lesion of the radial nerve at any site, or of the superficial radial sensory branch. Normal responses are obtained in patients with the posterior interosseous syndrome.

CLINICAL APPLICATIONS

Electrophysiologic studies may help to localize the lesion by the pattern of affected muscles on needle electromyography, and by the nerve conduction findings. They also provide a guide to the severity of the lesion and thus to the prognosis.

Trojaborg found that, in patients with radial nerve lesions in the spiral groove secondary to fractures of the humerus, responses could not be evoked in the brachioradialis or the extensors of the wrist and fingers, and sensory potentials could not be recorded after nerve stimulation.[61] In patients with compressive lesions of the nerve, such as occur in "Saturday night palsies," there may be marked slowing of motor conduction across the site of the lesion in the upper arm, but the distal motor latency and sensory conduction velocity in the forearm are usually normal.

Downie and Scott have suggested that the measurement of conduction velocity in the distal portion of the sensory branches of the radial nerve may help in selecting patients with chronic peripheral neuropathies for biopsy.[59]

MUSCULOCUTANEOUS NERVE

Clinical Aspects

The musculocutaneous nerve, which arises from the lateral cord of the brachial plexus, contains fibers originating from the C5, C6, and C7 segments of the cord. It supplies the coracobrachialis muscle, both heads of the biceps, and the brachialis muscle. As the lateral cutaneous nerve of the forearm, it also supplies the skin on both aspects of the radial border of the forearm and a variable area on the front and back of the hand.

Isolated lesions of the musculocutaneous nerve are rare, may occur at any point along the course of the nerve, and are usually secondary to trauma. They lead to weakness or paralysis of the muscles supplied by the nerve and to sensory loss along the radial border of the forearm. Before it enters the coracobrachialis muscle, however, the nerve is closely related to the lateral cord of the plexus, and both structures are usually involved by trauma in this region.

Electrophysiologic Aspects

Electromyographic sampling procedures can be used to determine whether denervation has occurred and whether it is restricted to the muscles supplied by the musculocutaneous nerve. Motor conduction velocity can be studied by stimulating the nerve at Erb's point and at the axilla while recording from the biceps muscle with a concentric needle electrode. Full details of the procedure are provided by Trojaborg,[62] who also describes a method of measuring sensory conduction velocity by stimulating, with needle electrodes, the lateral cutaneous nerve of the forearm at the elbow between the biceps tendon and brachioradialis muscle while recording, with needles placed close to the nerve, the response at the axilla and at Erb's point. He found maximal motor and sensory conduction velocity to be similar.

An antidromic technique for measuring conduction in the lateral cutaneous nerve of the forearm has also been described.[63] The nerve is stimulated percutaneously just lateral to the tendon of the biceps muscle at the elbow, while surface recordings are made some 12 cm distal to this site along a straight line between the stimulating cathode and the radial artery at the wrist (Fig. 9.15). By this means, a mean conduction velocity of 65 m/sec (standard deviation of 3.6) was obtained.

The diagnostic value of studying the musculocutaneous nerve has been stressed by Trojaborg,[62] who emphasized that, in patients with traction injuries of the brachial plexus, motor and sensory conduction studies of the musculocutaneous nerve may be a valuable addition to the other detailed electrophysiologic studies that are undertaken. This is because sensory conduction studies of the median, ulnar, and radial nerves provide information concerning the functional integrity of fibers derived from the C6 to C8 segments, whereas the musculocutaneous nerve covers the C5 segment.

scapular notch, passing below the superior transverse scapular ligament. It supplies the supraspinatus muscle, and then passes around the spine of the scapula and through the spinoglenoid notch (which is frequently covered by the inferior transverse scapular or spinoglenoid ligament) to the infraspinous fossa, supplying the infraspinatus muscle.

Lesions of the suprascapular nerve may result from trauma, including dislocation of the shoulder.[64] Entrapment of the nerve may also occur in the suprascapular notch beneath the transverse scapular ligament, or at the spinoglenoid notch.[65–67] In either case, there is pain about the shoulder, which is exacerbated by movement, as well as weakness, especially of external rotation of the arm. Treatment involves division of the superior or inferior transverse scapular ligament,[65,67] depending on the site of entrapment.

SUPRASCAPULAR NERVE

The suprascapular nerve, which branches off the upper trunk of the brachial plexus, contains fibers originating from C5 and C6, with a variable contribution from C4. The nerve passes beneath the trapezius, and enters the supraspinous fossa via the supra-

Electrophysiologic Aspects

Needle electromyography of the spinati muscles and recording, with a needle electrode, the muscle responses to stimulation of the nerve at Erb's point can be helpful in determining the presence and extent of injury to the suprascapular nerve, and in

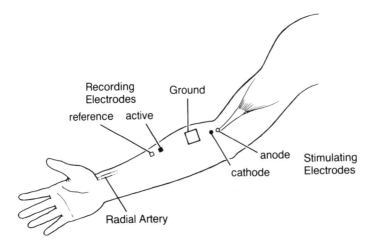

Fig. 9.15 Arrangement for antidromic conduction studies in the lateral cutaneous nerve of the forearm. The nerve is stimulated just lateral to the tendon of the biceps muscle at the elbow, and the response is recorded approximately 12 cm more distally by surface electrodes placed along a straight line between the stimulating cathode and the radial artery at the wrist.

providing a guide to prognosis. Kraft found that the motor response of the supraspinatus muscle normally ranged in latency between 1.7 and 3.7 msec (mean: 2.7) and that the latency of the infraspinatus muscle response ranged between 2.4 and 4.2 msec (mean: 3.3), with the distance between stimulating and recording electrodes ranging between 7.4 and 12 cm in the former instance and 10.6 and 15.0 cm in the latter instance, when measured with calipers.[68] An increase in latency has been reported in entrapment of the nerve.[69]

AXILLARY NERVE

The circumflex or axillary nerve, which contains fibers derived from C5 and C6, is one of the two terminal divisions of the posterior cord of the brachial plexus. It descends on the anterior aspect of the subscapularis muscle, escapes from the axilla, and eventually—when deep to the deltoid muscle—divides. Its anterior branch winds round the surgical neck of the humerus and is then closely applied to the anterior and intermediate fibers of the deltoid muscles which it supplies, whereas the posterior branch supplies teres minor and the posterior portion of the deltoid muscle. The tight attachment of the nerve to the deltoid for much of its length makes it liable to stretch injury, as occurs in shoulder dislocations.[70] The nerve supplies branches to the shoulder joint, to the deltoid and teres minor muscles, and to the skin of the upper, outer border of the arm.

Isolated injury to the nerve is uncommon, but may occur as a result of dislocation of the shoulder, fracture of the humeral neck or acromion,[71] or blunt trauma to the shoulder region. Incomplete or delayed recovery is said to be especially common with palsy following blunt trauma.[70] The nerve may

also be involved by penetrating injuries or as a feature of a more diffuse brachial plexopathy.

Electrophysiologic Aspects

The axillary nerve can be stimulated at Erb's point while the response of the deltoid muscle is recorded with a needle or surface electrode. Gassel reported a mean latency of 4.3 msec with distances between stimulating and recording electrodes of 15 to 16 cm, and a mean latency of 4.4 msec with distances between the electrodes of 18 to 19 cm.[72] Kraft reported latencies ranging from 2.8 to 5.0 msec (mean: 3.9 msec) at distances between electrodes of 14.8 to 21.0 cm, as measured with calipers.[68] Needle electromyography of the deltoid may reveal evidence of partial or complete denervation, with subsequent evidence of recovery in patients examined sequentially over a period of months. Examination of other muscles supplied from the C5 or C6 segments (such as the spinati, biceps, and brachioradialis muscles) shows no abnormality in patients with isolated axillary nerve lesions, which fact may be helpful if a radiculopathy is suspected.

LONG THORACIC NERVE

The long thoracic nerve contains fibers arising directly from the C5, C6, and C7 roots, and it passes behind the brachial plexus (which it is not a part of) to supply the serratus anterior muscle. Paralysis of this muscle results in weakness of shoulder abduction and in winging of the scapula. The nerve is liable to traction injury that is sometimes occupationally related, as in slaughterhouse workers, golfers, and tennis players.

Electrophysiologic Aspects

Needle electromyography of the serratus anterior muscle is useful in confirming that denervation has occurred, and in determining its degree of severity. Kaplan stimulated the nerve at Erb's point and recorded the motor response with needle electrodes inserted into the serratus anterior muscle at the T5 level in the midaxillary line.[73] The mean latency in normal subjects was 3.9 msec (standard deviation of 0.6 msec) over distances of between 17 and 23 cm (as measured with obstetric calipers). Prolonged latency was reported in subjects with palsies secondary to dysfunction of the nerve.

More recently, Petrera and Trojaborg studied 24 patients with unilateral serratus anterior weakness attributed, in 17 cases, to injury of the long thoracic nerve.[74] They stimulated the nerve in the supraclavicular fossa while the response of the serratus anterior muscle was recorded with a concentric needle electrode over the fifth or sixth rib, between the anterior and midaxillary lines. Mean latency on the asymptomatic side was 4.5 msec (standard deviation of 0.7 msec). The latency correlated with the distance between stimulating and recording electrodes so that a conduction velocity of 67 m/sec was estimated from the relationship between the two. On the affected side, motor responses were either completely absent (with complete lesions), of prolonged latency (with some partial lesions), or of normal latency. The occurrence of polyphasic responses of prolonged duration, reduced amplitude, and markedly increased latency was taken to imply that reinnervation was occurring after complete axonal degeneration.

REFERENCES

1. Rowntree T: Anomalous innervation of the hand muscles. J Bone Joint Surg 31B:505, 1949

2. Wilbourn AJ, Lambert EH: The forearm median-to-ulnar nerve communication. Electrodiagnostic aspects. Neurology 26:368, 1976

3. Crutchfield CA, Gutmann L: Hereditary aspects of median-ulnar nerve communications. J Neurol Neurosurg Psychiatry 43:53, 1980

4. Feindel W, Stratford J: The role of the cubital tunnel in tardy ulnar palsy. Can J Surg 1:287, 1958

5. Neary D, Ochoa J, Gilliatt RW: Sub-clinical entrapment neuropathy in man. J Neurol Sci 24:283, 1975

6. Ebeling P, Gilliatt RW, Thomas PK: A clinical and electrical study of ulnar nerve lesions in the hand. J Neurol Neurosurg Psychiatry 23:1, 1960

7. Olney RK, Wilbourn AJ, Miller RG: Ulnar neuropathy at or distal to the wrist. Neurology 33:suppl. 2, 185, 1983

8. Hayes JR, Mulholland RC, O'Connor BT: Compression of the deep palmar branch of the ulnar nerve. J Bone Joint Surg 51B:469, 1969

9. Mayer RF: Nerve conduction studies in man. Neurology 13:1021, 1963

10. Thomas PK, Sears TA, Gilliatt RW: The range of conduction velocity in normal motor nerve fibres to the small muscles of the hand and foot. J Neurol Neurosurg Psychiatry 22:175, 1959

11. Trojaborg W: Motor nerve conduction velocities in normal subjects with particular reference to the conduction in proximal and distal segments of median and ulnar nerve. Electroencephalogr Clin Neurophysiol 17:314, 1964

12. Eisen A: Early diagnosis of ulnar nerve palsy. An electrophysiologic study. Neurology 24:256, 1974

13. Checkles NS, Russakov AD, Piero DL: Ulnar nerve conduction velocity—Effect of elbow position on measurement. Arch Phys Med Rehabil 52:362, 1971

14. Payan J: Electrophysiological localization of ulnar nerve lesions. J Neurol Neurosurg Psychiatry 32:208, 1969

15. Gilliatt RW, Sears TA: Sensory nerve action potentials in patients with peripheral nerve lesions. J Neurol Neurosurg Psychiatry 21:109, 1958

16. Gilliatt RW, Thomas PK: Changes in nerve conduction with ulnar lesions at the elbow. J Neurol Neurosurg Psychiatry 23:312, 1960

17. Kaeser HE: Nerve conduction velocity measurements. p. 116. In Vinken PJ, Bruyn GW (eds): Handbook of Clinical Neurology. Vol. 7. North-Holland, Amsterdam, 1970

18. Harding C, Halar E: Motor and sensory ulnar nerve conduction velocities: Effect of elbow position. Arch Phys Med Rehabil 64:227, 1983

19. Dawson GD, Scott JW: The recording of nerve action potentials through skin in man. J Neurol Neurosurg Psychiatry 12:259, 1949

20. Jabre JF: Ulnar nerve lesions at the wrist: New technique for recording from the sensory dorsal branch of the ulnar nerve. Neurology 30:873, 1980

21. Kim D-J, Kalantri A, Guha S, Wainapel SF: Dorsal cutaneous ulnar nerve conduction: Diagnostic aid in ulnar neuropathy. Arch Neurol 38:321, 1981

22. Odusote K, Eisen A: An electrophysiological quantitation of the cubital tunnel syndrome. Can J Neurol Sci 6:403, 1979

23. Simpson JA: Electrical signs in the diagnosis of carpal tunnel and related syndromes. J Neurol Neurosurg Psychiatry 19:275, 1956

24. Miller RG: The cubital tunnel syndrome: Diagnosis and precise localization. Ann Neurol 6:56, 1979

25. Payan J: Anterior transposition of the ulnar nerve: An electrophysiological study. J Neurol Neurosurg Psychiatry 33:157, 1970

26. Miller RG, Hummel EE: The cubital tunnel syndrome: Treatment with simple decompression. Ann Neurol 7:567, 1980

27. Marquis JW, Bruwer AJ, Keith HM: Supracondyloid process of the humerus. Proc Staff Meet Mayo Clin 32:691, 1957

28. Laha RK, Dujovny M, DeCastro C: Entrapment of median nerve by supracondylar process of the humerus. J Neurosurg 46:252, 1977

29. Morris HH, Peters BH: Pronator syndrome: Clinical and electrophysiological features in seven cases. J Neurol Neurosurg Psychiatry 39:461, 1976

30. Hartz CR, Linscheid RL, Gramse RR, Daube JR: The pronator teres syndrome: Compressive neuropathy of the median nerve. J Bone Joint Surg 63A:885, 1981

31. Kopell HP, Thompson WAL: Pronator syndrome: A confirmed case and its diagnosis. N Engl J Med 259:713, 1958

32. Rennels GD, Ochoa J: Neuralgic amyotrophy manifesting as anterior interosseous nerve palsy. Muscle Nerve 3:160, 1980

33. Wertsch JJ, Sanger JR, Matloub HS: Pseudo-anterior interosseous nerve syndrome. Muscle Nerve 8:68, 1985

34. Phalen GS: The carpal-tunnel syndrome. Seventeen years' experience in diagnosis and treatment of six hundred fifty-four hands. J Bone Joint Surg 48A:211, 1966

35. Gilliatt RW, Wilson TG: Ischaemic sensory loss in patients with peripheral nerve lesions. J Neurol Neurosurg Psychiatry 17:104, 1954

36. Fullerton PM: The effect of ischaemia on nerve conduction in the carpal tunnel syndrome. J Neurol Neurosurg Psychiatry 26:385, 1963

37. Kimura J: The carpal tunnel syndrome: Localization of conduction abnormalities within the distal segment of the median nerve. Brain 102:619, 1979

38. Nakano KK, Lundergan C, Okihiro MM: Anterior interosseous nerve syndromes: Diagnostic methods and alternative treatments. Arch Neurol 34:477, 1977

39. Buchthal F, Rosenfalck A, Trojaborg W: Electrophysiological findings in entrapment of the median nerve at wrist and elbow. J Neurol Neurosurg Psychiatry 37:340, 1974

40. Thomas JE, Lambert EH, Cseuz KA: Electrodiagnostic aspects of the carpal tunnel syndrome. Arch Neurol 16:635, 1967

41. Johnson RK, Shrewsbury MM: Anatomical course of the thenar branch of the median nerve—usually in a separate tunnel through the transverse carpal ligament. J Bone Joint Surg 52A:269, 1970

42. Schwartz MS, Gordon JA, Swash M: Slowed nerve conduction with wrist flexion in carpal tunnel syndrome. Ann Neurol 8:69, 1980

43. Johnson EW, Kukla RD, Wongsam PE, Piedmont A: Sensory latencies to the ring finger: Normal values and relation to carpal tunnel syndrome. Arch Phys Med Rehabil 62:206, 1981

44. Shahani BT, Young RR, Potts F, Maccabee

P: Terminal latency index (TLI) and late response studies in motor neuron disease (MND), peripheral neuropathies and entrapment syndromes. Acta Neurol Scand, 60:suppl. 73, 118, 1979

45. Buchthal F, Rosenfalck A: Sensory conduction from digit to palm and from palm to wrist in the carpal tunnel syndrome. J Neurol Neurosurg Psychiatry 34:243, 1971

46. Kimura J: A method for determining median nerve conduction velocity across the carpal tunnel. J Neurol Sci 38:1, 1978

47. Daube JR: Percutaneous palmar median nerve stimulation for carpal tunnel syndrome. Electroencephalogr Clin Neurophysiol 43:139, 1977

48. Gutmann L: Median-ulnar nerve communications and carpal tunnel syndrome. J Neurol Neurosurg Psychiatry 40:982, 1977

49. Kimura J: Collision technique. Neurology 26:680, 1976

50. Iyer V, Fenichel GM: Normal median nerve proximal latency in carpal tunnel syndrome: A clue to coexisting Martin-Gruber anastomosis. J Neurol Neurosurg Psychiatry 39:449, 1976

51. Goodman HV, Gilliatt RW: The effect of treatment on median nerve conduction in patients with the carpal tunnel syndrome. Ann Phys Med 6:137, 1961

52. Hongell A, Mattsson HS: Neurographic studies before, after, and during operation for median nerve compression in the carpal tunnel. Scand J Plast Reconstr Surg 5:103, 1971

53. Melvin JL, Johnson EW, Duran R: Electrodiagnosis after surgery for the carpal tunnel syndrome. Arch Phys Med Rehabil 49:502, 1968

54. Lotem M, Fried A, Levy M, Solzi P, Najenson T, Nathan H: Radial palsy following muscular effort: A nerve compression syndrome possibly related to a fibrous arch of the lateral head of the triceps. J Bone Joint Surg 53B:500, 1971

55. Sunderland S: Nerves and Nerve Injuries. 2nd Ed. Churchill Livingstone, Edinburgh, 1978

56. Dawson DM, Hallett M, Millender LH: Entrapment Neuropathies. Little, Brown & Co., Boston, 1983

57. Gassel MM, Diamantopoulos E: Pattern of conduction times in the distribution of the radial nerve. A clinical and electrophysiological study. Neurology 14:222, 1964.

58. Jebsen RH: Motor conduction velocity of distal radial nerve. Arch Phys Med Rehabil 47:12, 1966

59. Downie AW, Scott TR: An improved technique for radial nerve conduction studies. J Neurol Neurosurg Psychiatry 30:332, 1967

60. Critchlow JF, Seybold ME, Jablecki CJ: The superficial radial nerve: Techniques for evaluation. J Neurol Neurosurg Psychiatry 43:929, 1980

61. Trojaborg W: Rate of recovery in motor and sensory fibres of the radial nerve: Clinical and electrophysiological aspects. J Neurol Neurosurg Psychiatry 33:625, 1970

62. Trojaborg W: Motor and sensory conduction in the musculocutaneous nerve. J Neurol Neurosurg Psychiatry 39:890, 1976

63. Spindler HA, Felsenthal G: Sensory conduction in the musculocutaneous nerve. Arch Phys Med Rehabil 59:20, 1978

64. Zoltan JD: Injury to the suprascapular nerve associated with anterior dislocation of the shoulder: Case report and review of the literature. J Trauma 19:203, 1979

65. Clein LJ: Suprascapular entrapment neuropathy. J Neurosurg 43:337, 1975

66. Rask MR: Suprascapular nerve entrapment: A report of two cases treated with suprascapular notch resection. Clin Orthop 123:73, 1977

67. Aiello I, Serra G, Traina GC, Tugnoli V: Entrapment of the suprascapular nerve at the spinoglenoid notch. Ann Neurol 12:314, 1982

68. Kraft GH: Axillary, musculocutaneous, and suprascapular nerve latency studies. Arch Phys Med Rehabil 53:383, 1972

69. Khalili AA: Neuromuscular electrodiagnostic studies in entrapment neuropathy of the suprascapular nerve. Orthop Rev 3:27, 1974

70. Berry H, Bril V: Axillary nerve palsy following blunt trauma to the shoulder region: A clinical and electrophysiological review. J Neurol Neurosurg Psychiatry 45:1027, 1982

71. McGahan JP, Rab GT: Fracture of the acromion associated with an axillary nerve deficit. Clin Orthop 147:216, 1980

72. Gassel MM: A test of nerve conduction to muscles of the shoulder girdle as an aid in the diagnosis of proximal neurogenic and muscular disease. J Neurol Neurosurg Psychiatry 27:200, 1964

73. Kaplan PE: Electrodiagnostic confirmation of long thoracic nerve palsy. J Neurol Neurosurg Psychiatry 43:50, 1980

74. Petrera JE, Trojaborg W: Conduction studies of the long thoracic nerve in serratus anterior palsy of different etiology. Neurology 34:1033, 1984

10

Nerves in the Lower Limb

A number of different techniques for assessing the function of peripheral nerves in the lower limb have been described. Attention in this chapter, however, will be focused on those that are in wide clinical use or that have established practical value.

FEMORAL NERVE

Clinical Aspects

The femoral nerve, which contains fibers derived from the L2, L3, and L4 segments, enters the lower limb by passing beneath the inguinal ligament, where it can sometimes be compressed if patients are maintained in the dorsal lithotomy position for long periods of time. This nerve innervates the iliacus, sartorius, pectineus, and quadriceps femoris muscles, and its cutaneous branches supply the anterior medial aspect of the thigh and—through the saphenous nerve—the medial part of the lower leg.

An isolated femoral neuropathy may occur in patients with diabetes mellitus, a bleeding diathesis, or retroperitoneal neoplasms involving the nerve. Trauma is sometimes responsible for such a neuropathy, and may relate to intrapelvic operations or attempts at femoral artery catheterization. Femoral neuropathy has also followed gynecologic or urologic operations, appendectomy, obstetric delivery maneuvers, correction of congenital dislocation of the hip, and other procedures. Among the mechanisms that may be responsible for such trauma is compression of the nerve by self-retaining retractors.[1] In a number of instances, however, no specific cause can be recognized.

The neuropathy is characterized by weakness and wasting of the quadriceps, sensory impairment over the front of the thigh and the medial aspect of the calf, and a depressed patellar reflex. Weakness and wasting of the quadriceps muscles may also occur in patients with a myopathy, radiculopathy, or myelopathy, and as a consequence of disuse. In distinguishing between these disorders, electromyographic sampling procedures are of considerable help in indicating the neurogenic basis of the wasting, and in localizing the probable level (site) of the lesion. Nerve conduction studies may be valuable in demonstrating femoral nerve involvement, with conduction slowing being anticipated in compressive or diabetic neuropathies, and a reduction in size of the compound muscle action potential being expected if there is axonal loss or a conduction block between the sites of stimulation and recording.

Electrophysiologic Aspects

Gassel stimulated the femoral nerve with a bipolar surface electrode placed just below the inguinal ligament and lateral to the femoral artery, and recorded the response of the rectus femoris muscle with needle electrodes inserted into it at increasing distances down the front of the thigh from the site of stimulation.[2] The latency of the response increased progressively with distance and, because of the anatomic organization of the end-plate zone of the bipennate rectus femoris muscle, he was able to determine nerve conduction velocity between the proximal and distal recording points. Using a similar technique but recording with surface electrodes, Schubert and Keil found that the calculated conduction velocity varied considerably in normal subjects. They therefore recommended that the motor latency alone be used for determining whether change in femoral nerve physiology has occurred.[3]

Johnson and co-workers subsequently described a different technique for determining motor conduction velocity in the femoral nerve; this technique may be used for determining whether there is disproportionate slowing in the segment of nerve that passes beneath the inguinal ligament.[4] The nerve is stimulated above and below the ligament and at Hunter's canal (the adductor or subsartorial canal) on the medial aspect of the thigh. Surface electrodes are used for recording, the active electrode being placed over the center of the vastus medialis and the reference electrode on the quadriceps tendon just proximal to the patella (Figs. 10.1 and 10.2). Conduction velocity is calculated for the portions of nerve running from above the ligament to Hunter's canal, and from below the ligament to the canal, so that the delay across the inguinal ligament may be determined by subtraction.

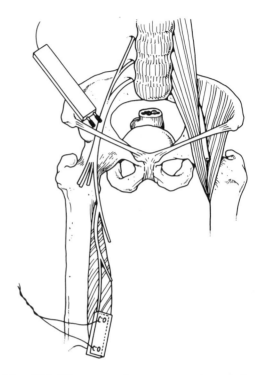

Fig. 10.1 Diagrammatic representation of electrode placements used for femoral nerve conduction studies. (Johnson EW, Wood PK, Powers JJ: Femoral nerve conduction studies. Arch Phys Med Rehabil 49:528, 1968.)

The values obtained from normal subjects by these techniques are shown in Table 10.1. However, unless needle electrodes are used for stimulation, responses may be small or hard to obtain in obese patients because of the distance between the stimulating electrodes and the subjacent nerve.

Sensory conduction studies can be performed on the saphenous nerve (p. 201), and the findings are particularly helpful when there is clinical uncertainty as to whether the lesion is at the root level or distal to the dorsal root ganglion.

Needle electromyography is helpful in distinguishing femoral neuropathy from disorders that resemble it. With involvement of the nerve itself, abnormalities are con-

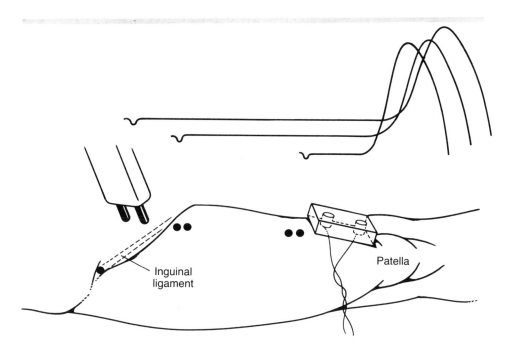

Fig. 10.2 Diagrammatic representation of the electrode placements used for femoral nerve conduction studies, showing the responses obtained to stimulation of the nerve above and below the inguinal ligament, and at Hunter's canal. (Johnson EW, Wood PK, Powers JJ: Femoral nerve conduction studies. Arch Phys Med Rehabil 49:528, 1968.)

fined to the muscles supplied by the nerve. With lumbar radiculopathies, the abnormalities found on needle examination are more extensive in distribution and include the paraspinal muscles, and the motor and sensory conduction velocities are normal. With a lesion at the lumbar plexus, the size of the saphenous nerve action potential may be reduced if axonal degeneration has occurred, but femoral motor conduction velocity is normal and the abnormal findings on needle examination extend beyond the femoral nerve territory.

SAPHENOUS NERVE

The saphenous nerve is a sensory branch of the femoral nerve that supplies the medial aspect of the calf, the medial malleolus, and a portion of the medial aspect of the foot. Lesions of the nerve may result from entrapment at the exit from Hunter's canal (about 6 inches above the medial condyle of the femur) or may follow trauma or surgery in which the nerve is damaged. Pain may be a conspicuous feature of saphenous neuropathy, and numbness and paresthesias occur in an appropriate distribution.

Electrophysiologic Aspects

Conduction in the saphenous nerve can be measured by the technique of Stohr and associates, in which needle electrodes are used for recording the sensory action potential.[5] The active electrode is placed near the femoral nerve at the inguinal ligament, with the reference one placed approxi-

Table 10.1. Femoral Nerve Conduction Studies—Normal Values

Terminal Latency

Mean Latency (msec)	Distance Between Stimulating and Recording Electrodes (cm)	Muscle Recorded from	Source
6.0 (SD 0.6)	30	Rectus femoris	Gassel[2]
5.5 (SD 0.47)	28	Rectus femoris	Schubert & Keil[3]
3.7 (SD 0.45)	14	Rectus femoris	Gassel[2]
3.29 (SD 0.36)	14	Rectus femoris	Schubert & Keil[3]

Motor Conduction Velocity

Mean Velocity (m/sec)	Site of Stimulation	Muscle Recorded from	Source
70 (SD 7.8)	Below inguinal ligament	Rectus femoris	Gassel[2]
64.3 (SD 8.0)	Below inguinal ligament	Rectus femoris	Schubert & Keil[3]
69.4 (SD 9.2)	Below inguinal ligament[a]	Vastus medialis	Johnson et al.[4]
66.7 (SD 7.4)	Above inguinal ligament[a]	Vastus medialis	johnson et al.[4]

[a] The mean conduction delay across the inguinal ligament was 1.1 msec (SD 0.4), with the mean distance between the points of stimulation above and below the ligament being 5.5 cm (SD 1.6).

mately 3 cm more laterally (Fig. 10.3). The position of the active electrode is then adjusted by using the electrode to stimulate the femoral nerve and determining the position that provides the lowest threshold for the motor response in the vastus medialis muscle. The saphenous nerve itself is then stimulated supramaximally on the medial aspect of the knee using surface electrodes, and then just above the medial malleolus. The latency to the onset of the negative deflection of the evoked nerve action potential is measured, as is the distance between the stimulating cathode and the active recording electrode. The reported mean velocity between the knee and inguinal ligament is 58.3 m/sec (standard deviation of 3.7) and the mean amplitude of the response is 5.3 μV (standard deviation of 2.7). The corresponding values for the ankle-to-knee segment of the nerve are 50.6 m/sec (standard deviation of 4.9), and 1.9 μV (standard deviation of 0.9), respectively.[5]

LATERAL FEMORAL CUTANEOUS NERVE

The lateral femoral cutaneous nerve, which has a variable derivation from some or all of the first three lumbar roots, enters the leg at the upper lateral end of the inguinal ligament, where entrapment can occur as it passes through or beneath the ligament. When it passes through the inguinal ligament, the nerve can be angulated by the posterior fascicle of the ligament, especially in patients who have an increased lumbar lordosis because of obesity, pregnancy, or other reasons. Other anatomic arrangements at this point have also been described, and may account for entrapment of the nerve. In one recent study, there were pathologic changes in 5 of 12 lateral femoral cutaneous nerves removed at autopsy from patients without disease of the peripheral nervous system. These changes included both wallerian degenera-

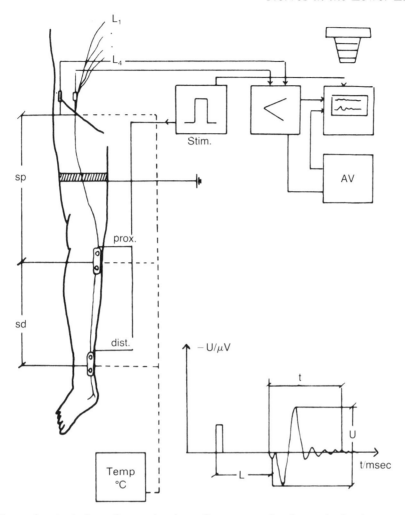

Fig. 10.3 Measuring technique for evaluation of nerve conduction velocity in upper and lower segments of the saphenous nerve. U, amplitude; L, latency; t, duration; sp, proximal segment of saphenous nerve; sd, distal segment of saphenous nerve. (Stöhr M, Schumm F, Ballier R: Normal sensory conduction in the saphenous nerve in man. Electroencephalogr Clin Neurophysiol 44:172, 1978.)

tion and local demyelination, and the fibers with the largest diameters were particularly affected.[6] Traumatic lesions involving the anterior thigh may also lead to dysfunction in this nerve.

The lateral femoral cutaneous nerve is purely sensory, and its entrapment leads to pain, paresthesias, and numbness over the anterolateral aspect of the thigh. The syndrome characterized by these symptoms is referred to as *meralgia paresthetica*.

Electrophysiologic Aspects

Electrophysiologic techniques have been used to confirm the diagnosis of meralgia paresthetica, the findings on the symptomatic and asymptomatic sides being compared. The only role of needle electromyography is in excluding other disorders that might be mistaken for meralgia paresthetica, such as an L2 or L3 radiculopathy or femoral neuropathy, but which lead to neu-

ANTERIOR SUPERIOR ILIAC SPINE

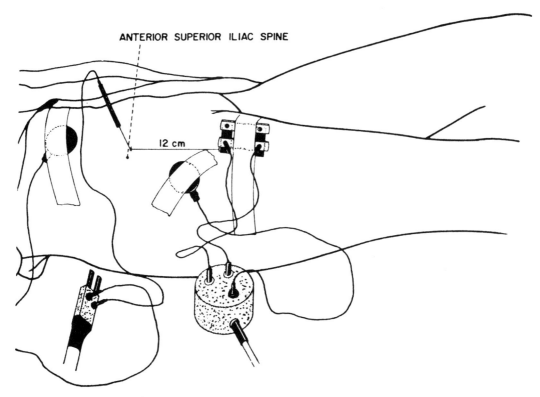

12 cm

Fig. 10.4 Electrode placement for antidromic stimulation of lateral femoral cutaneous nerve. (Butler ET, Johnson EW, Kaye ZA: Normal conduction velocity in the lateral femoral cutaneous nerve. Arch Phys Med Rehabil 55:31, 1974.)

rogenic weakness of the hip flexors or quadriceps muscles.

The functional integrity of the nerve itself can be tested by the technique advanced by Butler and co-workers.[7] The nerve is stimulated above the inguinal ligament with a needle electrode placed 1 cm medial to the anterior superior iliac spine, and the nerve action potential is recorded antidromically with surface electrodes placed 12 cm more distally, directly inferior to the anterior superior iliac spine on the anterior aspect of the thigh (Fig. 10.4). An orthodromic technique may be tolerated more easily by patients; the surface electrodes are used to stimulate the nerve and the needle electrodes are used to record the response. A mean latency (to peak of the negative deflection) of 2.6 msec (range, 2.3 to 3.1 msec;

standard deviation, 0.2 msec) has been reported with this technique,[7] which yields a conduction velocity of 47.9 m/sec (range, 43 to 55 m/sec; standard deviation, 3.7 m/sec). Amplitude of the nerve action potential varied between 10 and 25 μV. Prolonged latency has been found in several patients with peripheral nerve pathology, and in one patient with unilateral meralgia paresthetica the nerve action potential was unobtainable on the affected side but normal on the other.[7]

Sarala and co-workers used a similar orthodromic technique but with surface electrodes.[8] They found that, among nine patients with meralgia paresthetica, the nerve action potential was absent in six and was characterized by a prolonged latency in three.

The integrity of the lateral femoral cutaneous nerve can also be evaluated by recording somatosensory evoked potentials over the scalp, as discussed in Chapter 8.

SCIATIC NERVE

Clinical Aspects

The sciatic nerve contains fibers from the L4, L5, S1, S2, and S3 segments of the cord. It leaves the pelvis through the greater sciatic notch and passes down the back of the thigh, supplying the biceps femoris, semitendinosus, semimembranous, and adductor magnus muscles. Above the popliteal fossa, it divides into the common peroneal (lateral popliteal) and tibial (medial popliteal) nerves, through which it supplies much of the skin and all the muscles below the knee. The division of its fibers between these two branches can actually be traced back to the sacral plexus. It is important to appreciate this because injuries to the sciatic nerve tend to be selective, affecting the common peroneal fibers more frequently and severely than the tibial fibers.

Sciatic nerve lesions may result from trauma or surgery to the pelvis, buttock, hip, or thigh, and from misplaced intramuscular injections in the buttock. External compression of the nerve during coma induced by drugs or alcohol is another important cause. Sciatic neuropathy may also present as a postoperative pressure palsy or may result from prolonged immobilization in bed.[9] Finally, the nerve may be involved by pelvic neoplasms, compressed by the fetal head, or stretched with the patient in the lithotomy position. The distribution of the resulting weakness and wasting depends upon whether the lesion has affected the entire nerve or is restricted to one or the other of its divisions. Sensory loss occurs in the appropriate distribution below the knee, and is usually extensive.

Electrophysiologic Aspects

The sciatic nerve may be stimulated proximally at the gluteal fold between the ischial tuberosity and the greater trochanter of the femur, and distally at the apex of the popliteal fossa. Bipolar surface electrodes can be used for this purpose, but needle electrodes are generally preferred at the proximal site and are less distressing to the patient. Responses can be recorded from the medial head of the gastrocnemius, the abductor hallucis, or the abductor digiti minimi muscle when conduction velocity is to be studied in fibers destined for the tibial nerve, and from the tibialis anterior or extensor digitorum brevis muscle when fibers destined for the common peroneal nerve are being investigated. Either surface or needle electrodes can be used for recording, but Yap and Hirota have stressed that more accurate results are obtained with needle electrodes when responses are being recorded from one of a group of large muscles, such as the gastrocnemius.[10] Normal values for conduction velocity in motor fibers of the sciatic nerve are presented in Table 10.2.

Conduction in more proximal segments of the sciatic nerve can be assessed using H reflexes, F waves, or somatosensory evoked potentials (Ch. 8), but these techniques do not permit localization of the lesion.

Conduction studies may be useful in the diagnosis and evaluation of post-traumatic lesions of the sciatic nerve. They may also help to distinguish a proximal lesion that selectively affects the fibers destined for one or other branch of the sciatic nerve from a lesion affecting the common peroneal or tibial nerves after their separation.

Needle electromyography is also helpful in distinguishing sciatic nerve lesions from other lesions producing a somewhat similar clinical disorder. In particular, an L5 or S1 root lesion can be recognized by the pattern of involved muscles, which is clearly beyond the territory of the sciatic nerve (Table

Table 10.2. Motor Conduction Velocity of the Sciatic Nerve in the Thigh—Normal Mean Values

Conduction Velocity (m/sec)	Muscle Recorded from	Source
55 (SD 4.5)	Tibialis anterior	Gassel & Trojaborg[11]
51 (SD 7.0)	Extensor digitorum brevis	Gassel & Trojaborg[11]
51 (SD 5.8)	Abductor hallucis	Gassel & Trojaborg[11]
56 (SD 5.6)	Gastrocnemius	Gassel & Trojaborg[11]
53.8 (SD 3.3)	Gastrocnemius	Yap & Hirota[10]
51.3 (SD 4.4)	Abductor digiti minimi	Yap & Hirota[10]

13.2). Distinction between lesions involving the sciatic nerve and those involving the peroneal nerve may not be possible clinically, and needle examination of the short head of the biceps femoris muscle is then very helpful. This muscle is supplied by the sciatic nerve, so the presence of electromyographic abnormalities would favor a sciatic nerve lesion.

COMMON PERONEAL NERVE

Clinical Aspects

The common peroneal nerve, which is derived from the posterior divisions of the L4, L5, S1, and S2 roots, separates from the sciatic nerve at or above the apex of the popliteal fossa. It passes down along the lateral aspect of the fossa, gives off one cutaneous branch that joins the sural nerve and another that passes to the anterolateral aspect of the leg, and winds round the neck of the fibula deep to the peroneus longus. It then divides into the superficial peroneal (musculocutaneous) and deep peroneal (anterior tibial) nerves. The former supplies the peroneus longus and brevis muscles and the skin over the dorsum of the foot and the lower anterior aspect of the leg. The latter supplies the muscles in the anterior compartment of the leg, the extensor digitorum brevis in the foot, and the skin on the adjacent sides of the first and second toes.

The common peroneal nerve is particularly vulnerable to compression or direct trauma in the region of the head and neck of the fibula. Damage to the nerve may follow total knee replacement surgery.[12] Compression may occur from the use of plaster casts, high boots, or tight garters and stockings. It may also occur from improper positioning of patients in the lithotomy position so that the brace is pressing on the nerve, and is especially likely to occur in patients who are intoxicated, stuporous, or comatose. Common peroneal nerve palsy may occur as an occupational hazard among farm workers or others required to squat for prolonged periods, and the designation *strawberry pickers' palsy* has been applied in such instances.[13] The nerve may be compressed between the biceps tendon, lateral head of the gastrocnemius, and head of the fibula, with the force of compression arising from the body weight resting on the gastrocnemius muscle during squatting.[14] Alternatively, or additionally, the nerve may be compressed by a well-formed tendinous arch of the peroneus longus mussicle.[15] Peroneal neuropathy from ganglia, cysts, or tumors is rare but well recognized.

The clinical deficit resulting from a lesion of the common peroneal nerve consists of weakness of dorsiflexion and eversion of the foot, accompanied by sensory loss in an appropriate distribution. The muscles inverting the foot are spared because they are not supplied by this nerve; this fact is useful in distinguishing clinically between peroneal nerve palsy and either a sciatic nerve or a lumbosacral root lesion.

Electrophysiologic Aspects

MOTOR CONDUCTION STUDIES

A bipolar surface electrode can be used to stimulate the fibers of the common peroneal nerve at the following sites:

1. The lateral part of the popliteal fossa
2. Just below and behind the head of the fibula
3. On the dorsum of the ankle, at the junction of the outer and middle thirds of a line joining the lateral and medial malleoli

Recordings can conveniently be made with either surface or concentric needle electrodes from the extensor digitorum brevis muscle. Normal values for conduction velocity and distal latency are shown in Table 10.3.

The response of the extensor digitorum brevis to maximal stimulation of the deep peroneal nerve at the ankle is smaller in some patients than its response to stimulation of the common peroneal nerve at the knee. This is because the extensor digitorum brevis sometimes receives part of its nerve supply from the superficial peroneal nerve through a branch, the accessory deep peroneal nerve, which runs behind the lateral malleolus. Lambert, who called attention to this, stimulated behind the lateral malleolus and found evidence for an accessory nerve supplying part of the extensor digitorum brevis in 22 percent of cases.[18]

Such an anomalous innervation may have a familial basis, occurring with a dominant mode of inheritance. In one study, it was present in 78 percent of the relatives of five subjects with the anomaly, as compared to only 22 percent of unrelated persons.[19] The anomaly may have important clinical implications.[18] For example, a complete lesion of the deep peroneal nerve may not be recognized in the presence of this accessory nerve, because part of the extensor digitorum brevis remains under voluntary control and continues to be excited by stimulation of the common peroneal nerve at the knee. Again, signs of chronic partial denervation in this muscle may mistakenly be attributed to a lesion of the deep peroneal nerve when, in fact, they result from involvement of either the accessory nerve or the superficial peroneal from which it originates. Finally, a partial conduction block at the knee may not be recognized in the presence of this anomaly because the response to stimulation at the ankle is smaller than that to stimulation above the head of the fibula.

When no response can be evoked in the extensor digitorum brevis, recordings may be made instead from the tibialis anterior using either surface or needle electrodes. An attempt has recently been made to standardize the methodology for recording from the tibialis anterior, as well as from the peroneus brevis, which is supplied by the superficial peroneal nerve.[20] Recordings were made about the motor points of

Table 10.3. Motor Conduction Studies of the Common Peroneal Nerve—Normal Mean Values

	Distal Latency (msec)	Conduction Velocity (m/sec)	Source
Recording from extensor digitorum brevis	4.3[a] (SD 0.9)	49.5[a] (SD 5.6)	Mayer[16]
	4.9 (SD 0.9)	45.5 (SD 3.2)	Yap & Hirota[10]
		49.7 (SD 7.1)	Thomas et al.[17]

[a] Data for subjects between 10 and 35 years of age.

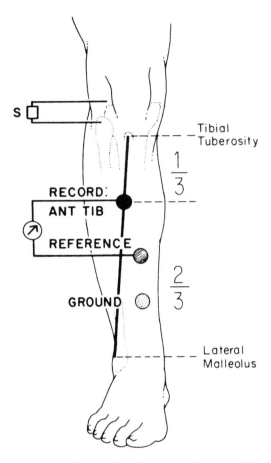

S

Tibial
Tuberosity

$\dfrac{1}{3}$

RECORD:
ANT TIB

REFERENCE

$\dfrac{2}{3}$

GROUND

Lateral
Malleolus

Fig. 10.5 Electrode placement for studying motor nerve conduction in the peroneal nerve by recording from the anterior tibial (ANT TIB) muscle. S, stimulator. (Devi S, Lovelace RE, Duarte N: Proximal peroneal nerve conduction velocity: Recording from anterior tibial and peroneus brevis muscles. Ann Neurol 2:116, 1977.)

these muscles. With the tibialis anterior, the recording surface electrode was placed at the junction of the upper one-third and lower two-thirds of the line between the tibial tuberosity and the tip of the lateral malleolus, with the reference point placed over the medial aspect of the tibia about 4 cm distal to the recording electrode (Fig. 10.5). For recording from the peroneus brevis the recording electrode was placed at the junction of the upper two-fifths and lower three-

fifths of a line between the fibular head and tip of the lateral malleolus, with a reference electrode placed on the muscle tendon some 4 cm distally (Fig. 10.6). The peroneal nerve was stimulated in the popliteal fossa and also 10 cm more distally, below the head of the fibula. With this technique, mean conduction velocity along the peroneal fibers to the tibialis anterior muscle was 66.3 m/sec (standard deviation of 12.9) and to the peroneus brevis was 55.3 m/sec (standard deviation of 10.2).

NERVE ACTION POTENTIAL

Surface electrodes may be used for stimulation. The cathode is placed over the anticipated position of the deep peroneal nerve on the dorsum of the ankle, and the anode is positioned more distally. Confirmation that the cathode is in the correct site is normally provided by the motor response of the extensor digitorum brevis muscle to stimulation of the nerve. Paired needle electrodes, inserted to a depth of 1.5 cm at right angles to the course of the nerve, are used for recording because of the small size of the potentials when surface electrodes are used. The distal needle is placed behind the neck of the fibula and the rostral one is positioned behind the tendon of the biceps femoris at its insertion into the head of the fibula, so that the interelectrode distance is about 3 to 4 cm.[21] The ground is placed between the stimulating and recording electrodes.

Using this technique, Gilliatt and associates found that the peak-to-peak amplitude of the potentials ranged from 2 to 15.5 μV in normal subjects.[21] They also measured the latency of the potentials and divided this into the conduction distance to obtain an estimate of conduction velocity. Latency was measured to the peak as well as to the onset of the main deflection of the potentials, because the latter measurement

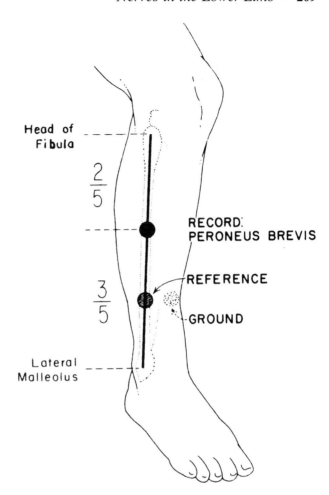

Fig. 10.6 Electrode placement for studying motor nerve conduction in the peroneal nerve by recording from peroneus brevis muscle. (Devi S, Lovelace RE, Duarte N: Proximal peroneal nerve conduction velocity: Recording from anterior tibial and peroneus brevis muscles. Ann Neurol 2:116, 1977.)

was unreliable in the case of small potentials. The normal conduction velocity was found to range between 39.8 and 51.8 m/sec (with a mean of 45.90 and standard deviation of 3.25) when calculated from measurements of latency to peak, and between 47.3 and 63.0 m/sec (with a mean of 53.0 and standard deviation of 3.85) when based on latency to onset. Potentials were absent or abnormal in patients with polyneuritis or localized lesions of the common peroneal nerve.

Sensory action potentials can also be recorded along the *superficial peroneal nerve*. The nerve is stimulated at the superior extensor retinaculum and responses are recorded about 1 or 2 cm distal to the head of the fibula, and then about 10 cm

more proximal to this site. The technique was described in detail by Behse and Buchthal, who used needle electrodes for both stimulation and recording.[22] At the head of the fibula, they placed the recording electrode near the superficial peroneal nerve by adjusting its position until the threshold for stimulation with it of the peroneus longus muscle was below 1 mA and lower than that of the tibialis anterior muscle. The more proximal recording electrode was placed in the popliteal fossa medial to the tendon of the biceps femoris muscle. The remote electrode for recording was placed at the same level, but at a transverse distance of 3 to 4 cm from the active one. A concentric needle electrode was inserted in the extensor digitorum brevis muscle to ensure that the stimulus did not activate the deep peroneal nerve. They found the mean maximal conduction velocity to be 56.5 m/sec (standard deviation of 3.4) using this technique.

Sensory conduction in the distal branches of the superficial peroneal nerve may also be measured antidromically using surface electrodes.[23,24] Recordings are made from the medial dorsal cutaneous branch[23] or the intermediate dorsal cutaneous branch,[24] while the nerve is stimulated some 12 or 14 cm more proximally (Fig. 10.7). Normal values are shown in Table 10.4. The technique is relatively simple to perform, does not require the use of an averager, and may be helpful as a means of testing the function of sensory fibers traversing the L5 nerve root. It may also aid in the study of early peripheral neuropathy.

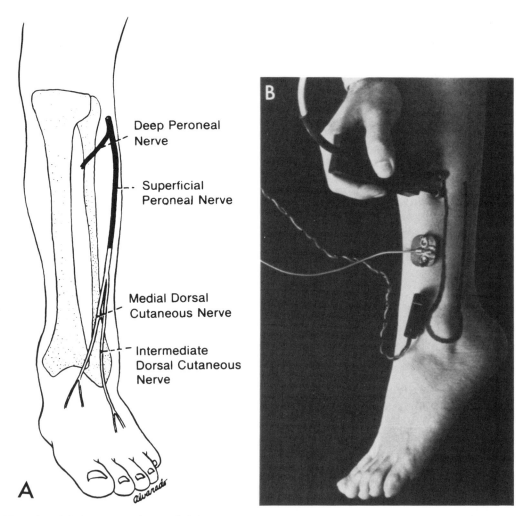

Fig. 10.7 (**A**) Anatomy of superficial peroneal nerve. (**B**) Stimulation and recording technique for studying the sensory response of the superficial peroneal nerve. (Jabre J: The superficial peroneal sensory nerve revisited. Arch Neurol 38:666, Copyright 1981 American Medical Association.)

Table 10.4. Sensory Conduction in Distal Branches of the Superficial Peroneal Nerve—Normal Mean Values Using an Antidromic Technique

	Latency to Peak (msec)	Conduction Velocity (msec)	Peak-to-Peak Amplitude of Sensory Action Potential (μV)	Source
Medial dorsal cutaneous branch	2.8[a] (SD 0.3)	51.2 (SD 5.7)	18.3 (SD 8.0)	Izzo et al.[23]
Intermediate dorsal cutaneous branch	2.8[a] (SD 0.3)	51.3 (SD 5.4)	15.1 (SD 8.2)	Izzo et al.[23]
	2.9[b] (SD 0.3)	65.7 (SD 3.7)	20.5 (SD 6.1)	Jabre[24]

[a] 14 cm between the stimulating and recording electrodes.
[b] 12 cm between the stimulating and recording electrodes.

PRESSURE PALSIES

The site of compression in pressure palsies is usually at the level of the head and neck of the fibula. Motor conduction velocity is sometimes reduced in the segment of nerve between knee and ankle, but in other cases it may be reduced only over the compressed segment about the knee. Redford found that the size of the response recorded from the tibialis anterior muscle with surface or subcutaneous needle electrodes was smaller when evoked by supramaximal stimulation of the nerve above the head of the fibula in the popliteal fossa than when evoked below it, whereas in normal subjects there was no difference in the amplitude of the responses.[25] He stressed the value of this approach, especially when—as occurs occasionally—no response can be recorded from the extensor digitorum brevis muscle. Pickett similarly found that amplitude of the compound muscle action potential was a good indicator for localizing the lesion, but used the response of the extensor digitorum brevis muscle and took as his criterion of abnormality a drop in amplitude of more than 20 percent across the knee segment.[26] The amplitude and conduction velocity of the nerve action potentials recorded at the head of the fibula after stimulation of the deep peroneal nerve at the ankle may also be reduced, even if the motor conduction velocity in this segment of the nerve is normal.[21]

Needle electromyography of muscles supplied by the peroneal nerve must be interpreted cautiously. Proximal lesions of the sciatic nerve may only involve the peroneal fibers, thereby producing electromyographic abnormalities in the same distribution as when the peroneal nerve itself is affected. Sampling of the short head of the biceps may, however, be useful in distinguishing between them, as discussed earlier. Needle examination of the extensor digitorum brevis muscle reveals signs of chronic partial denervation in 10 to 20 percent of normal healthy subjects,[27–29] so that examination of this muscle is generally not very helpful.

Singh and co-workers compared the diagnostic yield of different electrophysiologic criteria for confirming the diagnosis of a compressive lesion of the peroneal nerve at the head of the fibula.[30] Slowing of sensory conduction in the superficial peroneal nerve localized the lesion in 64 percent of patients, and there were no false-positive findings among patients whose peroneal palsy was not a result of compression at this site. In 20 percent of the patients with slowing along the segment of nerve across the fibular head, conduction velocity was normal when measured from the ankle to the popliteal fossa—that is, along a longer length of normal nerve encompassing the site of the lesion. Differences in amplitude, and temporal dispersion of the sensory responses recorded in the popliteal fossa and compared with those recorded below the head of the fibula were of limited value because of many false-positive findings in patients whose nerve lesion was not at that site. Slowing of motor conduction velocity across the head of the fibula localized the site of the lesion in one-third of patients, and was found to be more sensitive for this purpose than measurements of the size of the motor response. However, Singh and associates used a 75 percent reduction in amplitude of the compound muscle action potential of the extensor digitorum brevis muscle as a cut-off point to separate normal patients from those with peroneal nerve lesions at the fibular head.[30] They also used needle electrodes for both stimulation and recording, and it is well known that small changes in electrode position may markedly influence the amplitude of the response, making any but a large decrease in amplitude across the knee an unreliable criterion. The criterion adopted by Pickett, using surface electrodes, was a decrement of 20 percent or more across the knee.[26] He found this to be a more sensitive indicator than a change in motor conduction velocity for localizing mild lesions.

TIBIAL NERVE

Clinical Aspects

Arising from the sciatic nerve above the popliteal fossa, the tibial nerve supplies the gastrocnemius, plantaris, soleus, and popliteus muscles, gives origin to the sural nerve, and then continues its descent as the posterior tibial nerve, supplying the soleus, tibialis posterior, flexor digitorum longus, and flexor hallucis longus muscles. Between the heel and medial malleolus just before, within, or immediately distal to the tarsal tunnel (Fig. 10.8), the posterior tibial nerve gives off calcaneal branches and divides into the medial and lateral plantar nerves which supply the small muscles of the foot and the skin on the plantar aspect of the foot and toes.[31]

The posterior tibial nerve or its branches may be compressed between the bony floor of the tarsal tunnel and the flexor retinaculum or lanciniate ligament, which forms its roof (see Fig. 10.8). This may occur as a result of trauma, such as occurs with fractures or dislocations of the ankle. Other etiologic factors include space-occupying lesions, thrombophlebitis, hypertrophy of the abductor hallucis muscle or an accessory muscle belly of the short flexors, abnormal calcaneal eversion relative to an adducted talus, and an abducted forefoot which puts tension on the ligaments and fibrous structures of the tarsal tunnel and the posterior tibial nerve.[32] Compressive lesions of the individual plantar nerves may also occur beyond the tarsal tunnel. The clinical features and electrophysiologic findings in such circumstances are similar to those associated with the tarsal tunnel syndrome itself.

The predominant symptoms of the tarsal tunnel syndrome are pain, paresthesias, and numbness involving the toes and sole of the foot. Symptoms may be exacerbated by standing, often become worse as the day progresses, may disturb sleep at night, and sometimes radiate proximally to the calf or leg. They may be relieved by elevating the foot or removing the shoes. Examination reveals a sensory disturbance of the sole (sometimes including the heel) and a positive Tinel's sign over the tarsal tunnel region. There may also be mild weakness of flexion at the metatarsophalangeal joints.

Electrophysiologic Aspects

Bipolar surface electrodes can be used to stimulate the fibers of the tibial nerve in the popliteal fossa and as they run behind and

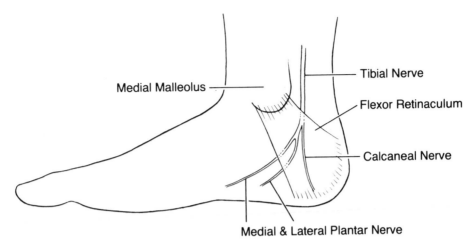

Fig. 10.8 Anatomy of the tarsal tunnel.

above the medial malleolus. Responses are recorded with surface disc electrodes from the abductor hallucis muscle when the function of the medial plantar nerve is being examined, and from the abductor digiti minimi when the lateral plantar nerve is under investigation.

In the case of the abductor hallucis muscle, the active electrode is placed about 1 cm behind and below the navicular tubercle on the medial aspect of the foot, and the reference is positioned over the first metatarsophalangeal joint. For recording from the abductor digiti minimi, the active electrode is placed beneath the anterior tip of the lateral malleolus at one-half the distance to the sole,[33] and the reference is placed at the base of the fifth toe. The ground electrode may be placed on the dorsum of the foot.

Normal values for motor conduction velocity and distal latency are shown in Table 10.5.

A technique for studying sensory conduction in the medial plantar nerve has been described.[35] Stimuli are delivered through

Table 10.5. Motor Conduction Studies of Tibial Nerve—Normal Mean Values

	Distal Latency (msec)	Conduction Velocity (m/sec)	Source
Recording from abductor hallucis	5.9[a] (SD 1.3)	45.5[a] (SD 3.8)	Mayer[16]
	4.4 (SD 0.9)		Goodgold et al.[34]
	5.32 (SD 0.82)		Johnson & Ortiz[33]
		43.2 (SD 4.9)	Thomas et al.[17]
Recording from abductor digiti minimi	6.3 (SD 1.1)	43.4 (SD 3.1)	Yap & Hirota[10]
	4.7 (SD 1.0)		Goodgold et al.[34]
	5.86 (SD 0.84)		Johnson & Ortiz[33]

[a] Data for subjects between 10 and 35 years of age.

two ring electrodes encircling the hallux, and responses are recorded from a distal electrode placed over a point at which the posterior tibial artery can be palpated close to the medial malleolus of the ankle. A proximal electrode is positioned on the medial edge of the Achilles tendon (Fig. 10.9). With this technique, the medial plantar sensory action potential usually consists of a negative wave, sometimes preceded or followed by a positive peak. In 69 control subjects, the potential was found to have a mean amplitude of 2.3 μV (standard deviation of 1.4), a mean latency to onset of 4.8 msec (standard deviation of 0.7), and a mean latency to peak of 5.7 msec (standard deviation of 1.1); maximal sensory conduction velocity in the nerve had a mean value of 35.6 m/sec (standard deviation of 5.6).[35] The small size of the response makes it necessary to use averaging techniques, but the single most important factor in obtaining a satisfactory record is careful positioning of the surface electrode where the posterior tibial pulse is palpable. The amplitude of

the response correlates well with that of the sural sensory action potential in the same subjects.[35]

Oh and co-workers studied sensory nerve conduction velocity in the medial and lateral plantar nerves in 20 normal control subjects.[36] Sensory potentials were again recorded orthodromically. The recording electrode was placed above the flexor retinaculum, and ring electrodes were used to stimulate the hallux for evaluating the medial plantar nerve and the little toe for examining the lateral plantar nerve. A signal averager was again used, and latency was measured to the negative peak of the nerve action potential in order to avoid the difficulty of recognizing the onset of small potentials. Sensory nerve conduction velocity was slower in the lateral than in the medial plantar nerve (with a mean and standard deviation of 31.68 ± 4.39 m/sec, compared to 35.22 ± 3.63 m/sec), and the amplitude of the nerve action potential was smaller (mean of 1.89 μV, compared to 3.61 μV).

Studies of sensory conduction are of

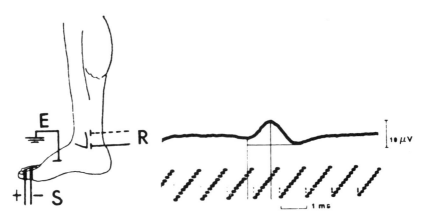

Fig. 10.9 Recording the medial plantar sensory nerve action potential. Placement of surface electrodes (R), ground or earth (E), and stimulating ring electrodes (S) is shown. On the right, an example of the averaged medial plantar sensory action potential obtained from a normal subject after 32 sweeps is shown. Vertical lines show measurements of latency to onset (3.8 msec) and peak (4.7 msec). Amplitude is 8.1 μV. Time scale of the staircases is 1 msec with ten 0.1-msec steps each. Stimulus occurs at sweep onset. (Guiloff RJ, Sherratt RM: Sensory conduction in medial plantar nerve. J Neurol Neurosurg Psychiatry 40:1168, 1977. Reproduced by permission of the Authors and Editors of the Journal of Neurology, Neurosurgery and Psychiatry.)

value in the investigation of patients with peripheral neuropathies or suspected tarsal tunnel syndrome. Recording the sensory action potential of the medial plantar nerve may also be helpful in the evaluation of patients with L4 or L5 nerve root or plexus lesions.[35]

The Tarsal Tunnel Syndrome

Motor conduction velocity of the tibial nerve and the terminal motor latencies of both its medial and lateral plantar branches must be measured on the affected side. These values can be compared with the corresponding figures on the clinically unaffected side (a difference in the latencies of more than 1 msec being significant),[37] and with the values obtained in normal subjects.

When conduction velocity in the tibial nerve is normal, a significantly prolonged latency in its medial or lateral plantar branches, or both, suggests that compression may have occurred within the tarsal tunnel. It is important, however, to ensure that the foot is warm when the study is performed because a profound increase in latency occurs in normal subjects as the temperature is reduced.[33] It must also be emphasized that, unless the stimulating cathode is positioned rostral to the proximal border of the flexor retinaculum, a falsely normal value for latency may be obtained.

In one study, a prolonged terminal motor latency in the medial or lateral plantar nerves was found in 11 of 21 patients (52 percent).[36] By contrast, abnormal sensory conduction was found in 19 patients (90 percent), along with either an absent or markedly attenuated sensory action potential or reduced conduction velocity. Such findings indicate the greater diagnostic sensitivity of the sensory studies, which should not be omitted from the evaluation of such patients.

Electromyographic sampling may show changes of chronic partial denervation in the intrinsic foot muscles, and the distribution of these changes may conform to that of the median or lateral plantar nerves. Abnormalities are not found in muscles supplied by the posterior tibial nerve above the ankle. However, electromyographic abnormalities may be found in the intrinsic muscles of asymptomatic feet, so their presence must be interpreted with caution.[27,29]

SURAL NERVE

Clinical Aspects

The earliest symptoms and signs of a polyneuropathy often arise as a result of involvement of distal sensory fibers in the legs; for this reason, it is important to have some means of evaluating objectively the functional integrity of these fibers. Although a number of techniques for studying sensory conduction in the legs have been described, only a few have achieved widespread use in clinical practice. The function of sensory fibers in the sural nerve can be evaluated by a relatively simple technique,[38,39] and this nerve, rather than the plantar nerves or distal branches of the superficial peroneal nerve, is usually examined when patients are being evaluated for suspected peripheral neuropathy.

The sural nerve, which is purely sensory, originates from the tibial nerve and receives a branch from the common peroneal about halfway down the leg. It then descends next to the lateral border of the Achilles tendon, supplying the posterolateral part of the lower leg, and winds round the lateral malleolus to supply the lateral aspect of the dorsum of the foot and the little toe.

Electrophysiologic Aspects

The sural sensory action potential can be recorded either antidromically or orthodromically, but the former is usually more

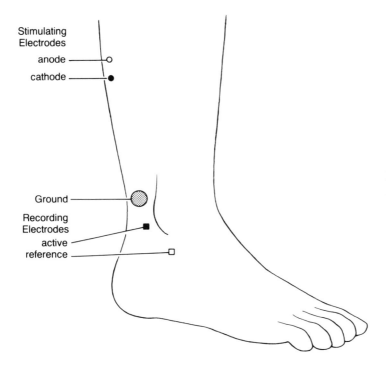

Stimulating
Electrodes

anode

cathode

Ground

Recording
Electrodes

active

reference

Fig. 10.10 Electrode placement for recording sural sensory action potentials.

convenient. Bipolar surface stimulating electrodes are placed slightly lateral to the midline on the posterior aspect of the calf at the junction of the middle and lower thirds of the leg, with the cathode distal to the anode (Fig. 10.10). The response is recorded by surface electrodes; the active one is placed just behind the lateral malleolus and the reference one is positioned below and behind the malleolus some 3 cm more distally. The ground lead is attached to the lower, lateral aspect of the calf between the stimulating and recording electrodes.

Measurements are made of the peak-to-peak amplitude of the response and the latency to onset of its negative phase. The latency will vary with conduction distance,

Table 10.6. Sural Nerve Conduction Studies—Normal Mean Values

Age (yr)	Conduction Velocity (m/sec)	Peak-to-Peak Amplitude of Sensory Action Potential (μV)	Source
1–15	52.1 (SD 5.1)	23.1 (SD 4.4)	Di Benedetto[38]
≥15	46.2 (SD 3.3)	23.7 (SD 3.8)	Di Benedetto[38]
0–20	46.9 (SD 3.0)	18.4 (SD 6.4)	Burke et al.[39]
21–40	46.2 (SD 3.7)	16.4 (SD 5.5)	Burke et al.[39]
41–60	46.4 (SD 3.7)	13.6 (SD 7.5)	Burke et al.[39]
61–80	45.5 (SD 3.1)	9.8 (SD 3.6)	Burke et al.[39]

but this can be corrected for by adjusting the position of the stimulating cathode so that the conduction distance is always the same (for example, 14 cm). Alternatively, the conduction distance can be divided by the latency in order to provide an estimate of conduction velocity. The results obtained from normal subjects are shown in Table 10.6, where it can be seen that the amplitude of the sural sensory action potential may diminish markedly with age in normal subjects.

Conduction can also be assessed in a more distal segment of the sural nerve. However, difficulty may sometimes be encountered in recording sensory action potentials in apparently normal subjects.[39]

SURAL CONDUCTION STUDIES IN THE DIAGNOSIS OF POLYNEUROPATHIES

Burke and colleagues compared the diagnostic yield from measuring sensory conduction in the median nerve with that from studying the sural nerve in 300 consecutive patients with symptoms suggestive of a sensory polyneuropathy.[39] Studies of the median nerve revealed no abnormality in 107 patients with electrical evidence of sural nerve involvement. The reverse case—normal sural but abnormal median studies—was uncommon, occurring in only 9 patients. They concluded that studies of sural nerve conduction are the most useful method for screening patients suspected of having a sensory polyneuropathy.

REFERENCES

1. Kourtopoulos H: Femoral nerve injury following appendectomy. J Neurosurg 57:714, 1982
2. Gassel MM: A study of femoral nerve conduction time. Arch Neurol 9:607, 1963
3. Schubert HA, Keil EW: Femoral nerve conduction velocity. Am J Phys Med 47:302, 1968
4. Johnson EW, Wood PK, Powers JJ: Femoral nerve conduction studies. Arch Phys Med Rehabil 49:528, 1968
5. Stöhr M, Schumm F, Ballier R: Normal sensory conduction in the saphenous nerve in man. Electroencephalogr Clin Neurophysiol 44:172, 1978
6. Jefferson D, Eames RA: Subclinical entrapment of the lateral femoral cutaneous nerve: An autopsy study. Muscle Nerve 2:145, 1979
7. Butler ET, Johnson EW, Kaye ZA: Normal conduction velocity in the lateral femoral cutaneous nerve. Arch Phys Med Rehabil 55:31, 1974
8. Sarala PK, Nishihara T, Oh SJ: Meralgia paresthetica: Electrophysiologic study. Arch Phys Med Rehabil 60:30, 1979
9. Stewart JD, Angus E, Gendron D: Sciatic neuropathies. Br Med J 287:1108, 1983
10. Yap CB, Hirota T: Sciatic nerve motor conduction velocity study. J Neurol Neurosurg Psychiatry 30:233, 1967
11. Gassel MM, Trojaborg W: Clinical and electrophysiological study of the pattern of conduction times in the distribution of the sciatic nerve. J Neurol Neurosurg Psychiatry 27:351, 1964
12. Kaushal SP, Galante JO, McKenna R, Backmann F: Complications following total knee replacement. Clin Orthop 121:181, 1976
13. Koller RL, Blank NK: Strawberry pickers' palsy. Arch Neurol 37:320, 1980
14. Sunderland S: Nerves and Nerve Injuries. 2nd Ed. Churchill Livingstone, Edinburgh, 1978
15. Sandhu HS, Sandhey BS: Occupational compression of the common peroneal nerve at the neck of the fibula. Aust NZ J Surg 46:160, 1976
16. Mayer RF: Nerve conduction studies in man. Neurology 13:1021, 1963
17. Thomas PK, Sears TA, Gilliatt RW: The range of conduction velocity in normal motor nerve fibres to the small muscles of the hand and foot. J Neurol Neurosurg Psychiatry 22:175, 1959
18. Lambert EH: The accessory deep peroneal nerve. A common variation in innervation

of extensor digitorum brevis. Neurology 19:1169, 1969

19. Crutchfield CA, Gutmann L: Hereditary aspects of accessory deep peroneal nerve. J Neurol Neurosurg Psychiatry 36:989, 1973

20. Devi S, Lovelace RE, Duarte N: Proximal peroneal nerve conduction velocity: Recording from anterior tibial and peroneus brevis muscles. Ann Neurol 2:116, 1977

21. Gilliatt RW, Goodman HV, Willison RG: The recording of lateral popliteal nerve action potentials in man. J Neurol Neurosurg Psychiatry 24:305, 1961

22. Behse F, Buchthal F: Normal sensory conduction in the nerves of the leg in man. J Neurol Neurosurg Psychiatry 34:404, 1971

23. Izzo KL, Sridhara CR, Rosenholtz H, Lemont H: Sensory conduction studies of the branches of the superficial peroneal nerve. Arch Phys Med Rehabil 62:24, 1981

24. Jabre JF: The superficial peroneal sensory nerve revisited. Arch Neurol 38:666, 1981

25. Redford JB: Nerve conduction in motor fibers to the anterior tibial muscle in peroneal palsy. Arch Phys Med Rehabil 45:500, 1964

26. Pickett JB: Localizing peroneal nerve lesions to the knee by motor conduction studies. Arch Neurol 41:192, 1984

27. Falck B, Alaranta H: Fibrillation potentials, positive sharp waves and fasciculation in the intrinsic muscles of the foot in healthy subjects. J Neurol Neurosurg Psychiatry 46:681, 1983

28. Wiechers D, Guyton JD, Johnson EW: Electromyographic findings in extensor digitorum brevis in normal population. Arch Phys Med Rehabil 57:84, 1976

29. Gatens PF, Saeed MA: Electromyographic findings in the intrinsic muscles of normal feet. Arch Phys Med Rehabil 63:317, 1982

30. Singh N, Behse F, Buchthal F: Electrophysiological study of peroneal palsy. J Neurol Neurosurg Psychiatry 37:1202, 1974

31. Dellon AL, Mackinnon SE: Tibial nerve branching in the tarsal tunnel. Arch Neurol 41:645, 1984

32. DeLisa JA, Saeed MA: AAEE Case Report No. 8: The Tarsal Tunnel Syndrome. American Association of Electromyography and Electrodiagnosis, Rochester, Minnesota, 1983

33. Johnson EW, Ortiz PR: Electrodiagnosis of tarsal tunnel syndrome. Arch Phys Med Rehabil 47:776, 1966

34. Goodgold J, Kopell HP, Spielholz NI: The tarsal-tunnel syndrome. N Engl J Med 273:742, 1965

35. Guiloff RJ, Sherratt RM: Sensory conduction in medial plantar nerve. J Neurol Neurosurg Psychiatry 40:1168, 1977

36. Oh SJ, Sarala PK, Kuba T, Elmore RS: Tarsal tunnel syndrome: Electrophysiological study. Ann Neurol 5:327, 1979

37. Lam SJS: Peripheral nerve compression syndromes in the lower limb. Guy's Hosp Rep 117:49, 1968

38. Di Benedetto M: Sensory nerve conduction in lower extremities. Arch Phys Med Rehabil 51:253, 1970

39. Burke D, Skuse NF, Lethlean AK: Sensory conduction of the sural nerve in polyneuropathy. J Neurol Neurosurg Psychiatry 37:647, 1974

11

Peripheral Nerve Disorders

Peripheral nerve disorders vary widely in their clinical manifestations, depending on the pattern of involvement. The function of a single, isolated peripheral nerve may be disturbed (*mononeuropathy*), or several nerves may be affected individually (*mononeuropathy multiplex* or *multiple mononeuropathy*). In other instances, peripheral nerve dysfunction is widespread and symmetric, and clinical deficits resulting from lesions of the individual nerves cannot be recognized (*polyneuropathy*).

Selective involvement of motor or sensory fibers occurs in some neuropathies, and the electrophysiologic findings may permit such selective involvement to be documented. For example, a sensory neuronopathy may characteristically be found in association with malignant disease and has a very distinctive electrophysiologic appearance. Certain other disorders are associated particularly with selective or predominant motor involvement, such as may occur with the use of dapsone, exposure to certain organophosphorus compounds, and lead toxicity.

In this chapter, the clinical and electrophysiologic features of certain peripheral nerve disorders are briefly reviewed, but no attempt is made to discuss them from every aspect or to consider every pathologic condition in which the peripheral nerves are involved. Other than a brief discussion on traumatic lesions, simple mononeuropathies and entrapment neuropathies—in which the function of individual nerves is impaired as a result of compression by neighboring anatomic structures—are not considered since they have already been discussed in Chapters 9 and 10.

TRAUMATIC LESIONS OF THE PERIPHERAL NERVES

Seddon divided peripheral nerve injuries into three different categories, depending on their severity.[1] The term *neurapraxia* was used to refer to injuries in which function is temporarily deranged but the structural integrity of the nerve is preserved. *Axonotmesis* was the term applied to injuries in which the functional and anatomic continuity of nerve fibers is interrupted but the connective tissue structure of the nerve remains intact; this type of injury is followed by good functional recovery as regeneration occurs. In contrast, recovery is delayed and incomplete after injuries in which both the connective tissue structure of the nerve and the continuity of the nerve fibers are disrupted, and such injuries were termed *neurotmesis*. The pathologic and electrophysiologic changes accompanying focal nerve lesions of differing severity and duration, ranging from mild, acute compression to nerve transection, have been presented in Chapter 7.

Electrophysiologic methods have a definite place in the evaluation of peripheral nerve injuries. They are helpful in determining the site of the focal nerve lesion, determining its severity, and providing a guide to prognosis. Electromyographic sampling procedures can be undertaken immediately after the onset of the lesion to determine whether or not any motor units remain under voluntary control in the affected muscles. If surviving units are found, the possibility that they are innervated anomalously must, however, be considered and excluded, if necessary, by nerve stimulation techniques (p. 265). Regardless of the nature of the lesion, insertion activity will be normal at this time and abnormal spontaneous activity will not be present unless it is a result of previous pathology. In neurapraxia, subsequent needle examinations reveal no abnormalities other than a reduction in the number of motor units under voluntary control. Following axonotmesis or neurotmesis, however, the amount of insertion activity becomes excessive after a few days, and spontaneous fibrillation potentials and positive sharp waves appear after a variable interval, sometimes as long as 5 weeks, depending upon the site of the muscle. In general, the more distal the muscle, the longer is the interval before these electromyographic abnormalities can be detected. The sequence of electromyographic changes that occur with regeneration and reinnervation were described earlier (p. 64), and the only point that warrants reiteration is that electromyographic signs of reinnervation are found long before there are any clinical signs of recovery.

Nerve stimulation techniques can also be used to assess the completeness or severity of a peripheral nerve lesion and to follow

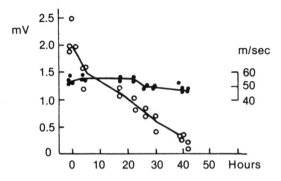

Fig. 11.1 The conduction velocity (*closed circles*) and muscle action potential amplitude (*open circles*) measured serially during the course of wallerian degeneration in guinea pigs. (Kaeser HE, Lambert EH: Nerve function studies in experimental polyneuritis. Electroencephalogr Clin Neurophysiol, Suppl. 22:29, 1962.)

the course of any regeneration. If a motor response can be recorded after stimulation of the nerve above the site of the lesion, the nerve must be in continuity, at least in part, with some functionally intact axons (provided that the possibility of anomalous innervation can be excluded). The presence of a response to stimulation below the lesion can also be used to document the integrity of axons if sufficient time has elapsed for conduction to fail in those fibers that are degenerating. Unfortunately, there is only a limited amount of information relating to the temporal course of wallerian degeneration in humans, and considerable variation occurs between different animal species.[2] However, the human facial nerve is known to remain excitable for 120 to 192 hours after it has been transected.[3] While the degenerating distal stump of a transected nerve remains excitable, there is little change in its conduction velocity, but the amplitude of the evoked motor response gradually declines, as shown in Figure 11.1.

After injuries leading solely to neurapraxia, conduction may be slowed across the affected segment of nerve or, in severe cases, may be blocked completely, but conduction below the level of the lesion is normal. Following axonotmesis or neurotmesis, no response can be recorded from the distal nerve or affected muscles to nerve stimulation above the level of injury (or to more distal stimulation once the nerve fibers have degenerated) when the lesion is complete. In a partial lesion, the amplitude of the response is reduced, but the conduction velocity and terminal latency may be normal if undamaged fibers are able to conduct normally.

With complete degeneration, once the motor responses to nerve stimulation are lost, no responses will be recorded until the affected muscles have become reinnervated. Conduction velocity during the early stages of regeneration is extremely slow; in order for it to be measured, the nerve may have to be stimulated proximal to the site of the lesion because the electric threshold for exciting the regenerating fibers is so high that percutaneous stimulation distally is not feasible. Although the conduction velocity gradually increases with time, it nevertheless remains lower than normal over periods of follow-up extending over several years.[4]

MONONEUROPATHY MULTIPLEX AND POLYNEUROPATHY

Electrodiagnostic studies are important in the evaluation of patients with polyneuropathy or mononeuropathy multiplex. Nerve conduction studies permit the extent of peripheral nerve involvement to be documented, and in some instances may permit recognition of widespread peripheral nerve dysfunction when patients present with an apparently isolated mononeuropathy. Again, as mononeuropathy multiplex advances, the neurologic deficit becomes confluent so that a polyneuropathy is simulated clinically. Electrodiagnostic studies may then be the sole means of distinguishing the two processes. Electrophysiologic techniques also provide a means of following

the course of peripheral nerve disorders and in guiding prognosis. There is some evidence that patients with a diffuse disorder affecting peripheral nerve function have an increased susceptibility to focal compressive neuropathies. Electrodiagnostic studies thus may be helpful in determining the extent to which clinical deficits relate to such superadded lesions, which may be amenable to specific therapeutic maneuvers. Finally, the electrophysiologic changes may suggest the nature of the underlying pathology.

Peripheral neuropathies can conveniently be characterized on the basis of the structure primarily affected by the disease process,[5] although their classification on these grounds is not absolute. In some, the predominant pathologic feature is axonal degeneration, and these disorders are therefore referred to as axonal neuropathies, even though some degree of demyelination may occur as a secondary phenomenon. Degeneration may commence distally and spread centripetally, as in the neuropathy of chronic alcoholism; such disorders are referred to as "dying back" neuropathies or distal axonopathies. Nerve conduction studies in the axonal neuropathies reveal that conduction velocity is normal or only mildly reduced,[6] and such reduction as does occur is usually attributable to loss of the fastest conducting fibers, although other factors may also be involved. Compound muscle action potentials and sensory action potentials are reduced in size, reflecting the axonal loss. In addition, electromyographic signs of denervation are usually found when affected muscles are sampled with a needle electrode. It may be difficult or even impossible to distinguish between an axonopathy and a motor or sensory neuronopathy on electrophysiologic grounds. Equal involvement both proximally and distally would favor the latter, especially if it occurs in a setting in which only motor or sensory function is affected.

In other neuropathies, the predominant pathologic change consists of demyelination, the axons themselves being relatively spared. The myelin may only be lost in the region of the nodes of Ranvier (paranodal demyelination), or it may be lost in the entire internodal segments (segmental demyelination). Conduction is slowed considerably in affected fibers; therefore, a reduction in maximal nerve conduction velocity of more than 40 percent has been taken to indicate the presence of segmental demyelination.[6] The compound muscle action potentials and sensory action potentials may be small and dispersed, and typically become increasingly attenuated and dispersed as the conduction distance is increased. In severe cases, conduction may be blocked completely. Needle electromyography reveals no abnormality other than a reduction in the number of motor units under voluntary control, unless some of the axons have degenerated.

The electrophysiologic findings may help to distinguish the cause of a demyelinative neuropathy. Chronic familial or hereditary demyelinative neuropathy is characterized by uniform slowing, whereas in the acquired neuropathies there is differential slowing of conduction velocity in different segments of the nerve and in corresponding segments of different nerves, with conduction block in some instances.[7] In general, the slowing of conduction velocity tends to be more extreme in patients with hereditary neuropathies. The F wave responses may be absent or markedly delayed in latency in patients with acquired demyelinative neuropathies, with considerable variation depending on the nerves studied. By contrast, F wave responses are delayed to an extent comparable to the reduced peripheral conduction velocity in the familial neuropathies.

Identification of the cause of a polyneuropathy or mononeuropathy multiplex may be difficult, and in a certain proportion of cases, no etiology can be identified. Intensive evaluation of a large series of patients referred with undiagnosed polyneuropathy to one large medical center permitted an etiologic classification to be reached in 76 percent of patients.[8] Inherited disorders were found to be the most common previously unrecognized cause, accounting for 42 percent of the patients in that series. The most common reason for failing to diagnose the disorder initially was failure to take an adequate history, failure by patient or physician to relate neurologic problems in relatives to those of the patient, or the presence of only mild involvement in other family members as a result of genetic heterogeneity.[8] Diagnostic yield is, therefore, increased by obtaining a more detailed family history—with particular reference to relatively minor abnormalities, such as high-arched feet—and by neurologically evaluating relatives who, for one reason or another, are suspected of having a neuropathy. In the series already alluded to, an inflammatory-demyelinating radiculoneuropathy was diagnosed in 21 percent of patients, and another 13 percent were found to have neuropathies associated with diverse medical disorders (e.g., metabolic disease, such as diabetes mellitus; malignant disease; paraproteinemia; leprosy; or exposure to some neurotoxic compound). In a more recent study, McLeod and coworkers reported that in only about 13 percent of patients with chronic polyneuropathy of a duration longer than 1 year did an etiologic diagnosis remain uncertain despite intensive investigation.[9] The authors emphasized that continued follow-up is worthwhile since a diagnosis may be established on re-examination of such patients.

Mononeuropathy multiplex implies a multifocal disorder of the peripheral nerves. Occlusive disease of the vasa nervorum, especially in association with diabetes, collagenosis, atherosclerosis, drug reactions, or amyloid vasculopathy, may be responsible.[10] Other disorders, such as neurofibromatosis; metastatic deposits; remote effects of malignant disease; infectious neuropathies, such as leprosy or Lyme disease; chronic inflammatory polyneuropathy; and hereditary liability to pressure palsy may present in this way.[10] Sometimes, no specific etiologic diagnosis can be made despite nerve biopsy. The electrodiagnostic findings in infarctive mononeuropathy multiplex is that of axonal loss with little, if any, demyelination. Accordingly, sensory and compound muscle action potentials are small or even absent, whereas nerve conduction velocities are normal or reduced only mildly. The needle examination may show evidence of denervation, with abnormal spontaneous activity and a reduction in the number of motor unit potentials under voluntary control. Electrophysiologic evidence of reinnervation may also be present in chronic cases. When the underlying pathology is segmental demyelination, there may be marked conduction slowing, dispersed sensory and compound muscle action potentials, and evidence of multifocal conduction block.

Multiple entrapment neuropathies can be considered forms of mononeuropathy multiplex, and patients with certain disorders, such as rheumatoid arthritis and diabetes, are at risk for both nerve infarction and multiple nerve entrapment. Electrophysiologic studies can help to differentiate these two processes and, therefore, guide management.

INHERITED NEUROPATHIES

Hereditary Motor and Sensory Neuropathy

Several different types of hereditary motor and sensory neuropathy (HMSN) are described. Types I and II (also referred to as the hypertrophic and neuronal forms of peroneal muscular atrophy or Charcot-Marie-Tooth disease) are clinically similar, but the age at onset of the former is commonly in the first decade; the latter usually occurs in the second decade or later. Inheritance of either type I or type II may occur as an autosomal dominant or, less commonly, a recessive trait, but occasional sporadic cases also occur. Clinically, there is a slowly progressive distal weakness, wasting, sensory loss, and areflexia, which is more prominent in the legs than the arms. Patients with HMSN type I, in particular, may present with foot deformities or gait disturbances in childhood or early adult life, and scoliosis is common in severe cases. The recessive form of either type is often clinically more severe than the dominant form, and type I tends to be clinically more severe than type II. The peripheral nerves may be thickened palpably in type I, which is sometimes designated the Roussy-Lévy syndrome when tremor is a conspicuous clinical feature. The electrophysiologic findings in the two types are quite dissimilar.[11,12]

In type I, needle electromyography shows evidence of chronic partial denervation in distal extremity muscles, especially in the legs. Fibrillation potentials and positive sharp waves are frequently found, and the interference pattern is reduced. However, complex repetitive discharges are rare, and fasciculation potentials are infrequent. In many patients, there is evidence of reinnervation with large, long-duration, polyphasic motor unit potentials.[13] Maximal motor and sensory conduction velocities are markedly reduced, typically to less than 60 percent of normal, and sensory action potentials are generally small and broken up, when they can be recorded at all.

In type II HMSN, electrophysiologic evidence of chronic partial denervation is also present in the distal muscles, but fasciculation potentials and complex repetitive discharges are encountered much more often than in type I,[13] motor conduction velocity is considerably less slowed than in type I and may, in fact, be in the normal range, and sensory conduction velocity is normal or slowed only slightly, although sensory action potentials may be small or absent.

Pathologic examination of nerve biopsy specimens confirms the distinction of HMSN types I and II. In the former, there is segmental demyelination, onion-bulb formations, an increase in the endoneurial space, and extensive loss of myelinated fibers. In type II HMSN, the endoneurial area is normal or increased only slightly, onion-bulb formations are virtually absent, demyelination is rare, and there is loss of the larger axons.[14] Further support of the genetic distinction of these two types of HMSN may be derived from the positive correlation that exists between index cases and their affected relatives for values of motor conduction velocity.[15,16] Moreover, HMSN type I but not type II has been shown to be linked to the Duffy blood group.[17]

A clinically similar disorder may occur in patients with a distal form of progressive spinal muscular atrophy, but there is no sensory loss and the peripheral nerves are not enlarged. Electrophysiologic investigation reveals that motor conduction velocity is normal or only slightly reduced, and sensory action potentials and conduction velocity are normal. It is best considered with the hereditary spinal muscular atrophies (p. 87).

HMSN type III is a recessively inherited disorder that is progressive from its onset in infancy or childhood. Sometimes referred to as Dejerine-Sottas disease, it is characterized by a motor and sensory polyneuropathy with weakness, impaired gait, sensory loss, and depressed or absent tendon reflexes. There may also be sensory ataxia. The peripheral nerves may be palpably enlarged, and histologic examination reveals marked segmental demyelination, onion-bulb formation, and thin myelin sheaths. Electrophysiologically, there is marked slowing of conduction, and sensory

action potentials may be unrecordable. The threshold for electrical stimulation may, however, be very high, and this must be remembered when conduction studies are performed. Cases with a dominant mode of inheritance are also well recognized, and in these, neurologic impairment is less severe and the prognosis is more favorable. Dyck and Lambert have emphasized that they are best classified with neuropathies of the Charcot-Marie-Tooth type.[11]

HMSN type IV, or Refsum's disease, is discussed separately on p. 228. Other types or variants of HMSN have also been described with such associated features as optic atrophy (type VI) or retinitis pigmentosa (type VII). A prednisone-responsive form has also been reported,[18] with nerve conduction velocity and electromyographic findings consistent with segmental demyelination and axonal degeneration. These patients may have had a superimposed chronic relapsing inflammatory demyelinative polyradiculoneuropathy attributable either to chance or to a causal association between the two disorders, or they may merely have had the inherited neuropathy alone. Certainly, however, they had definite features of the hereditary disorder, including pes cavus, and bony abnormalities or asymptomatic neuropathies were found in their relatives.

Hereditary Sensory and Autonomic Neuropathies

The classification of these disorders has recently undergone revision.[19] Type I, which is dominantly inherited, usually has its onset in the second decade. There is impaired appreciation of pain and temperature distally in the limbs, plantar ulcers may be present, and spontaneous pain is often especially troublesome. Motor involvement may occur, with pes cavus and muscle atrophy, but is usually mild. Maximal motor conduction velocity is generally within or only just below the normal range, whereas sensory action potentials are small or unrecordable. There may be evidence of chronic partial denervation distally in the legs.

Type II is recessively inherited and is associated with impairment of all sensory modalities. The disturbance is usually present from birth or early infancy, and is associated with mutilating acropathy and reduced or absent tendon reflexes. The electrophysiologic findings may include signs of chronic partial denervation in distal muscles, normal or only slightly reduced motor conduction velocity, and absent sensory action potentials.

Type III, the so-called Riley-Day syndrome, is recessively inherited and is characterized by feeding difficulties in infancy, recurrent pulmonary infections, impaired lacrimation, hypotension and hypertension, abnormalities of sweating, areflexia, and impaired response to painful stimuli. There is a loss of unmyelinated and small myelinated fibers from the peripheral nerves. Motor conduction velocity may be slightly reduced and sensory action potentials are small or absent.[20]

Types IV and V hereditary sensory and autonomic neuropathies have also been described, as have other variants, but these are so rare that they merit no description here. Rather, the reader is referred to the comprehensive account provided by Dyck.[19]

Susceptibility to Pressure Palsies

Hereditary neuropathy with a susceptibility to pressure palsies seems to be inherited as an autosomal dominant trait with total penetrance but variable expression.[21,22] It has been described in a number of different families since the first English-language report in 1954 by Davies,[23] and occurs at any age from the first to the seventh decade.

Earl and co-workers described in detail the clinical features of the disorder in members of four families in whom the peripheral nerves were particularly susceptible to pressure or traction.[24] Many family members gave a history suggestive of recurrent, transient, peripheral nerve lesions, and persistent palsies developed in some of them. Nerve conduction studies not only provided evidence of abnormal function in peripheral nerves that had been clinically involved, but also in some that had not, and similar changes were found in clinically unaffected family members as well. Measurement of nerve action potentials seemed much more sensitive than measurement of motor conduction velocity for detecting slight abnormalities of peripheral nerve function and was, therefore, thought to be particularly valuable in genetic studies. In another noteworthy and more recent report, 19 of 87 family members in four generations were affected.[21]

Histopathologic studies may reveal tomaculous neuropathy (i.e., randomly distributed, focal thickenings of the myelin sheaths with apparent compression and flattening of axons at such sites). Moreover, there may be extensive demyelination with remyelination,[25] abnormal distribution in the diameter of myelinated fibers,[26] and onion-bulb formations.[25]

Clinical presentation is typically with an isolated mononeuropathy or a mononeuropathy multiplex of variable severity, occurring after mild compression or traction of the nerves. The median, ulnar, radial, and peroneal nerves are commonly affected, whereas the cranial nerves are only infrequently involved. Symptoms may disappear after weeks or months, but neurologic abnormalities may persist in patients who have had frequent episodes. The relationship of this syndrome to hereditary susceptibility to plexopathies (p. 280) is controversial, but in both disorders the morphologic findings may be similar, with tomaculae in the nerves.[25]

Leukodystrophies

METACHROMATIC LEUKODYSTROPHY

Several distinct types of metachromatic leukodystrophy, an inherited sphingolipid storage disease, have been described, classified according to age at onset, clinical features, and course of the disorder. Generally, demyelination occurs in the central and peripheral nervous systems. The most common type of the disorder is inherited as an autosomal recessive trait and becomes clinically manifest between 1 and 4 years of age. Signs include impaired motor activity, followed by mental regression and then by ataxia, weakness, dysarthria, dysphagia, optic atrophy, and other deficits. Patients eventually become demented, quadriplegic, and speechless before death supervenes.

Peripheral nerve dysfunction is manifest initially by depressed tendon reflexes. Nerve conduction studies may reveal a marked reduction in motor[27] or sensory conduction velocity,[28] and the size of the compound muscle action potentials and sensory action potentials may be reduced.[27,28] Thus, in patients with a central nervous system degenerative disorder, nerve conduction studies may help in the differential diagnosis of leukodystrophy. In some patients, however, motor and sensory conduction studies are normal. When the disorder develops at a somewhat late age, electrophysiologic studies may also show a reduced motor conduction velocity, small compound muscle action potentials, and unrecordable nerve action potentials.[29] Electrophysiologic abnormalities may also occur in the absence of clinical abnormalities.[29,30]

GLOBOID CELL LEUKODYSTROPHY

Globoid cell leukodystrophy, or Krabbe's disease, is another degenerative central nervous system disorder that affects the peripheral nerves. It has an autosomal recessive mode of inheritance, and usually is manifested clinically in the first 6 months of postnatal life by a regression of motor activity, generalized rigidity, pyramidal signs, and mental deterioration. Seizures and tonic spasms may occur. The end stage is characterized by blindness, deafness, irritability, and profound mental withdrawal, and is followed by death, usually before 2 years of age. Peripheral nerve involvement may be manifested by depressed or absent tendon reflexes, but in other patients there are hyperactive tendon reflexes because of the central nervous system pathology. Nevertheless, maximal motor conduction velocity is often reduced, although to a variable degree in different patients, and sensory conduction velocities may also be reduced or distal sensory latencies prolonged.[31] Thus, the electrophysiologic findings may be helpful in identifying the peripheral nerve dysfunction, although in some cases the findings may be normal.[32] Electrophysiologic abnormalities may be present in asymptomatic subjects, and have been reported in patients as young as 7 weeks of age.[33]

ADRENOLEUKODYSTROPHY

Adrenoleukodystrophy has a sex-linked male inheritance, and is characterized by the occurrence of Addison's disease, progressive mental deterioration, quadriparesis, dysarthria, dysphagia, and a pseudobulbar syndrome, leading ultimately to a decerebrate state before death finally occurs. Cortical blindness is sometimes a feature, and increasing skin pigmentation is characteristic. In some patients, there is neurogenic atrophy and depressed tendon reflexes. Nerve conduction studies may be normal or may show a reduction in motor and sensory conduction velocity, and somatosensory evoked potentials recorded over the scalp may be delayed and of abnormal morphology.[34]

Spinocerebellar Degenerations

FRIEDREICH'S ATAXIA

Friedreich's ataxia is usually inherited in an autosomal recessive manner, and patients generally present in childhood or early adult life. The development of an ataxic gait is followed by clumsiness of the hands and other signs of cerebellar dysfunction. Involvement of the corticospinal fibers leads to weakness of the legs and extensor plantar responses, whereas involvement of the peripheral sensory fibers leads to sensory disturbances in the limbs and depressed or absent tendon reflexes. Pes cavus is also present. On pathologic examination, posterior root fibers and sensory fibers in the peripheral nerves are found to have degenerated and there is marked loss of cells in the posterior root ganglia. Changes also occur in the CNS, being most conspicuous in the posterior and lateral columns of the cord, but description of such changes is beyond the scope of this book.

There may be a marked discrepancy between the clinical state and the severity of the electrophysiologic findings. Dyck and Lambert found that the most impressive electrophysiologic abnormality in 12 patients was sensory action potentials that were either absent or grossly reduced in amplitude when recorded at the wrist after stimulation of digital nerve fibers.[12] Conduction velocity in motor fibers was normal or only mildly reduced. The findings in several other studies were similar.[35,36]

OTHER SPINOCEREBELLAR DEGENERATIONS

The peripheral nerve changes that occur in the other spinocerebellar degenerations have received less attention. In one study of 19 patients with either olivopontocerebellar atrophy or cerebello-olivary degeneration, motor and sensory conduction studies were within normal limits in 10. In six other patients, there was mild slowing of motor conduction in at least one nerve, and in three, there was impaired sensory conduction.[37] In three of five patients undergoing sural nerve biopsy, there was a reduction in density of myelinated fibers of all sizes. However, the electrophysiologic and pathologic findings were less marked than in Friedreich's ataxia.

In patients with familial spastic paraplegia who are younger than 40 years of age, normal motor and sensory conduction studies have been reported.[38] However, in other instances, a reduction in amplitude of the sural sensory action potential has been described.[19]

Porphyria

Peripheral nerve involvement may occur clinically during acute attacks in both variegate porphyria and acute intermittent porphyria. Motor symptoms usually precede sensory ones, with weakness often being more pronounced proximally than distally and in the upper limbs rather than the lower. There may also be facial weakness and a bulbar palsy. Similarly, sensory symptoms and signs may be predominantly proximal in distribution, but in other cases they occur in the extremities.[39] Symptoms may occur during discrete paralytic episodes that are often precipitated by drugs, such as barbiturates. Attacks may be associated with psychiatric disturbances and abdominal pain.

Signs of denervation are found if the affected muscles are sampled with a needle electrode, but nerve conduction velocity is normal.[40–42] Albers and co-workers described the electrophysiologic findings in eight patients with an episode of acute quadriparesis.[43] There was evidence, on needle examination, of partial denervation, especially in the proximal muscles, with reduced recruitment of motor units and profuse, spontaneous fibrillation potentials. With time, the motor unit potentials tended to become polyphasic and their amplitude and duration increased. Some compound muscle action potentials were small, but motor conduction velocity was normal; sensory conduction velocity was also normal, but sensory action potentials were sometimes small or absent. The electrophysiologic findings are thus in keeping with the results of neuropathologic studies that suggest that the neuropathy is of the axonal type, with more selective involvement of motor fibers than of sensory ones.[44]

Miscellaneous Hereditary Disorders

ABETALIPOPROTEINEMIA (Bassen-Kornzweig Syndrome)

Abetalipoproteinemia is an autosomal recessive disorder characterized by the absence of betalipoproteins and low levels of cholesterol in the serum, accompanied by acanthocytosis, malabsorption in infancy, retarded growth, and a neurologic disorder manifested by ataxia and peripheral neuropathy. Electrophysiologic studies typically show signs of chronic partial denervation in the distal limb muscles, a normal conduction velocity, and small or absent sensory action potentials[45] that are consistent with an axonal large-fiber neuropathy, although weakness has sometimes been ascribed to myopathy.[46]

FABRY'S DISEASE

Fabry's disease is inherited as a sex-linked recessive trait and is caused by α-galactosidase A deficiency. Clinical manifestations include a skin rash, cerebral and cardiac ischemic complications, renal failure, and a neurologic disorder characterized predominantly by burning pain in the limbs, which is often stabbing in character. Pathologic studies demonstrate a loss of small myelinated and unmyelinated fibers in the peripheral nerves. Electrophysiologic studies sometimes reveal a reduced motor conduction velocity and increased terminal motor latency, but abnormalities may only be found in some of the nerves that are tested.[47] In other instances, nerve conduction studies are normal.[47,48]

NIEMANN-PICK DISEASE

Peripheral neuropathy occasionally occurs in some types of Niemann-Pick disease. Electrophysiologically, there may be evidence of denervation and a reduced conduction velocity in the peripheral nerves.

REFSUM'S DISEASE

Refsum's disease is inherited in an autosomal recessive manner and is caused by a disturbance in the metabolism of phytanic acid that produces an increase in the level of phytanic acid in the blood.[49] Clinical onset usually occurs in late childhood or adolescence. The disease is characterized by pigmentary retinal degeneration; symmetric, progressive motor and sensory polyneuropathy; and a cerebellar syndrome. Auditory dysfunction, cardiomyopathy, and ichthyotic skin changes may also occur, as may anosmia, pupillary abnormalities, and cataracts.

The peripheral nerves may be palpably enlarged. On histopathologic examination, there is a loss of myelinated axons and segmental demyelination. Electrophysiologic studies reveal that motor and sensory conduction velocity is often markedly reduced and sensory action potentials are frequently lost; there may also be electromyographic evidence of denervation in affected muscles.[50] Dietary treatment may lead to clinical and electrophysiologic improvement.[51]

TANGIER DISEASE

Tangier disease is inherited as a recessive trait, and is characterized by a near absence of high-density lipoproteins and their major protein constituents, apolipoproteins.[52,53] A reportedly consistent clinical finding is enlarged, yellowish tonsils secondary to storage of cholesterol esters. More than half of the reported cases have peripheral nerve involvement, which may take the form of a relapsing and remitting mononeuropathy multiplex[52] or a pseudosyringomyelic syndrome with selective loss of pain and temperature appreciation.[52–54] In either case, there may be neurogenic weakness, and electromyographic sampling may show signs of chronic partial denervation in affected muscles. Maximal motor or sensory conduction velocity may be mildly reduced when there is mononeuropathy multiplex, but sensory nerve action potentials usually are normal; the findings are consistent with the primary pathology being demyelinative. By contrast, in the pseudosyringomyelic form, maximal nerve conduction velocities may be normal or reduced only slightly, which is consistent with selective involvement of small myelinated and unmyelinated fibers, and sensory nerve action potentials are small or absent (reflecting axonal loss).

METABOLIC DISORDERS

Uremia

Diseases causing renal failure, such as diabetes, amyloidosis, multiple myeloma, or the vasculitides, may lead to peripheral nerve dysfunction with features typical of the primary pathology. Furthermore, peripheral neuropathy may relate to medication (such as nitrofurantoin) in patients with kidney disease. In such instances, and especially in patients with diabetic nephropathy, it is generally impossible to determine on electrophysiologic grounds whether the diabetes or uremia is primarily responsible for the peripheral nerve dysfunction. The first clear description of the neuropathy that occurs in patients with chronic renal failure was provided by Asbury and co-workers,[55] and it is now widely recognized that motor conduction velocity may be slightly reduced in such patients even if clinical signs of neuropathy are absent.[56]

On clinical grounds, the peripheral nerve disorder is characterized by a symmetric, sensorimotor polyneuropathy that tends to affect the lower limbs more than the upper limbs and that is more marked distally than proximally. The pathologic basis of this neuropathy has been the subject of some controversy. Axonal degeneration seems to be the most conspicuous feature,[55,57] with some demyelinative changes occurring perhaps as a secondary phenomenon, but some authors have been more impressed by the segmental demyelination that occurs.[58] Associated syndromes include muscle cramps, restless legs, and burning feet.

Motor and sensory conduction velocity is moderately reduced, and the sensory action potentials may be dispersed, but electromyographic evidence of denervation in the distal muscles is usually inconspicuous except in advanced cases. Nevertheless, quantitative studies of the changes in motor unit potential parameters and a reduction in the number of functioning motor units support the diagnosis of a distal axonal neuropathy, accompanied by a relatively impaired capacity for collateral reinnervation and compensatory increase in size of surviving motor units.[59]

Jebsen and associates found that the extent of any disturbance in peripheral nerve function is related to the severity of impaired renal function.[60] A single dialysis session has no significant effect on conduction velocity.[60] The neuropathy may improve clinically but shows little change electrophysiologically with prolonged dialysis.[61] Moreover, the neuropathy may worsen despite continuing hemodialysis,[62] and a large proportion of patients undergoing hemodialysis who have no clinical evidence of neuropathy are found to have a mild neuropathy when studied electrophysiologically.[63]

With renal transplantation, the neuropathy may markedly improve.[64,65] Improvement, attributed to remyelination, has been reported over many months, depending on the severity of the neuropathy.[66] In other instances, improvement has been described as occurring in two stages, an early rapid phase within a few weeks, and a later, more prolonged improvement over a number of months. Recovery tends to be more rapid and complete in distal nerve segments than in proximal ones.[65] However, in patients receiving transplants from either cadavers or related living donors, Oh and co-workers found that motor and sensory conduction velocities improved rapidly, usually within a few days, and that the improvement in sensory conduction velocity in the median nerve showed a negative linear correlation with the acute metabolic alterations that follow renal transplantation, especially the decline in serum creatinine and myoinositol concentrations.[67] They therefore suggested that metabolic alterations, especially in myoinositol, may be related to the decreased conduction velocities associated with uremic polyneuropathy.

F wave studies may also be helpful in evaluating peripheral nerve dysfunction in patients with uremia. Abnormalities may sometimes be found at an earlier stage with such methods than with conduction studies of distal segments of nerves.[68]

The carpal tunnel syndrome has also been described in patients with renal disease. In particular, it may occur distal to arteriovenous fistulae placed in the forearm for access during hemodialysis,[69] possibly because of nerve ischemia induced by a vascular steal mechanism. Other compressive or entrapment neuropathies, such as ulnar nerve lesions at the elbow, may occur in bedridden patients.

Other abnormalities in the peripheral nerves have been reported to occur with chronic renal failure. First, a reversible membrane abnormality that may result in a decreased resting membrane potential has been described[70] and is thought to be responsible for extension of the refractory period and an impairment of repetitive impulse conduction. Second, there may be a resistance of the nerves to ischemia so that, during 30 minutes of sustained ischemia of the limbs, the nerve action potential persists for longer than in normal subjects, sometimes persisting to the end of the test.[71]

Diabetes Mellitus

Involvement of the peripheral nervous system in diabetes may be manifested clinically by a symmetric sensory, motor, or mixed polyneuropathy, an asymmetric motor neuropathy, an autonomic neuropathy, a polyradiculopathy, or by isolated lesions of individual nerves. These manifestations occur either singly or in combination with each other. Their incidence may be influenced by the duration, severity, and adequacy of control of the diabetes, but discussion of their pathogenesis is beyond the scope of this text.

The primary pathologic change in diabetic neuropathy appears to be axonal degeneration,[72] so that even at an early stage there may be fibrillation potentials in affected muscles, as well as small sensory action potentials. In general, the size of the compound muscle action potential is affected only later. Not suprisingly, maximal motor or sensory conduction velocity, as measured in the clinical neurophysiology laboratory, may be normal or reduced only slightly as a result of degeneration of the fastest-conducting fibers (as emphasized in Chapter 7, where the differences between axonal and demyelinative neuropathies were stressed). However, nerve conduction studies sometimes show that velocities are slowed to a greater degree than can be accounted for by axonal loss, and this slowing has been attributed to segmental demyelination.[73] Conspicuous segmental demyelination is found in some diabetic nerves,[74] and although the relationship of this to axonal loss is unclear, Sugimura and Dyck believe that, in some cases, it is not a secondary response but a selective abnormality of the Schwann cells.[75]

A *distal sensory or mixed polyneuropathy* is the most common manifestation of diabetic neuropathy. It may be asymptomatic, with the diagnosis being made on the basis of depressed tendon reflexes and impaired appreciation of vibration in the legs. Clinical onset sometimes appears to relate either to an exacerbation of the diabetes or, curiously, to the initiation of treatment with hypoglycemic agents, but the mechanisms involved are unclear and the relationship may be fortuitous. Symptoms, which occur more frequently in the lower limbs than in the upper limbs, consist of pain, paresthesias, or numbness, or all three. In severe cases, distal sensory loss occurs in all limbs, and motor deficits are evident. In some instances, sensory loss involves predominantly the appreciation of pain and temperature, and leads to distal ulceration and neuropathic joint degeneration. In other cases, postural loss is so severe that there is marked sensory ataxia. Autonomic symptoms also occur and are sometimes conspicuous, especially in patients with the pseudosyringomyelic form of neuropathy.

In general, the electrophysiologic findings correlate with the particular clinical features of individual cases. In five patients with a predominantly sensory neuropathy affecting the legs, Gilliatt and Willison reported that the most consistent finding was reduction or loss of peroneal nerve action potentials, with motor conduction velocity being less constantly affected.[76] In two patients with a mixed motor and sensory neuropathy, they found that motor conduction velocity was markedly reduced, and in five patients with isolated peripheral nerve lesions, electrophysiologic abnormalities were confined to the clinically affected nerves.

Abnormalities of sensory[77] or motor[78,79] conduction may be found in diabetics without clinical evidence of neuropathy. In their study of 30 patients with diabetic neuropathy, Lamontagne and Buchthal examined sensory conduction in the median nerve, as well as motor conduction in this nerve and in the common peroneal nerve.[80] They found that the most sensitive indicator of subclinical neuropathy was involvement of sensory fibers. Abnormalities were present in 24 patients, 12 of whom had no sensory symptoms or signs and 5 of whom had no other evidence of neuropathy in the arms. All patients with slowed conduction in motor fibers also had disturbances of sensory conduction, consisting of a reduced conduction velocity and abnormalities in the amplitude and shape of the sensory action potential. Motor conduction velocity was reduced in some patients who had no clinical evidence of motor involvement and, in general, was more pronounced distally than proximally. A correlation was found between the degree to which motor conduction was slowed in the common peroneal nerve and the clinical severity of the neuropathy. Electromyographic sampling of muscles frequently revealed evidence of denervation, with such changes occurring more frequently in distal than in proximal muscles, and in the lower limb than in the upper limb.

In diabetics, the peripheral nerves exhibit a greater resistance to ischemia than do the nerves of normal persons, as has also been described in uremic patients and those with certain other conditions (p. 230). The significance of this finding is not clear.

Several problems arise when electrophysiologic techniques are used to screen for peripheral nerve involvement in diabetes. First, sensory action potentials tend to decline in size with advancing age, regardless of whether the patient is diabetic. Second, it is not uncommon to find evidence of abnormal spontaneous activity, suggestive of denervation, on needle examination of the intrinsic foot muscles of asymptomatic, apparently healthy subjects.[81–83] Third, the electrophysiologic changes may be so mild that they remain within the bounds of normality for individual subjects; minor abnormalities may only become apparent when data from a group of diabetic subjects are compared to data from a group of normal persons. As with all clinical and electrophysiologic work, no single factor may be relied upon in reaching a final conclusion; rather, diagnosis must be based on the total clinical and electrophysiologic context.

Some laboratories have recently been involved in electrophysiologic studies performed to monitor changes in peripheral nerve function among patients undergoing experimental forms of treatment for diabetes. The validity of such an approach is not established, the clinical relevance of any changes that occur is unclear, and not all populations of fibers comprising the nerve are evaluated by the electrophysiologic techniques in current use.

The concept of *diabetic amyotrophy* is both controversial and confusing. It is defined differently by different authors. For example, some have stressed the rapidity of its onset, whereas others have emphasized its insidiousness; both symmetry and asymmetry of clinical deficit have been held to be typical; and the presence of pain or other sensory disturbance is regarded as characteristic by some but not by others.

Asbury, in an eloquent editorial, pleaded for the term to be discarded, believing that diabetic amyotrophy is neither a distinct clinical syndrome nor a well-defined term.[84] It now seems likely that the motor deficit labeled by this term is a reflection of diabetic polyradiculopathy, which is discussed below. Brown and Asbury have distinguished between symmetric and asymmetric forms of diabetic "proximal motor neuronopathy," and have attributed a different pathologic basis to them, but the validity of this is unclear.[72]

The clinical manifestations of *diabetic polyradiculoneuropathy* have been reported by Bastron and Thomas.[85] In most cases, this disorder becomes manifest as an asymmetric thoracolumbar polyradiculopathy with pain and unilateral weakness of the thigh, often accompanied by weight loss. These researchers believed that the same syndrome had been subsumed by such terms as diabetic amyotrophy, lumbar plexopathy, mononeuropathy multiplex, femoral neuropathy, neuropathic cachexia, and diabetic myopathy. Among 105 diabetic patients who had undergone neurologic examination and comprehensive electrophysiologic studies leading to a diagnosis of polyradiculopathy, the most common initial symptom was pain, followed by dysesthesia and weakness. The most common sites of involvement with the presenting symptom were the chest wall, abdomen, or back (in 42 patients); the anterior thigh or leg (in 41 patients); the buttocks, posterior thigh, or calf (in 7 patients); the foot (in 9 patients); and the entire leg (in 6 patients). Unilateral onset, whether as pain or weakness, occurred in three out of every four patients. The disorder often advanced by spreading from its localized site of onset. On examination, weakness was present in 84 patients, and was bilateral but asymmetric in 59. Often, it was clearly myotomal in distribution, but sometimes it was more focal. Sensation was impaired in 85 patients, but this impairment was usually mild and often peripheral, suggesting an associated polyneuropathy. In fact, in 80 of the 105 patients (76 percent), there was evidence of either clinical or subclinical polyneuropathy, in addition to the polyradiculopathy. Follow-up information was limited, but most patients seemed to improve after a period of several months, and some recovered completely.

The electrophysiologic findings were of some interest. All patients with polyradiculopathy had abnormalities in the paraspinal muscles on needle examination, with increased insertion activity and abnormal spontaneous activity often being found in multiple areas bilaterally. There was a common discrepancy between the profusion of spontaneous activity in the paraspinal muscles and the relative paucity of similar activity in the limbs. There was no reliable means of predicting whether the disease would remain confined to a few adjacent nerve roots or become increasingly widespread and disabling.[85]

Although a polyradiculopathy seems to be the most unifying and satisfactory explanation currently available for "diabetic amyotrophy," it has not met with universal acceptance, and need not be the sole basis for the syndrome. Hypothetical alternatives will continue to be advanced until detailed autopsy studies settle the issue. In a published study of one patient, small infarcts were found in proximal major nerve trunks of the leg, the left lumbosacral plexus (the more symptomatic side), and the L5 root, but the extent to which the other nerve roots were examined pathologically remains unclear.[86]

In distinguishing proximal neurogenic atrophy secondary to polyradiculopathy from other disorders that may simulate it clinically, electrophysiologic techniques have an important role. In patients with diabetic amyotrophy, conduction time in the femoral nerve may be prolonged[80,87,88] and the size of the compound muscle action potential of the rectus femoris, as elicited by

nerve stimulation, may be reduced,[88] but the distribution of abnormalities revealed at needle electromyography is clearly more extensive than just femoral nerve involvement. With a focal plexus lesion, the paraspinal muscles are spared and the limb changes are unilateral; these findings were encountered in several of the patients studied by Subramony and Wilbourn.[88] The selective distribution of changes found at needle electromyography is helpful in excluding proximal myopathies accompanied by conspicuous, abnormal, spontaneous activity, such as polymyositis. A degenerative disorder, like amyotrophic lateral sclerosis or progressive spinal muscular atrophy, should not be diagnosed on electrophysiologic grounds unless there is evidence of denervation that cannot be accounted for by a lesion at a single major level of the central nervous system.

In the last few years, several papers have outlined the clinical and electrophysiologic features of diabetic *thoracoabdominal radiculopathy*.[89–91] Patients typically present with severe chest or abdominal pain that may not be radicular in character, and with dysesthesias. Sensory abnormalities may be present over the trunk on clinical examination. Weakness may also be present, but is harder to evaluate. The findings on electrophysiologic needle examination of the paraspinal muscles are generally abnormal, and abnormalities may also be present in the abdominal or intercostal muscles if these are examined. (Although I have recorded from the intercostal muscles using needle electrodes without any complications, the procedure is not without risk.) The electrophysiologic changes may be wider in distribution than is the pain. Some patients may also have evidence of a concurrent diabetic polyneuropathy or entrapment neuropathy.

The possibility of diabetic thoracoabdominal radiculopathy is not excluded if needle electromyography fails to reveal any abnormalities. Abnormalities may be sparse and, if an appreciable interval of time has elapsed since clinical onset of the disorder, reinnervation may result in the disappearance of spontaneous activity.

Diabetic truncal polyneuropathy, characterized clinically by sensory deficits in the distribution of the thoracic intercostal nerves, occurs in patients with rostrally advancing, distal polyneuropathy involving the limbs. The sensory loss is relatively symmetric and involves multiple thoracic dermatomes starting close to the midline anteriorly. Waxman and Sabin recently emphasized that this disorder is distinct from the truncal thoracoabdominal radiculopathies just described, and that its occurrence is not limited to diabetes; it may also occur, for example, in nutritional polyneuropathies, in the polyneuropathy of dominantly inherited amyloidosis, and in hereditary sensory neuropathy.[92] Its recognition in diabetes may be aided by its frequent association with autonomic neuropathy.

A variety of *simple mononeuropathies* may occur in patients with diabetes. Common cranial neuropathies involve the third, fourth, sixth, or seventh nerve, and the fifth nerve may also be affected, as evidenced by blink reflex studies.[93] The study of the facial nerve is considered separately in Chapter 12. Patients with diabetes (or other systemic disorders affecting peripheral nerve function) seem more likely than normal persons to develop *entrapment neuropathies* (p. 119). In addition, an acute mononeuropathy may occur due to *infarction*; it is often accompanied by pain, is associated with a poorer prognosis than entrapment neuropathy, and does not require decompressive surgery. The electrophysiologic findings in diabetic patients with focal mononeuropathies do not differ significantly from those in nondiabetic patients with similar mononeuropathies, and the reader is, therefore, referred to Chapters 9 and 10 for a discussion of the findings in the individual nerves. However, evaluation may be complicated by the co-existence or superimposition of other peripheral nerve complications of diabetes.

Diabetes is a common cause for *mononeuropathy multiplex,* which usually has a vascular basis. Accordingly, the electrophysiologic findings generally reflect axonal degeneration. In patients with *autonomic neuropathy*, disorders of vasomotor, sudomotor, gastrointestinal, sphincter, or sexual function may occur, and abnormal pupillary responses may be evident. The investigation of autonomic function is discussed in detail in Chapter 15 and elsewhere.[94]

Hypoglycemic Neuropathy or Neuronopathy

Motor symptoms, sensory symptoms, or both may occur distally in the extremities, sometimes predominantly in the arms, in patients with profound or episodic hypoglycemia, but whether the site of pathology is the peripheral nerves or the spinal cord is unclear.[95–98] The precise etiology of the disorder is also uncertain, but it is generally related to the presence of an insulin-producing tumor rather than to the taking of hypoglycemic agents for the treatment of diabetes. Depending on the time of the study, electromyography may reveal signs of denervation (and subsequently, of reinnervation) distally in the limbs, with little change in motor and sensory conduction velocities.

Alcoholism and Nutritional Deficiency

Symptoms of alcoholic peripheral neuropathy were first recognized more than 200 years ago, but the precise pathogenesis is unclear. Some authors have suggested that the disorder relates to nutritional deficiency, especially of vitamins, but Behse and Buchthal found no evidence of malnutrition, hepatic dysfunction, or reduced blood levels of vitamins B_1, B_6, or B_{12} in a number of their patients, and suggested instead that a direct toxic effect of the alcohol was the cause.[99] The disorder is characterized by distal sensorimotor neuropathy which is frequently accompanied by painful cramps, muscle tenderness, and painful paresthesias, and which is often more pronounced in the legs than in the arms. The main pathologic feature of the disorder is axonal degeneration.[99] Electrophysiologic investigation reveals that motor and sensory conduction velocity may be mildly reduced, even when clinical evidence of peripheral nerve involvement is lacking,[99–101] but marked slowing of conduction is uncommon. The amplitude of the sensory or compound muscle action potentials may also be reduced,[99,101] and this may be the sole abnormality. Casey and LeQuesne used an elegant technique to measure sensory conduction between the tip and base of the middle finger, and between the base of this finger and the wrist in alcoholic subjects.[102] An abnormality in the amplitude of the potentials recorded at the base of the finger was found in 7 of 16 subjects, but only one patient had an abnormality in the potential elicited at the wrist. This technique enabled them to obtain evidence of peripheral nerve involvement when routine investigative procedures revealed no abnormality, and to demonstrate the distal nature of the lesion.

Needle electromyography generally shows evidence of denervation with some reinnervation, especially in the distal muscles of the legs, even if there is no clinical evidence of motor impairment.[99] Proximal muscle weakness and muscle wasting is seen in some alcoholic patients and has sometimes been attributed to myopathy.

The prognosis of alcoholic peripheral neuropathy was studied by Hillbom and Wennberg, who found that 7 of 10 patients—all of whom had managed to stop drinking alcohol—showed almost complete clinical and electrophysiologic recovery from their polyneuropathy over a 3- to 5-year period.[103] Others have found the outlook to be much gloomier, even among patients eating a nutritious diet and abstaining from alcohol.[99]

Peripheral nerve involvement may occur in patients with nutritional deficiencies of various sorts. A sensorimotor polyneuropathy, which is more marked distally than proximally and is more pronounced in the legs than in the arms, is a well-recognized feature of beriberi and is similar to the neuropathy that occurs in alcoholism.

Neuropathy after gastrectomy-induced malnutrition is clinically similar to alcoholic neuropathy, but Behse and Buchthal found motor and sensory conduction velocities to be markedly slowed in the legs, and segmental demyelination was evident on pathologic examination of biopsy specimens.[99] The degree of conduction slowing in such patients was greater than in patients with severe alcoholic neuropathy.

In vitamin B_{12} deficiency, a distal sensory neuropathy may develop, characterized electrophysiologically by a mild, distal slowing of sensory conduction that may revert to normal with treatment.[104] Sensory action potentials are often small or unrecordable. Nerve conduction studies and sural nerve biopsy were performed by McCombe and McLeod in three patients with pernicious anemia and symptoms of peripheral neuropathy, and both studies suggested that the underlying pathology was axonal degeneration.[105] In one study, 13 of 20 patients (65 percent) with untreated pernicious anemia showed signs of peripheral nerve dysfunction with reduced conduction velocities.[106] Somatosensory and other modality evoked potential studies may also be abnormal in vitamin B_{12} deficiency.

Vitamin E deficiency may occur in patients with malabsorption syndrome, and leads to a neurologic disorder characterized by dysarthria, cerebellar ataxia, and peripheral neuropathy with proprioceptive loss and reduced or absent tendon reflexes. Motor and sensory conduction velocity may be normal, but sensory action potentials are sometimes small or absent. Somatosensory evoked potential studies may also be abnormal, suggesting dysfunction of the posterior columns.[107]

Hepatic Disease

A sensory neuropathy may occur with primary biliary cirrhosis.[108,109] Although motor conduction studies may show no abnormality, sensory or nerve action potentials are small or absent, suggesting that the neuropathy is of the axonal type with selective involvement of sensory fibers.

A polyneuropathy which is predominantly demyelinative in type may also occur in patients with chronic liver disease.[110-112] Detailed studies by Kardel and Nielsen of patients with hepatic neuropathy showed no correlation between neurologic findings and the results of liver function tests or measures of the functioning liver mass,[113] and neurologic findings occurred with the same frequency in patients with or without chronic alcoholism or a diabetic glucose tolerance test. Electrophysiologically, there were small dispersed sensory action potentials, and a mild reduction in sensory conduction velocity.

Endocrinopathies

Median nerve compression may occur at the wrist in patients with hypothyroidism.[114,115] Symptoms may be bilateral, and clinical and electrophysiologic improvement often occurs with treatment of the underlying thyroid disorder. Less commonly, a sensory–motor polyneuropathy occurs with hypothyroidism and is sometimes its presenting feature. It is characterized by slowing of motor conduction velocity and

loss or reduction in amplitude of sensory action potentials.[116,117] The neuropathy has been ascribed to axonal degeneration,[117] but segmental demyelination has also been implicated.[116] In patients with acromegaly, bilateral carpal tunnel syndrome[118] or a mild motor and sensory polyneuropathy may also occur,[119] with the latter being characterized by mildly reduced motor conduction velocity and small sensory action potentials.

INFECTIOUS AND INFLAMMATORY NEUROPATHIES

Leprosy

Leprosy is extremely common in some parts of the world, and its peripheral nerve aspects are important. The short clinical account given here is based largely on the recent review by Sabin and Swift.[120] In this disease, sensory disturbances precede motor deficits and are mainly due to involvement of intracutaneous nerves. In tuberculoid leprosy, these disturbances develop at the same time and in the same distribution as the skin lesion, but they may be more extensive if nerve trunks lying beneath the lesion are also involved. Sensory loss is more widespread in lepromatous leprosy, and seems to develop earlier and to a greater extent in the coolest regions of the body, such as the dorsal surfaces of the hands and feet, where the bacilli proliferate most actively. Motor deficits result from the involvement of nerves in sites where they run superficially, and therefore, where their temperature is lowest. In the arms, the ulnar nerve is usually affected first, with involvement being most pronounced in the region proximal to the olecranon groove, where the nerve is superficial. The median nerve may be affected, particularly that segment of it which emerges from beneath the forearm flexor muscle to run toward the carpal tunnel, and in some cases the motor fibers of the radial nerve are involved just above the elbow. Motor disturbances occur in the legs as a result of involvement of the peroneal nerve at the head of the fibula and the posterior tibial nerve in the lower part of the leg, and patchy facial weakness may result from involvement of the superficial branches of the seventh cranial nerve.

Motor disturbances in leprosy are confined to the distribution of the individual peripheral nerves that are affected, and are thus suggestive of a multiple mononeuropathy. The distribution of the sensory changes simulates that of a distal polyneuropathy, but careful assessment reveals that it corresponds instead to the temperature of the tissues. In the legs, for example, the area between the toes and in the popliteal fossae, where the temperature is higher, is often spared. A superadded sensory deficit may, however, be present as a result of involvement of the main nerve trunks.

Electromyographic examination of paretic muscles usually provides evidence of denervation in all forms of leprosy. Verghese and co-workers examined motor conduction velocity in the median and ulnar nerves in a large series of patients.[121] They found marked slowing in a large number of patients with clinical evidence of nerve involvement (that is, thickening or tenderness of the nerve, or muscle weakness), regardless of the type of leprosy they had.[121] Conduction in the ulnar nerve is slowed particularly in the upper arm, whereas in the median nerve, there is marked slowing in the forearm but not in the carpal tunnel or distally. Abnormalities of sensory conduction, such as small or absent sensory action potentials and prolonged conduction times, may also be found in both tuberculoid[122] and lepromatous[123] leprosy. The conduction time of the facial nerve may be increased in patients with facial weakness, and electromyographic signs of denervation are often found in affected muscles.[124] Electrophysiologic abnormalities may improve after appropriate drug treatment of the leprosy.[123]

A detailed account of the neuropathologic findings in leprosy is beyond the scope of this book, but segmental demyelination is probably responsible for the slowing of nerve conduction that occurs.

Acute Acquired Demyelinative Polyradiculoneuropathy (Guillain-Barré syndrome)

Acquired demyelinative neuropathy, or Guillain-Barré syndrome, is an acute, monophasic, immunologically mediated disorder that is diagnosed on clinical, laboratory, and electrophysiologic grounds.[125] Progressive weakness and areflexia are prerequisites for diagnosis. In fact, the most common initial complaint is weakness, often beginning in the legs and ascending to involve the arms and face. Facial weakness occurs in about 50 percent of patients, and is often bilateral. Sensory complaints are also common, consisting usually of distal numbness or paresthesias, but the findings on sensory examination may be relatively inconspicuous. The neurologic deficit is often symmetric. Autonomic disturbances may include hypertension, hypotension, respiratory impairment, cardiac irregularities, and impaired thermoregulatory sweating, and a fatal outcome may result from respiratory failure or cardiac arrhythmias. The neurologic deficit progresses at a variable rate, but most patients are at their worst within 4 weeks, and many reach this point sooner. The deficit then remains stable for days or weeks before recovery begins. Most patients completely recover within weeks or months, and less than 20 percent are left with any permanent deficit. The Miller-Fisher variant of the disease has a temporal course similar to that just described, but is characterized by ophthalmoplegia, ataxia, and areflexia.

Examination of the cerebrospinal fluid reveals characteristic changes. There is a marked increase in protein content, but the cell count is normal. Abnormalities may not, however, be found if the fluid is examined in the first few days, as they develop at varying intervals from disease onset in different patients.

Pathologic examination reveals perivascular inflammatory infiltrates in the peripheral nerves, and segmental demyelination of nerve fibers is seen, accompanied in severe cases by a certain amount of axonal degeneration. These changes may be diffuse or focal, and in the latter case, may be restricted to the proximal or distal segments of the affected nerves. When they occur primarily in the nerve roots or proximal portions of the peripheral nerves, measurement of conduction velocity in more distal segments may reveal no significant abnormality. Accordingly, although nerve conduction studies may help to establish the diagnosis, the diagnosis is not excluded if the electrophysiologic findings are normal.

Motor and sensory conduction velocity is usually reduced, and slowing is sometimes pronounced at common sites of compression or entrapment.[126] In a study of 114 patients, McLeod found abnormalities of motor and sensory conduction in about 90 percent of patients, with the likelihood of detecting abnormalities increasing with the number of nerves studied.[127] Marked slowing of conduction velocity or an abnormally prolonged distal motor latency, consistent with demyelination, was evident in at least one nerve in 50 percent of the patients. Abnormalities of sensory conduction in the median or ulnar nerves, or both, were found in 76 percent of patients by McLeod[127] and in 58 percent of patients studied by Eisen and Humphreys.[128] Commonly, median sensory studies are abnormal, whereas sural studies are normal.[129] In many patients, there is evidence of partial conduction block, with temporal dispersion of muscle or nerve action potentials.

Electromyographic sampling of weak muscles initially shows no abnormality other than a reduced number of motor units under voluntary control. After a variable time (depending on the muscle examined and the site of the nerve lesion), however, abnormal spontaneous activity indicative of denervation may be found. This finding is consistent with pathologic observations that both axonal degeneration and segmental demyelination may occur.

The electrophysiologic findings depend on the time that the examination is performed in relation to the course of the clinical disorder. However, electrophysiologic changes do not necessarily parallel the clinical disorder, and abnormalities may first appear as the patient is clinically improving.[127] Lambert and Mulder found conduction velocity to be normal in 14 percent of the patients they examined during the first 3 weeks of illness, even though the clinical features of these patients were typical of the disease and their cerebrospinal fluids were abnormal.[126] Furthermore, conduction velocity may remain abnormal when clinical recovery is complete and for a considerable time thereafter.[130–132]

Abnormalities are initially more common in motor fibers than in sensory ones; sensory abnormalities, which are often patchy in distribution, become most prominent about 4 weeks or so after onset of disease.[129] Conduction block or small compound muscle action potentials, or both, are more characteristic early findings than is reduced motor conduction velocity, being found in 74 percent of patients within 2 weeks of onset of paralysis in one study.[133] This suggests that conduction block tends to affect slow-conducting motor axons sooner than the fastest-conducting axons,[133] a view which has recently received experimental support.[134] Small compound muscle potentials may relate to primary demyelination and conduction block between the sites of stimulation and recording, or to axonal loss. Demyelination and axonal degeneration may occur in the terminal arborizations of motor axons beyond the site of distal stimulation. Conduction abnormalities commonly begin to resolve about 6 to 10 weeks after onset.[129]

Early in the course of the disorder, when distal sensory conduction studies are likely to be normal, recordings of somatosensory evoked potentials following median nerve stimulation may document conduction delay between Erb's point and the cervical cord.[135] However, in some patients, the findings obtained with this technique are normal.[136] Similarly, F wave latency measurements may detect proximal lesions in motor fibers when conventional nerve conduction studies are normal,[136,137] although the yield is generally disappointing.

The mechanisms that best account for the clinical weakness and sensory loss that accompany the disease are conduction block and, to a lesser extent, axonal loss.[133] Axonal degeneration is, however, the main cause of residual muscle weakness or wasting. Several authors have found a good correlation between the size of the compound muscle action potentials in distal muscles and the subsequent development of denervation or the clinical outcome.[129,133] A prognostic role for electrophysiologic studies was also stressed by Peterson and coworkers.[138] They found that clinical recovery correlated with preservation of the size of the compound muscle action potentials in response to distal stimulation, prolonged distal motor latencies, and lack or scarcity of fibrillation potentials. These electrophysiologic abnormalities permit the outcome of the disease to be predicted with some confidence, presumably because they reflect demyelination rather than axonal degeneration. When the electrophysiologic findings suggest that there has been conspicuous axonal loss (i.e., when there is profuse fibrillation, only slight slowing in maximal conduction velocity, and a marked reduction in size of compound muscle action potentials), clinical recovery is likely to be prolonged, and there may be a severe residual neurologic deficit.[138]

It is of some interest that, in the Miller-Fisher variant of the disease, which was described earlier, nerve conduction studies may also show abnormal conduction in peripheral sensory fibers from initial stages of the disorder.[139]

Treatment of the Guillain-Barré syndrome is supportive, coupled with plasmapheresis in severe cases, especially those of recent onset.[140] Steroids have no role in the management of the disease.

Chronic Inflammatory Demyelinating Polyradiculoneuropathy

Chronic inflammatory demyelinating polyradiculoneuropathy is similar to the Guillain-Barré syndrome except that it shows no improvement within 6 months of onset, and it follows a chronic progressive course, or a course punctuated by relapses.[141,142] The etiology is unknown, but the disorder is often responsive to treatment with steroids and sometimes to plasmapheresis. Cerebrospinal fluid examination reveals findings that resemble those in the Guillain-Barré syndrome. The electrophysiologic findings similarly indicate a demyelinative neuropathy with superimposed axonal degeneration. Sensory action potentials may be absent, whereas a marked slowing of motor conduction velocity, a prolonged distal motor latency, and small, dispersed compound muscle action potentials are present. The electrophysiologic abnormalities may not reflect the severity of clinical involvement, but usually, by the time patients present for evaluation, multifocal conduction block or slowed conduction velocities, or both, are evident.

Sarcoidosis

Multiple cranial nerve palsies, which are often fluctuating and remitting, may occur in sarcoidosis, with the seventh nerve being affected most commonly. Other peripheral nerve disorders that may occur include a multiple mononeuropathy and, less commonly, a symmetric polyneuropathy that may sometimes preferentially affect either motor or sensory fibers. The multiple mononeuropathy may be accompanied by pain, dysesthesias, and sensory loss in large areas of bizarre outline on the trunk,[143] and an erroneous diagnosis of visceral disease is often made initially. Onset and progression may be subacute. The multiple mononeuropathy sometimes coexists with the polyneuropathy. The polyneuropathy may resemble the Guillain-Barré syndrome except that it evolves more slowly and has a more progressive course.[143]

The peripheral nerve complications of sarcoidosis frequently remit spontaneously, but treatment with steroids may hasten recovery and prevent further complications.

Silverstein and Siltzbach reported that conduction velocity was reduced in clinically affected nerves and that electromyographic signs of denervation were present in affected muscles.[144] Slowing of nerve conduction velocity was also found by Wells,[145] and was sometimes of a severity usually ascribed to segmental demyelination, but others have found no reduction, at least in motor conduction velocity.[143] The pathophysiologic basis of the neuropathy awaits adequate delineation.

Rheumatoid Arthritis and Other Collagen-Vascular Diseases

In addition to compressive or entrapment neuropathies, an isolated ischemic mononeuropathy of acute onset, with pain and sensory complaints, followed by weakness, may occur in patients with rheumatoid arthritis. Sometimes, several nerves may be involved by one or another of these mechanisms, so that the clinical picture is of a mononeuropathy multiplex. The electrophysiologic abnormalities resulting from focal nerve lesions were discussed in Chapters 9 and 10, and the only points that need emphasis here are that ischemic lesions may be localized to sites that are not typical of compressive lesions (such as the middle of the upper arm or the midthigh region) and that the findings with ischemic lesions are more suggestive of axonal than demyelinative pathology.

A mild, distal, predominantly sensory neuropathy and a severe, progressive sensorimotor neuropathy can also occur in patients with rheumatoid arthritis. Both of these are predominantly axonal in type, although segmental demyelination also occurs to some extent, and they are probably ischemic in etiology. Electromyographic signs of denervation may be found and sensory action potentials may be unrecordable, but little slowing of conduction occurs except in nerves that are least affected. Thus, motor conduction velocity usually shows little reduction in patients with a sensorimotor neuropathy, but may be markedly slowed in patients who, on clinical grounds, have a purely sensory neuropathy.[146]

Mononeuropathy multiplex or symmetric polyneuropathy, or both, have been described in patients with systemic lupus erythematosus, Churg-Strauss syndrome, polyarteritis, giant cell arteritis, and Wegener's granulomatosis; the recent literature is reviewed elsewhere.[147,148] However, it is often not possible to distinguish in the original published accounts between a mononeuropathy multiplex that is so advanced that a widespread confluent deficit is present, and a symmetric polyneuropathy.

Lyme Disease

Lyme disease, which is carried by ticks, is characterized by cutaneous lesions, arthropathy, and neurologic disturbances, which may include cranial neuropathies, mononeuropathy multiplex, and radiculoneuropathy, as well as signs of central nervous system dysfunction.[147] The neuropathy is sometimes characterized by axonal degeneration, and electrophysiologic findings depend on the nature and severity of the underlying pathology.

TOXIC NEUROPATHIES

The possibility of an occupationally related toxic disorder merits particular consideration when several patients with similar neurologic disturbances of uncertain cause are seen. Since patients will probably have different primary physicians, such a clustering of cases may not be evident until referral for electrodiagnostic evaluation, when an attempt should be made to find some factor common to these patients, such as place or nature of work.

Electrophysiologic techniques permit detection of subclinical neurologic damage in subjects known to have been exposed to neurotoxic substances and may also help in characterizing neurotoxic disorders. Furthermore, they permit the findings in different subjects, or in the same subjects at different times, to be compared.

LeQuesne stressed that the most useful electrophysiologic technique for detecting subclinical toxic neuropathies depends on the condition under suspicion.[149] For example, although measurements of maximal motor conduction velocity are usually of little help in screening for suspected toxic neuropathies because these are axonal in type, they may be very helpful in screening for the neuropathy induced by some hexacarbon solvents. Unfortunately, the most appropriate electrophysiologic test is not always clear, however, as in lead-exposed patients.

Organic Neurotoxins

HEXACARBON SOLVENTS

The solvent *n*-hexane is used in the furniture, printing, and footwear industries, and is also present in certain glues and con-

tact cements. A subacute, progressive, distal, axonal, sensorimotor polyneuropathy may result from industrial exposure to it or from its inhalation for recreational purposes,[150–152] and may worsen for some time even after exposure is stopped. Sensory nerve action potentials are small or absent, and signs of chronic partial denervation may be found in weak muscles. However, maximal motor conduction velocities are characteristically reduced and distal motor latencies are increased, presumably because of secondary demyelinative changes. These electrophysiologic findings are helpful for diagnostic and comparative purposes, and for minimizing exposure. Median- and peroneal-derived somatosensory evoked potentials in patients with *n*-hexane polyneuropathy are reportedly normal,[153] providing no evidence of central somatosensory pathology.

The electrophysiologic findings in the polyneuropathy caused by methyl *n*-butyl ketone are similar to those associated with *n*-hexane neuropathy. The fact that they may be obtained when the clinical deficit is minimal and there are no objective neurologic signs suggests that electrodiagnostic evaluation can detect subclinical pathology.[154]

ORGANOPHOSPHORUS INSECTICIDES

In addition to their acute cholinergic toxicity, some organophosphates can induce a polyneuropathy that relates to inhibition of an enzyme called neuropathy target esterase, or neurotoxic esterase (NTE). Outbreaks of this neuropathy affecting thousands of patients have occurred even in recent years.[155,156] Symptoms begin 1 to 3 weeks after acute exposure, and generally follow acute cholinergic symptoms. Examination reveals a distal, symmetric, predominantly motor polyneuropathy, but mild pyramidal signs may also be present. Partial recovery of peripheral nerve function may eventually occur, but central nervous system signs often then become more evident,[157] determining the ultimate prognosis for functional recovery.[155,158] Objective evidence of sensory loss is usually slight or absent. The initial functional and structural damage occurs in the distal segments of the largest and longest axons. There are also central abnormalities, especially in the cord.

Electromyographic sampling indicates that there is partial denervation of affected muscles but, after a few weeks, large polyphasic motor unit potentials may also be found. With supramaximal stimulation of motor nerves, compound muscle action potentials may be small and terminal motor latencies delayed; maximal motor conduction velocity is usually normal or only slightly reduced. Sensory action potentials are generally small or absent, distinguishing the disorder from motor neuron disease, which it may clinically resemble.

Some have emphasized the importance of the size of the M wave as a monitor of organophosphate exposure, asserting that it increases with mild exposure and diminishes with greater exposure, without detectable inhibition of blood cholinesterase activity.[159,160] Others have been unable to reproduce these findings in humans[161–163] or rats,[164] and in patients with suspected organophosphorus-induced neuropathy, the amplitude of sensory action potentials seems to be the best electrophysiologic parameter to monitor, despite the lack of clinical evidence of sensory involvement.[149]

Neuropathy target esterase is present in peripheral lymphocytes, as well as in the nervous system. In one study, lymphocyte NTE was measured in an attempt to monitor chronic occupational exposure to organophosphates causing neuropathy.[162] The intensity and length of exposure correlated with the inhibition of lymphocytic NTE, but none of the subjects studied developed a peripheral neuropathy.

ACRYLAMIDE

Nontoxic acrylamide polymer is used as a flocculator; as a strengthener of chipboard, paper, and cardboard; and as a grouting agent in the waterproofing of mines, tunnels, and foundations. It is prepared from the neurotoxic monomer, exposure to which may lead to a distal sensorimotor polyneuropathy, with the motor deficit usually being especially conspicuous. Other signs may include ataxia, hyperhidrosis, and skin changes. The electrophysiologic findings are well described. There is little, if any, change in motor conduction velocity, but M waves may be markedly dispersed.[165,166] Sensory nerve action potentials are usually small or absent,[166] and this is the most sensitive electrophysiologic parameter with which patients may be screened for early development of the disorder.

Animal studies show that axonal function (especially of the large-diameter axons) is disturbed in the short intramuscular segment of the stretch receptor afferent.[167] Further, there is an elevated threshold and reduced response to stretch of both primary and secondary spindle endings prior to loss of responsiveness, implying a primary abnormality of the receptor itself.[168] Early recognition of acrylamide neurotoxicity in those at risk may, therefore, depend on testing the function of sensory receptors and the most distal portions of axons.

In the distal axonopathies, degeneration commences distally in long, large-diameter, peripheral and central axons. The distal segments of the rostral projections of sensory neurons in the lumbar dorsal root ganglia, which ascend in the cord to end in the gracile nuclei, are especially vulnerable. Studies of the short-latency somatosensory evoked potential elicited by stimulation of leg nerves in humans may, therefore, permit neurotoxic damage to be detected at an early stage, as has been reported in studies on monkeys.[169]

Heavy Metals

Toxic neuropathies produced by heavy metals have usually been related either to occupational use or to deliberate administration for homicidal or suicidal purposes. Peripheral neuropathy of the axonal type occurs, usually in the context of some systemic disturbance. The precise neurologic manifestations depend upon a variety of factors, including the age of the patient, the duration and extent of the exposure, and the form of the metal to which exposure has occurred.[170,171]

ARSENIC

Neurotoxicity may relate to attempted suicide or homicide, or to industrial exposure (e.g., in copper and lead smelting processes, or with the use of pesticides). A symmetric, distal, sensorimotor polyneuropathy, accompanied or preceded by systemic disturbances, may develop slowly following chronic low-level exposure, or the onset may be rapid following acute massive exposure, and may result in irreversible disability. The electrodiagnostic findings are usually typical of an axonal polyneuropathy. However, in patients with subacute arsenic polyneuropathy, electrodiagnostic findings may be more suggestive of an acquired segmental demyelinating polyradiculoneuropathy.[170] Thus, there may be a progressive decrement in motor amplitude on proximal stimulation, nonuniform slowing in motor conduction velocity and prolonged F waves, and widespread signs of denervation on needle examination. Patients may also have a modestly elevated protein level in the cerebrospinal fluid, with normal glucose and cell count, simulating the Guillain-Barré syndrome.[170] Increased urinary concentrations of arsenic, or an increased arsenic concentration in hair or nails, confirm the diagnosis.

GOLD

Gold, which is used in treating rheumatoid arthritis, may cause a symmetric polyneuropathy, regional or generalized myokymia, or some combination of these abnormalities.

The polyneuropathy is sometimes accompanied by stomatitis, dermatitis, and other manifestations. It may progress rapidly, or may develop gradually over several weeks or longer. Distal sensory complaints are common early features, especially burning dysesthesias in the feet. Weakness then develops and may overshadow the sensory complaints. The electrodiagnostic findings are poorly characterized.

Myokymia and muscle aching may also occur, together with autonomic disturbances (postural hypotension, hyperhidrosis, hypertension, or cardiac dysrhythmias) and mental changes. Motor and sensory conduction studies are normal, and needle examination reveals no abnormalities except myokymia and fasciculations which may be either widespread or restricted in distribution.

INORGANIC LEAD

There is a risk of lead toxicity among those involved in the manufacture or repair of batteries or other lead-containing products, the smelting of lead or lead-containing ores, and the ship-breaking industry. It also occurs in those using lead-containing paints or consuming contaminated illicit alcohol.

Exposure to inorganic lead may produce dysfunction of both the central and peripheral nervous systems, and may be accompanied by a variety of systemic manifesta-tions. The peripheral neuropathy is pre-dominantly motor, and in adults, is char-acteristically more severe in the arms than in the legs. It typically affects the radial nerves, although other nerves may also be affected, and it leads to an asymmetric, pro-gressive motor deficit. Sensory loss is usu-ally inconspicuous or absent. The tendon reflexes may be absent or depressed. Elec-trophysiologic studies indicate that the neu-ropathy is of the axonal type,[172–174] although in certain animal species, it is demyelinative in nature.[175–177] However, the possibility cannot be excluded that it is the motor neuron cell body in the cord that is the primary site of pathology.[178]

Clinical abnormalities generally do not occur with blood lead levels of less than 90 to 100 μg/100 ml in adults. Catton and co-workers reported a minimal subclinical de-fect of peripheral nerve function in lead ac-cumulator workers, finding that, despite normal maximal motor conduction velocity, the ratio of the amplitude of the compound muscle action potential elicited by stimu-lation of the peroneal nerve at the knee and ankle was sometimes smaller than that elic-ited in control subjects.[179] This may have been caused by dispersion of the response, but conduction blocking may also have con-tributed. There was little correlation be-tween peripheral nerve damage and blood lead level. By contrast, Seppalainen and as-sociates reported subclinical slowing of nerve conduction velocities in exposed workers, even if blood levels of lead were less than 70 μg/100 ml, and regarded this as a warning of incipient neuropathy.[180] Sim-ilarly, in lead-exposed workers with a max-imal blood lead level of 70 to 140 μg/100 ml, Buchthal and Behse found slight slowing in motor and sensory conduction velocity in some nerves, which was unrelated to the blood lead level.[173] Because there were no associated histopathologic changes in sural nerve biopsy specimens, the slowed con-duction was attributed to a minor defect in the excitable membrane of the nerve fibers and was not considered to be evidence of subclinical neuropathy.[173]

MERCURY

Inorganic mercury can produce a periph-eral neuropathy, usually in addition to cen-tral manifestations (e.g., tremor or mental impairment). It may affect the motor or sen-sory fibers predominantly, or it may cause a more symmetric motor and sensory dis-turbance. Subclinical polyneuropathy may be recognized by electrodiagnostic means. Albers and co-workers studied 138 workers exposed to inorganic mercury vapor.[181] In 18 patients, there was clinical evidence of a primarily sensory polyneuropathy. These patients had elevated urine mercury in-dexes, were significantly older than the other workers, and had worked in the plant for longer than the others. Electrodiagnos-tic findings suggested that the neuropathy was predominantly axonal, affecting the sensory fibers initially.

Organic (methyl) mercury can cause major outbreaks of poisoning, as in Mina-mata disease, if mercury is discharged into water as an industrial waste product and then methylated by small organisms; the concentration of organic mercury increases in fish, and eventually the fish become toxic to humans. Toxic effects may also result from the use of methyl mercury as a fun-gicide if treated seeds are eaten instead of planted. The resulting disorder is charac-terized by a variety of symptoms secondary to central nervous system dysfunction, and also by distal paresthesias and superficial sensory disturbances simulating peripheral neuropathy. However, electrophysiologic studies generally show no evidence of pe-ripheral sensory neuropathy.[182] Further-more, the N20 component of the somato-sensory evoked potential is absent because of preferential pathologic involvement of the precentral and postcentral cerebral cortex,[183] suggesting that sensory symptoms arise centrally. However, Cinca and associates reported two patients with definitely abnormal peripheral sensory conduction and normal motor conduction during the acute stages of intoxication, whereas sensory conduction velocity was normal 6 months later.[184] This finding suggests that peripheral sensory neuropathy may be detectable electrophysiologically in the early stages of severe organic mercury intoxication.

PLATINUM

Cisplatin, an anticancer agent, may produce a sensory polyneuropathy, beginning usually with numbness and tingling in the hands and feet, and followed by distal sensory loss, with little evidence of any motor disturbance. Remission may occur if administration of cisplatin is discontinued. Electrophysiologic studies show that sensory nerve action potentials become attenuated or lost, whereas motor conduction velocity and terminal motor latency are unaffected.[170,171]

THALLIUM

Until its toxicity became evident, thallium was used to produce hair loss over the scalp in the treatment of various fungal infections. It has also been used as a rodenticide or insecticide and as a homicidal or suicidal agent. It may cause a combination of cutaneous, gastrointestinal, and neurologic symptoms and signs. Neurologic manifestations include cranial neuropathies, diverse dyskinesias, dysautonomias, and mental abnormalities. A generalized polyneuropathy may occur and usually commences with painful distal paresthesias. The electrodiagnostic findings in patients are poorly described, but in animal studies, axonal degeneration occurs, with progres-

Table 11.1. Drug-Induced Peripheral Neuropathy[a]

Sensory	Chloramphenicol
	Cisplatin
	Pyridoxine
Motor	Dapsone
	? Imipramine
	Certain sulfonamides
Mixed	Amiodarone
	Chloroquine
	Disulfiram
	Ethambutol[b]
	Gold
	Hydralazine[b]
	Indomethacin
	Isoniazid
	Misonidazole[b]
	Metronidazole[b]
	Nitrofurantoin
	Nitrous oxide
	Penicillamine
	Perhexilene maleate
	Phenytoin
	Thalidomide
	Vincristine

[a] Only a limited number of drugs is shown.
[b] Predominantly sensory.

sive reduction in the size of the compound muscle action potential and little change in motor conduction velocity or terminal latency.[170,171]

Drugs

A wide variety of drugs have been reported to cause peripheral nerve dysfunction; some of the more important are listed in Table 11.1. A detailed review is provided elsewhere.[185,186]

Diphtheria

Diphtheritic neuropathy, which occurs as a result of a neurotoxin released by the causative organisms, is relatively common in many parts of the world. Palatal weakness may develop 2 to 4 weeks after infection of the throat, and infection of the skin may similarly be followed by focal weakness of the neighboring muscles. Disturbances of accommodation may occur about 4 or 5 weeks after infection, and a generalized polyneuropathy may be seen after 1 to 3 months. Both motor and sensory disturbances occur with the polyneuropathy, and are more pronounced distally than proximally. Pathologic examination reveals that the lesion is characterized by segmental demyelination, with sparing of the axons. Nerve conduction studies show that motor and sensory conduction velocity is reduced, as is the amplitude of nerve action potentials, and in severe cases a complete block of conduction may occur.

MALIGNANT DISEASE

Neoplastic disease may directly involve the spinal cord or the individual (often multiple) nerve roots, may infiltrate much of a limb plexus, or rarely may affect individual peripheral nerves. The findings in patients with spinal lesions are considered on p. 84, and the electrophysiologic features of plexopathies are reviewed on p. 276. Involvement of a single peripheral nerve may be the result of a primary tumor of that nerve; the lack of an electrophysiologic abnormality despite detailed examination does not exclude this possibility when it is suspected on clinical grounds.[187] If abnormalities are found, these commonly reflect axonal loss rather than focal demyelination, but are never pathognomonic of the underlying cause.[187] Typically, then, fibrillation potentials are found on needle examination of affected muscles, and there is a reduction in the size of sensory action potentials or, less often, of compound muscle action potentials.

Several types of neuromuscular disorder may occur as paraneoplastic syndromes in patients with known malignant disease, and their true incidence is uncertain. Similarly unclear is the number of patients with polyneuropathy of obscure etiology in whom investigations reveal an occult malignant disease.

One important paraneoplastic neuromuscular disorder is a subacute sensory polyneuropathy of axonal type. This may be clinically conspicuous and precede discovery of the underlying malignant process by many months. The findings are typified by loss or marked attenuation of sensory action potentials in the extremities, but no abnormality of sensory conduction velocity (when this can be measured). Motor conduction and F wave studies are normal, but H reflexes are unrecordable. The needle examination may show poor activation of motor units, attributed to deafferentation.[188] This disorder typically follows a subacute course, is most commonly associated with bronchial (oat cell) carcinoma, is without effective treatment, and is more properly regarded as a *sensory neuronopathy* than an axonopathy.[189]

More commonly, patients with neoplastic diseases are found to have a mixed (sensory and motor), slowly progressive, distal, axonal *polyneuropathy* that is without any special distinguishing features. The electrophysiologic findings are those associated with any axonal neuropathy, with small or absent sensory action potentials and, in more severe cases, some reduction in the size of the compound muscle potentials. Conduction velocities are usually normal or only slightly reduced. Needle examination may reveal evidence of denervation, together with some reinnervation, in the extremities.

Guillain-Barré syndrome has been associated with Hodgkin's disease,[190] but the electrophysiologic features are unremarkable (p. 237). A *mononeuropathy multiplex* may also occur in patients with malignant disease and has been attributed to a paraneoplastic vasculitis limited mainly to the peripheral nerves.[191]

A subacute, predominantly motor neuronopathy has been described in some patients with lymphomas,[192] and clinically may be mistaken for motor neuron disease. Indeed, there is pathologic evidence of degeneration of anterior horn cells. However, the bulbar muscles are spared, there is no pyramidal deficit, mild sensory disturbances may occur, and the disorder usually follows a benign course that is independent of the course of the underlying neoplasm. Electromyographic needle examination shows evidence of denervation in affected muscles, whereas motor and sensory conduction velocities are generally normal. Whether *amyotrophic lateral sclerosis* occurs more commonly in patients with neoplastic disease than otherwise now seems unlikely, despite early suggestions to the contrary, but in any event the electrophysiologic features of that disorder (p. 86) are not altered by the context in which it arises.

The *Lambert-Eaton myasthenic syndrome* is a well-recognized, nonmetastatic complication of malignant disease. It is discussed in Chapter 14.

In some patients with malignant disease, there may be signs of a *proximal myopathy.* This may be attributable to coexisting *polymyositis,* which is discussed on p. 76. Proximal motor deficits can also arise from polyradiculopathy associated with malignant disease (p. 246), mononeuropathy multiplex involving the nerves to the proximal muscles, or a pure myopathic syndrome. Occasionally, proximal weakness and wasting are found in patients with known malignant neoplastic disease and sensory loss or depressed tendon reflexes in the legs, and the term *neuromyopathy* is sometimes used in this context. No specific electrodiagnostic findings have emerged in connection with this ill-defined complex.

Plasma Cell Dyscrasias

In a number of patients with polyneuropathy, serum protein electrophoresis or immunoelectrophoresis and studies of the urine reveal abnormalities that suggest disorders such as myeloma, benign monoclonal gammopathy, amyloidosis, and Waldenström's macroglobulinemia. An excellent review is provided by Kelly.[193] In *benign monoclonal gammopathy*, the polyneuropathy is characterized by a mixed motor and sensory deficit and is associated with an increased protein concentration in the cerebrospinal fluid. Marked slowing of conduction velocities is especially conspicuous in the IgM gammopathies.[194] The size of sensory and compound muscle action potentials may be reduced, and signs of denervation may be present in the distal muscles of the extremities. Treatment with immunosuppressant drugs and plasmapheresis may be helpful.

In *primary systemic amyloidosis*, the neuropathy is predominantly sensory in type, at least initially, and tends to involve primarily the small fibers comprising the nerve. There is disproportionate impairment of pain and temperature appreciation, and spontaneous stabbing pain may be very troublesome. As the disorder advances, however, a broader spectrum of fibers becomes involved, and autonomic dysfunction often becomes disabling.[195] The electrophysiologic findings indicate an axonal neuropathy. Sensory action potentials are small or absent, and in more advanced cases the compound muscle action potentials may also be of low voltage. Nerve conduction velocity is usually normal or reduced only slightly. Signs of acute or chronic partial denervation, sometimes with reinnervation, are found on needle examination of the distal muscles. Electrophysiologic signs of carpal tunnel syndrome may be superimposed upon the polyneuropathy. The response to treatment is generally disappointing. Immunosuppressive therapy and plasmapheresis are of uncertain value but worthy of trial. The mortality rate associated with amyloid infiltration of vital organs is high.[193]

In patients with *multiple myeloma*, either

an axonal or, in rare instances, a demyelinating neuropathy may occur. The axonal neuropathy may involve both sensory and motor fibers, or it may take the form of a sensory neuropathy, such as occurs in some patients with bronchial carcinoma. Electrophysiologic findings are often indistinguishable from those described above for amyloid neuropathy.[196] The demyelinating neuropathy simulates acute or chronic idiopathic polyradiculoneuropathy (p. 237).

Osteosclerotic myeloma may be associated with a chronic, symmetric, distal, progressive neuropathy involving both motor and sensory fibers. On both pathologic and electrophysiologic examination, the neuropathy appears to be a mixed one, with axonal degeneration and demyelinative changes. The findings include slowing of motor and sensory conduction velocities; small, dispersed, sensory and compound muscle action potentials; and evidence of denervation in the distal muscles on needle examination. The neuropathy may improve with radiotherapy to, or excision of, solitary bone lesions.

A demyelinative sensorimotor neuropathy with marked slowing of conduction velocities has been described in *Waldenström's macroglobulinemia.*

A motor neuropathy or neuronopathy may rarely be associated with a *gammopathy*. In one autopsied case, the primary pathology was in the anterior roots, and it was not possible to distinguish the disorder from motor neuron disease on clinical or electrophysiologic grounds. In this patient, treatment with plasmapheresis and immunosuppression led to clinical improvement and a reduction of serum IgM to normal levels.[197]

MISCELLANEOUS DISORDERS

Neuropathy in Critically III Patients

Bolton and co-workers recently reported on five patients who developed a severe motor and sensory polyneuropathy while critically ill with sepsis and multiorgan dysfunction complicating a variety of primary illnesses.[198] Recognition of the peripheral nerve pathology may be difficult, but early clinical signs include a difficulty in weaning patients from ventilators as the major illness subsides, or the development of hypotonic, areflexic limbs. Electrophysiologic examination reveals that the polyneuropathy is axonal in type, with marked reduction in the size of compound muscle and sensory nerve action potentials, but normal or only slight slowing of nerve conduction velocities. The precise cause of the polyneuropathy is unknown, but nutritional factors may play a role and potentially neurotoxic substances (such as aminoglycoside antibiotics) should be discontinued, if possible.

In this context, it should be emphasized that critically ill patients who are confined to bed may also develop compressive neuropathies, such as ulnar nerve lesions at the elbow. Care must be taken to avoid such neuropathies by good nursing care.

Acquired Immunodeficiency Syndrome

A variety of cranial and peripheral nerve complications may occur in patients with acquired immunodeficiency syndrome (AIDS) or AIDS-related complex.[199] Such complications include a distal, symmetric, sensorimotor polyneuropathy with electrophysiologic evidence of mild slowing of nerve conduction velocities and minimal evidence of denervation. Chronic inflammatory polyneuropathy may also occur in this clinical context, as may a mononeuropathy multiplex, a variety of cranial nerve syndromes, herpes zoster radiculitis, and muscular pathology[200,201].

REFERENCES

1. Seddon HJ: Three types of nerve injury. Brain 66:237, 1943
2. Gilliatt RW: Recent advances in the path-

ophysiology of nerve conduction. p. 2. In Desmedt JE (ed): New Developments in Electromyography and Clinical Neurophysiology. Vol. 2. S. Karger AG, Basel, 1973

3. Gilliatt RW, Taylor JC: Electrical changes following section of the facial nerve. Proc R Soc Med 52:1080, 1959

4. Hodes R, Larrabee MG, German W: The human electromyogram in response to nerve stimulation and the conduction velocity of motor axons. Studies on normal and on injured peripheral nerves. Arch Neurol Psychiatry 69:340, 1948

5. Thomas PK: The peripheral neuropathies. p. 323. In Williams R (ed): Fifth Symposium on Advanced Medicine. Pitman Medical, London, 1969

6. Gilliatt RW: Nerve conduction in human and experimental neuropathies. Proc R Soc Med 59:989, 1966

7. Lewis RA, Sumner AJ: The electrodiagnostic distinctions between chronic familial and acquired demyelinative neuropathies. Neurology 32:592, 1982

8. Dyck PJ, Oviatt KF, Lambert EH: Intensive evaluation of referred unclassified neuropathies yields improved diagnosis. Ann Neurol 10:222, 1981

9. McLeod JG, Tuck RR, Pollard JD, Cameron J, Walsh JC: Chronic polyneuropathy of undetermined cause. J Neurol Neurosurg Psychiatry 47:530, 1984

10. Parry GJ: Mononeuropathy multiplex (AAEE case report No. 11). Muscle Nerve 8:493, 1985

11. Dyck PJ, Lambert EH: Lower motor and primary sensory neuron diseases with peroneal muscular atrophy. I. Neurologic, genetic and electrophysiologic findings in hereditary polyneuropathies. Arch Neurol 18:603, 1968

12. Dyck PJ, Lambert EH: Lower motor and primary sensory neuron diseases with peroneal muscular atrophy. II. Neurologic, genetic and electrophysiologic findings in various neuronal degenerations. Arch Neurol 18:619, 1968

13. Behse F, Buchthal F: Peroneal muscular atrophy (PMA) and related disorders. I. Clinical manifestations as related to biopsy findings, nerve conduction and electromyography. Brain 100:41, 1977

14. Behse F, Buchthal F: Peroneal muscular atrophy (PMA) and related disorders. II. Histological findings in sural nerves. Brain 100:67, 1977

15. Thomas PK, Calne DB: Motor nerve conduction velocity in peroneal muscular atrophy: Evidence for genetic heterogeneity. J Neurol Neurosurg Psychiatry 37:68, 1974

16. Harding AE, Thomas PK: The clinical features of hereditary motor and sensory neuropathy types I and II. Brain 103:259, 1980

17. Guiloff RJ, Thomas PK, Contreras M, Armitage S, Schwarz G, Sedgwick EM: Linkage of autosomal dominant type I hereditary motor and sensory neuropathy to the Duffy locus on chromosome 1. J Neurol Neurosurg Psychiatry 45:669, 1982

18. Dyck PJ, Swanson CJ, Low PA, Bartelson JD, Lambert EH: Prednisone-responsive hereditary motor and sensory neuropathy. Mayo Clin Proc 57:239, 1982

19. Dyck PJ: Inherited neuronal degeneration and atrophy affecting peripheral motor, sensory and autonomic neurons. p. 1600. In Dyck PJ, Thomas PK, Lambert EH, Bunge R (eds): Peripheral Neuropathy. 2nd Ed. W.B. Saunders, Philadelphia, 1984

20. Brown JC, Johns RJ: Nerve conduction in familial dysautonomia (Riley Day syndrome). JAMA 201:200, 1967

21. Debruyne J, Dehaene I, Martin JJ: Hereditary pressure-sensitive neuropathy. J Neurol Sci 47:385, 1980

22. Meier C, Moll C: Hereditary neuropathy with liability to pressure palsies. J Neurol 228:73, 1982

23. Davies DM: Recurrent peripheral-nerve palsies in a family. Lancet 2:266, 1954

24. Earl CJ, Fullerton PM, Wakefield GS, Schutta HS: Hereditary neuropathy, with liability to pressure palsies. A clinical and electrophysiological study of four families. Q J Med 33:481, 1964

25. Madrid R, Bradley WG: The pathology of neuropathies with focal thickening of the myelin sheath (tomaculous neuropathy). Studies on the formation of the abnormal myelin sheath. J Neurol Sci 25:415, 1975

26. Behse F, Buchthal F, Carlsen F, Knappeis GG: Hereditary neuropathy with liability to pressure palsies. Electrophysiological and histopathological aspects. Brain 95:777, 1972

27. Fullerton PM: Peripheral nerve conduction in metachromatic leucodystrophy (sulphatide lipidosis). J Neurol Neurosurg Psychiatry 27:100, 1964

28. Yudell A, Gomez MR, Lambert EH, Dockerty MB: The neuropathy of sulfatide lipidosis (metachromatic leukodystrophy). Neurology 17:103, 1967

29. Clark JR, Miller RG, Vidgoff JM: Juvenile-onset metachromatic leukodystrophy: Biochemical and electrophysiologic studies. Neurology 29:346, 1979

30. Pilz H, Hopf HC: A preclinical case of late adult metachromatic leukodystrophy? Manifestation only with lipid abnormalities in urine, enzyme deficiency, and decrease of nerve conduction velocity. J Neurol Neurosurg Psychiatry 35:360, 1972

31. Hogan GR, Gutmann L, Chou SM: The peripheral neuropathy of Krabbe's (globoid) leukodystrophy. Neurology 19:1094, 1969

32. Bischoff A: Neuropathy in leukodystrophies. p. 891. In Dyck PJ, Thomas PK, Lambert EH (eds): Peripheral Neuropathy. W.B. Saunders, Philadelphia, 1975

33. Lieberman JS, Oshtory M, Taylor RG, Dreyfus PM: Perinatal neuropathy as an early manifestation of Krabbe's disease. Arch Neurol 37:446, 1980

34. Vercruyssen A, Martin JJ, Mercelis R: Neurophysiological studies in adrenomyeloneuropathy. A report on five cases. J Neurol Sci 56:327, 1982

35. McLeod JG: An electrophysiological and pathological study of peripheral nerves in Friedreich's ataxia. J Neurol Sci 12:333, 1971

36. Oh SJ, Halsey JH, Jr: Abnormality in nerve potentials in Friedreich's ataxia. Neurology 23:52, 1973

37. McLeod JG, Evans WA: Peripheral neuropathy in spinocerebellar degenerations. Muscle Nerve 4:51, 1981

38. McLeod JG, Morgan JA, Reye C: Electrophysiological studies in familial spastic paraplegia. J Neurol Neurosurg Psychiatry 40:611, 1977

39. Ridley A: The neuropathy of acute intermittent porphyria. Q J Med 38:307, 1969

40. Lambert EH: Diagnostic value of electrical stimulation of motor nerves. Electroencephalogr Clin Neurophysiol, suppl. 22:9, 1962

41. Maytham DV, Eales L: Electrodiagnostic findings in porphyria. S Afr Med J [Special Issue of 25 September]:99, 1971

42. Nagler W: Peripheral neuropathy in acute intermittent porphyria. Arch Phys Med Rehabil 51:426, 1971

43. Albers JW, Robertson WC, Daube JR: Electrodiagnostic findings in acute porphyric neuropathy. Muscle Nerve 1:292, 1978

44. Cavanagh JB, Mellick RS. On the nature of the peripheral nerve lesions associated with acute intermittent porphyria. J Neurol Neurosurg Psychiatry 28:320, 1965

45. Miller RG, David CJF, Illingworth DR, Bradley W: The neuropathy of abetalipoproteinemia. Neurology 30:1286, 1980

46. Schwartz JF, Rowland LP, Eder H, Marks PA, Osserman EF, Hirschberg E, Anderson H: Bassen-Kornzweig syndrome: Deficiency of serum β-lipoprotein. Arch Neurol 8:438, 1963

47. Sheth KJ, Swick HM: Peripheral nerve conduction in Fabry disease. Ann Neurol 7:319, 1980

48. Kocen RS, Thomas PK: Peripheral nerve involvement in Fabry's disease. Arch Neurol 22:81, 1970

49. Refsum S, Stokke O, Eldjarn L, Fardeau M: Heredopathia atactica polyneuritiformis (Refsum disease). p. 1680. In Dyck PJ, Thomas PK, Lambert EH, Bunge R (eds): Peripheral Neuropathy. 2nd Ed. W.B. Saunders, Philadelphia, 1984

50. Engel WK: In Steinberg D, Vroom FQ, Engel WK, Cammermeyer J, Mize CE, Avigan J: Refsum's disease—A recently characterized lipidosis involving the nervous system. Combined clinical staff conference at the National Institutes of Health. Ann Intern Med 66:365, 1967

51. Lundberg A, Lilja LG, Lundberg PO, Try K: Heredopathia atactica polyneuritiformis (Refsum's disease). Experiences of dietary treatment and plasmapheresis. Eur Neurol 8:309, 1972

52. Pollock M, Nukada H, Frith RW, Simcock JP, Allpress S: Peripheral neuropathy in Tangier disease. Brain 106:911, 1983

53. Haas LF, Austad WI, Bergin JD: Tangier disease. Brain 97:351, 1974

54. Kocen RS, Lloyd JK, Lascelles PT, Fosbrooke AS, Williams D: Familial α-lipoprotein deficiency (Tangier disease) with neurological abnormalities. Lancet 1:1341, 1967

55. Asbury AK, Victor M, Adams RD: Uremic polyneuropathy. Arch Neurol 8:413, 1963

56. Preswick G, Jeremy D: Subclinical polyneuropathy in renal insufficiency. Lancet 2:731, 1964

57. Thomas PK, Hollinrake K, Lascelles RG, O'Sullivan DJ, Baillod RA, Moorhead JF, Mackenzie JC: The polyneuropathy of chronic renal failure. Brain 94:761, 1971

58. Dinn JJ, Crane DL: Schwann cell dysfunction in uraemia. J Neurol Neurosurg Psychiatry 33:605, 1970

59. Hansen S, Ballantyne JP: A quantitative electrophysiological study of uraemic neuropathy. Diabetic and renal neuropathies compared. J Neurol Neurosurg Psychiatry 41:128, 1978

60. Jebsen RH, Tenckhoff H, Honet JC: Natural history of uremic polyneuropathy and effects of dialysis. N Engl J Med 277:327, 1967

61. Nielsen VK: The peripheral nerve function in chronic renal failure. VII. Longitudinal course during terminal renal failure and regular hemodialysis. Acta Med Scand 195:155, 1974

62. Bakke L: Uraemic polyneuropathy. Acta Neurol Scand 46:suppl. 43, 205, 1970

63. Dyck PJ, Johnson WJ, Lambert EH, Bushek W, Pollock M: Detection and evaluation of uremic peripheral neuropathy in patients on hemodialysis. Kidney Int 7:201, 1975

64. Bolton CF, Baltzan MA, Baltzan RB: Effects of renal transplantation on uremic neuropathy. A clinical and electrophysiologic study. N Engl J Med 284:1170, 1971

65. Nielsen VK: The peripheral nerve function in chronic renal failure: IX. Recovery after renal transplantation. Electrophysiological aspects (sensory and motor nerve conduction). Acta Med Scand 195:171, 1974

66. Bolton CF: Electrophysiologic changes in uremic neuropathy after successful renal transplantation. Neurology 26:152, 1976

67. Oh SJ, Clements RS Jr, Lee YW, Diethelm AG: Rapid improvement in nerve conduction velocity following renal transplantation. Ann Neurol 4:369, 1978

68. Ackil AA, Shahani BT, Young RR, Rubin NE: Late response and sural conduction studies. Usefulness in patients with chronic renal failure. Arch Neurol 38:482, 1981

69. Harding AE, Le Fanu J: Carpal tunnel syndrome related to antebrachial Cimino-Brescia fistula. J Neurol Neurosurg Psychiatry 40:511, 1977

70. Lowitzsch K, Göhring U, Hecking E, Köhler H: Refractory period, sensory conduction velocity and visual evoked potentials before and after haemodialysis. J Neurol Neurosurg Psychiatry 44:121, 1981

71. Castaigne P, Cathala H-P, Beaussart-Boulengé L, Petrover M: Effect of ischaemia on peripheral nerve function in patients with chronic renal failure undergoing dialysis treatment. J Neurol Neurosurg Psychiatry 35:631, 1972

72. Brown MJ, Asbury AK: Diabetic neuropathy. Ann Neurol 15:2, 1984

73. Behse F, Buchthal F, Carlsen F: Nerve biopsy and conduction studies in diabetic neuropathy. J Neurol Neurosurg Psychiatry 40:1072, 1977

74. Thomas PK, Lascelles RG: The pathology of diabetic neuropathy. Q J Med 35:489, 1966

75. Sugimura K, Dyck PJ: Sural nerve myelin thickness and axis cylinder caliber in human diabetes. Neurology 31:1087, 1981

76. Gilliatt RW, Willison RG: Peripheral nerve conduction in diabetic neuropathy. J Neurol Neurosurg Psychiatry 25:11, 1962

77. Downie AW, Newell DJ: Sensory nerve conduction in patients with diabetes mellitus and controls. Neurology 11:876, 1961

78. Lawrence DG, Locke S: Motor nerve conduction velocity in diabetes. Arch Neurol 5:483, 1961

79. Mulder DW, Lambert EH, Bastron JA, Sprague RG: The neuropathies associated with diabetes mellitus. A clinical and electromyographic study of 103 unselected diabetic patients. Neurology 11:275, 1961

80. Lamontagne A, Buchthal F: Electrophysiological studies in diabetic neuropathy. J Neurol Neurosurg Psychiatry 33:442, 1970

81. Wiechers D, Guyton JD, Johnson EW: Electromyographic findings in extensor

digitorum brevis in normal population. Arch Phys Med Rehabil 57:84, 1976

82. Gatens PF, Saeed MA: Electromyographic findings in the intrinsic muscles of normal feet. Arch Phys Med Rehabil 63:317, 1982

83. Falck B, Alaranta H: Fibrillation potentials, positive sharp waves and fasciculation in the intrinsic muscles of the foot in healthy subjects. J Neurol Neurosurg Psychiatry 46:681, 1983

84. Asbury AK: Proximal diabetic neuropathy. Ann Neurol 2:179, 1977

85. Bastron JA, Thomas JE: Diabetic polyradiculopathy. Clinical and electromyographic findings in 105 patients. Mayo Clin Proc 56:725, 1981

86. Raff MC, Sangalang V, Asbury AK: Ischemic mononeuropathy multiplex associated with diabetes mellitus. Arch Neurol 18:487, 1968

87. Chopra JS, Hurwitz LJ: Femoral nerve conduction in diabetes and chronic occlusive vascular disease. J Neurol Neurosurg Psychiatry 31:28, 1968

88. Subramony SH, Wilbourn AJ: Diabetic proximal neuropathy. Clinical and electromyographic studies. J Neurol Sci 53:293, 1982

89. Sun SF, Streib EW: Diabetic thoracoabdominal neuropathy: Clinical and electrodiagnostic features. Ann Neurol 9:75, 1981

90. Kikta DG, Breuer AC, Wilbourn AJ: Thoracic root pain in diabetes: The spectrum of clinical and electromyographic findings. Ann Neurol 11:80, 1982

91. Longstreth GF, Newcomer AD: Abdominal pain caused by diabetic radiculopathy. Ann Intern Med 86:166, 1977

92. Waxman SG, Sabin TD: Diabetic truncal polyneuropathy. Arch Neurol 38:46, 1981

93. Kimura J: An evaluation of the facial and trigeminal nerves in polyneuropathy: Electrodiagnostic study in Charcot-Marie-Tooth disease, Guillain-Barré syndrome, and diabetic neuropathy. Neurology 21:745, 1971

94. Aminoff MJ: Autonomic insufficiency and its evaluation. Medicine (N Am) 34:4863, 1986

95. Harrison MJG: Muscle wasting after prolonged hypoglycaemic coma: Case report with electrophysiological data. J Neurol Neurosurg Psychiatry 39:465, 1976

96. Jaspan JB, Wollman RL, Bernstein L, Rubinstein AH: Hypoglycemic peripheral neuropathy in association with insulinoma: Implication of glucopenia rather than hyperinsulinism. Medicine 61:33, 1982

97. Danta G: Hypoglycemic peripheral neuropathy. Arch Neurol 21:121, 1969

98. Mulder DW, Bastron JA, Lambert EH: Hyperinsulin neuronopathy. Neurology 6:627, 1956

99. Behse F, Buchthal F: Alcoholic neuropathy: Clinical, electrophysiological, and biopsy findings. Ann Neurol 2:95, 1977

100. Mawdsley C, Mayer RF: Nerve conduction in alcoholic polyneuropathy. Brain 88:335, 1965

101. Walsh JC, McLeod JG: Alcoholic neuropathy. An electrophysiological and histological study. J Neurol Sci 10:457, 1970

102. Casey EB, LeQuesne PM: Electrophysiological evidence for a distal lesion in alcoholic neuropathy. J Neurol Neurosurg Psychiatry 35:624, 1972

103. Hillbom M, Wennberg A: Prognosis of alcoholic peripheral neuropathy. J Neurol Neurosurg Psychiatry 47:699, 1984

104. Mayer RF: Peripheral nerve function in vitamin B_{12} deficiency. Arch Neurol 13:355, 1965

105. McCombe PA, McLeod JG: The peripheral neuropathy of vitamin B_{12} deficiency. J Neurol Sci 66:117, 1984

106. Cox-Klazinga M, Endtz LJ: Peripheral nerve involvement in pernicious anaemia. J Neurol Sci 45:367, 1980

107. Harding AE, Muller DPR, Thomas PK, Willison HJ: Spinocerebellar degeneration secondary to chronic intestinal malabsorption: A vitamin E deficiency syndrome. Ann Neurol 12:419, 1982

108. Thomas PK, Walker JG: Xanthomatous neuropathy in primary biliary cirrhosis. Brain 88:1079, 1965

109. Charron L, Peyronnard J-M, Marchand L: Sensory neuropathy associated with primary biliary cirrhosis. Histologic and morphometric studies. Arch Neurol 37:84, 1980

110. Dayan AD, Williams R: Demyelinating peripheral neuropathy and liver disease. Lancet 2:133, 1967

111. Seneviratne KN, Peiris OA: Peripheral nerve function in chronic liver disease. J Neurol Neurosurg Psychiatry 33:609, 1970

112. Knill-Jones RP, Goodwin CJ, Dayan AD, Williams R: Peripheral neuropathy in chronic liver disease: Clinical, electrodiagnostic, and nerve biopsy findings. J Neurol Neurosurg Psychiatry 35:22, 1972

113. Kardel T, Nielsen VK: Hepatic neuropathy: A clinical and electrophysiological study. Acta Neurol Scand 50:513, 1974

114. Murray IPC, Simpson JA: Acroparaesthesia in myxoedema. A clinical and electromyographic study. Lancet 1:1360, 1958

115. Purnell DC, Daly DD, Lipscomb PR: Carpal-tunnel syndrome associated with myxedema. Arch Intern Med 108:751, 1961

116. Dyck PJ, Lambert EH: Polyneuropathy associated with hypothyroidism. J Neuropathol Exp Neurol 29:631, 1970

117. Pollard JD, McLeod JG, Angel Honnibal TG, Verheijden MA: Hypothyroid polyneuropathy. J Neurol Sci 53:461, 1982

118. O'Duffy JD, Randall RV, MacCarty CS: Median neuropathy (carpal-tunnel syndrome) in acromegaly. A sign of endocrine overactivity. Ann Intern Med 78:379, 1973

119. Low PA, McLeod JG, Turtle JR, Donnelly P, Wright RG: Peripheral neuropathy in acromegaly. Brain 97:139, 1974

120. Sabin TD, Swift TR: Leprosy. p. 1955. In Dyck PJ, Thomas PK, Lambert EH, Bunge R (eds): Peripheral Neuropathy. 2nd Ed. W.B. Saunders, Philadelphia, 1984

121. Verghese M, Ittimani KV, Satyanarayan IR, Mathai R, Bhakthaviziam C: A study of the conduction velocity of the motor fibers of ulnar and median nerves in leprosy. Int J Lepr 38:271, 1970

122. Jopling WH, Morgan-Hughes JA: Pure neural tuberculoid leprosy. Br Med J 2:799, 1965

123. Rosenberg RN, Lovelace RE: Mononeuritis multiplex in lepromatous leprosy. Arch Neurol 19:310, 1968

124. Dastur DK, Antia NH, Divekar SC: The facial nerve in leprosy. 2. Pathology, pathogenesis, electromyography and clinical correlations. Int J Lepr 34:118, 1966

125. Asbury AK: Diagnostic considerations in Guillain-Barré syndrome. Ann Neurol 9, suppl.:1, 1981

126. Lambert EH, Mulder DW: Nerve conduction in the Guillain-Barré syndrome. Electroencephalogr Clin Neurophysiol 17:86, 1964

127. McLeod JG: Electrophysiological studies in the Guillain-Barré syndrome. Ann Neurol 9, suppl.:20, 1981

128. Eisen A, Humphreys P: The Guillain-Barré syndrome. A clinical and electrodiagnostic study of 25 cases. Arch Neurol 30:438, 1974

129. Albers JW, Donofrio PD, McGonagle TK: Sequential electrodiagnostic abnormalities in acute inflammatory demyelinating polyradiculoneuropathy. Muscle Nerve 8:528, 1985

130. Cerra D, Johnson EW: Motor nerve conduction velocity in "idiopathic" polyneuritis. Arch Phys Med Rehabil 42:159, 1961

131. Bannister RG, Sears TA: The changes in nerve conduction in acute idiopathic polyneuritis. J Neurol Neurosurg Psychiatry 25:321, 1962

132. Pleasure DE, Lovelace RE, Duvoisin RC: The prognosis of acute polyradiculoneuritis. Neurology 18:1143, 1968

133. Brown WF, Feasby TE: Conduction block and denervation in Guillain-Barré polyneuropathy. Brain 107:219, 1984

134. Lafontaine S, Rasminsky M, Saida T, Sumner AJ: Conduction block in rat myelinated fibres following acute exposure to anti-galactocerebroside serum. J Physiol 323:287, 1982

135. Brown WF, Feasby TE: Sensory evoked potentials in Guillain-Barré polyneuropathy. J Neurol Neurosurg Psychiatry 47:288, 1984

136. Walsh JC, Yiannikas C, McLeod JG: Abnormalities of proximal conduction in acute idiopathic polyneuritis: Comparison of short latency evoked potentials and F-waves. J Neurol Neurosurg Psychiatry 47:197, 1984

137. King D, Ashby P: Conduction velocity in the proximal segments of a motor nerve in the Guillain-Barré syndrome. J Neurol Neurosurg Psychiatry 39:538, 1976

138. Peterson GW, Miller RG, Albers JW, Daube JR: Prognostic value of electrodiagnosis in acute Guillain-Barré syndrome. Muscle Nerve 5:556, 1982

139. Guiloff RJ: Peripheral nerve conduction in Miller Fisher syndrome. J Neurol Neurosurg Psychiatry 40:801, 1977

140. Guillain-Barré Syndrome Study Group: Plasmapheresis and acute Guillain-Barré syndrome. Neurology 35:1096, 1985

141. Dyck PJ, Lais AC, Ohta M, Bastron JA, Okazaki H, Groover RV: Chronic inflammatory polyradiculoneuropathy. Mayo Clin Proc 50:621, 1975

142. Prineas JW, McLeod JG: Chronic relapsing polyneuritis. J Neurol Sci 27:427, 1976

143. Matthews WB: Sarcoid neuropathy. p. 2018. In Dyck PJ, Thomas PK, Lambert EH, Bunge R (eds): Peripheral Neuropathy. 2nd Ed. W.B. Saunders, Philadelphia, 1984

144. Silverstein A, Siltzbach LE: Neurologic sarcoidosis. Study of 18 cases. Arch Neurol 12:1, 1965

145. Wells CEC: The natural history of neurosarcoidosis. Proc R Soc Med 60:1172, 1967

146. Weller RO, Bruckner FE, Chamberlain MA: Rheumatoid neuropathy: A histological and electrophysiological study. J Neurol Neurosurg Psychiatry 33:592, 1970

147. Layzer RB: Neuromuscular Manifestations of Systemic Disease. F.A. Davis, Philadelphia, 1985

148. Conn DL, Dyck PJ: Angiopathic neuropathy in connective tissue diseases. p. 2027. In Dyck PJ, Thomas PK, Lambert EH, Bunge R (eds): Peripheral Neuropathy. 2nd Ed. W.B. Saunders, Philadelphia, 1984

149. LeQuesne PM: Neurophysiological investigation of subclinical and minimal toxic neuropathies. Muscle Nerve 1:392, 1978

150. Herskowitz A, Ishii N, Schaumburg H: n-Hexane neuropathy: A syndrome occurring as a result of industrial exposure. N Engl J Med 285:82, 1971

151. Korobkin R, Asbury AK, Sumner AJ, Nielsen SL: Glue-sniffing neuropathy. Arch Neurol 32:158, 1975

152. Shirabe T, Tsuda T, Terao A, Araki S: Toxic polyneuropathy due to glue-sniffing. Report of two cases with a light and electron-microscopic study of the peripheral nerves and muscles. J Neurol Sci 21:101, 1974

153. Zappoli R, Giuliano G, Rossi L, Papini M, Ronchi O, Ragazzoni A, Amantini A: CNV and SEP in shoe industry workers with neuropathy resulting from toxic effect of adhesive solvents. p. 476. In Otta DA (ed): Multidisciplinary Perspectives in Event-Related Brain Potential Research. U.S. Environmental Protection Agency, Cincinnati, 1978

154. Allen N, Mendell JR, Billmaier DJ, Fontaine RE, O'Neill J: Toxic polyneuropathy due to methyl n-butyl ketone. An industrial outbreak. Arch Neurol 32:209, 1975

155. Senanayake N: Tri-cresyl phosphate neuropathy in Sri Lanka: A clinical and neurophysiological study with a three year follow up. J Neurol Neurosurg Psychiatry 44:775, 1981

156. Senanayake N, Johnson MK: Acute polyneuropathy after poisoning by a new organophosphate insecticide. N Engl J Med 306:155, 1982

157. Morgan JP, Penovich P: Jamaica ginger paralysis. Forty-seven-year follow-up. Arch Neurol 35:530, 1978

158. Vasilescu C: Triorthocresyl phosphate neuropathy. Arch Neurol 36:455, 1979

159. Roberts DV: A longitudinal electromyographic study of six men occupationally exposed to organophosphorus compounds. Int Arch Occup Environ Health 38:221, 1977

160. Roberts DV: Theoretical and practical consequences of the use of organophosphorus compounds in industry. J Soc Occup Med 29:15, 1979

161. Kimura J: Electrodiagnostic study of pesticide toxicity. p. 174. In Xintaras C, Johnson BL, DeGroot I (eds): Behavioral Toxicology. Vol. I. (NIOSH publication No. 74-126). National Institute for Occupational Safety and Health, Cincinnati, 1974

162. Lotti M, Becker CE, Aminoff MJ, Woodrow JE, Seiber JN, Talcott RE, Richardson RJ: Occupational exposure to the cotton defoliants DEF and merphos. A rational approach to monitoring organophosphorous-induced delayed neurotoxicity. J Occup Med 25:517, 1983

163. Stalberg E, Hilton-Brown P, Kolmodin-Hedman B, Holmstedt B, Augustinsson K-B: Effect of occupational exposure to organophosphorus insecticides on neuromuscular function. Scand J Work Environ Health 4:255, 1978

164. Maxwell IC, LeQuesne PM: Neuromuscular effects of chronic administration of two organophosphorus insecticides to rats. Neurotoxicology 3:1, 1982

165. Fullerton PM: Electrophysiological and histological observations on peripheral nerves in acrylamide poisoning in man. J Neurol Neurosurg Psychiatry 32:186, 1969

166. Takahashi M, Ohara T, Hashimoto K: Electrophysiological study of nerve injuries in workers handling acrylamide. Int Arch Arbeitsmed 28:1, 1971

167. Sumner AJ, Asbury AK: Physiological studies of the dying-back phenomenon. Muscle stretch afferents in acrylamide neuropathy. Brain 98:91, 1975

168. Lowndes HE, Baker T, Cho E-S, Jortner BS: Position sensitivity of de-efferented muscle spindles in experimental acrylamide neuropathy. J Pharmacol Exp Ther 205:40, 1978

169. Arezzo JC, Schaumburg HH, Vaughan HG, Spencer PS, Barna J: Hind limb somatosensory evoked potentials in the monkey: The effects of distal axonopathy. Ann Neurol 12:24, 1982

170. Wilbourn AJ: Metal neuropathies. Syllabus from Course on Toxic Neuropathies. American Association of Electromyography and Electrodiagnosis, 1984

171. Windebank AJ, McCall JT, Dyck PJ: Metal neuropathy. p. 2133. In Dyck PJ, Thomas PK, Lambert EH, Bunge R (eds): Peripheral Neuropathy. 2nd Ed. W.B. Saunders, Philadelphia, 1984

172. Oh SJ: Lead neuropathy: Case report. Arch Phys Med Rehabil 56:312, 1975

173. Buchthal F, Behse F: Electrophysiology and nerve biopsy in men exposed to lead. Br J Ind Med 36:135, 1979

174. Simpson JA, Seaton DA, Adams JF: Response to treatment with chelating agents of anaemia, chronic encephalopathy, and myelopathy due to lead poisoning. J Neurol Neurosurg Psychiatry 27:536, 1964

175. Fullerton PM: Chronic peripheral neuropathy produced by lead poisoning in guinea-pigs. J Neuropathol Exp Neurol 25:214, 1966

176. Dyck PJ, O'Brien PC, Ohnishi A: Lead neuropathy: 2. Random distribution of segmental demyelination among "old internodes" of myelinated fibers. J Neuropathol Exp Neurol 36:570, 1977

177. Schlaepfer WW: Experimental lead neuropathy: A disease of the supporting cells in the peripheral nervous system. J Neuropathol Exp Neurol 28:401, 1969

178. Rowland LP: Peripheral neuropathy, motor neuron disease, or neuronopathy? p. 27. In Battistin L, Hashim GA, Lajtha A (eds): Clinical and Biological Aspects of Peripheral Nerve Diseases. Alan R. Liss, New York, 1983

179. Catton MJ, Harrison MJG, Fullerton PM, Kazantzis G: Subclinical neuropathy in lead workers. Br Med J 2:80, 1970

180. Seppalainen AM, Hernberg S, Kock B: Relationship between blood lead levels and nerve conduction velocities. Neurotoxicology 1:313, 1979

181. Albers JW, Cavender GD, Levine SP, Langolf GD: A symptomatic sensorimotor neuropathy in workers exposed to elemental mercury. Neurology 32:1168, 1982

182. LeQuesne PM, Damluji SF, Rustam H: Electrophysiological studies of peripheral nerves in patients with organic mercury poisoning. J Neurol Neurosurg Psychiatry 37:333, 1974

183. Tokuomi J, Uchino M, Imamura S, Yamanaga H, Nakanishi R, Ideta T: Minamata disease (organic mercury poisoning): Neuroradiologic and electrophysiologic studies. Neurology 32:1369, 1982

184. Cinca I, Dumitrescu I, Onaca P, Serbanescu A, Nestorescu B: Accidental ethyl mercury poisoning with nervous system, skeletal muscle, and myocardium injury. J Neurol Neurosurg Psychiatry 43:143, 1979

185. Argov Z, Mastaglia FL: Drug-induced peripheral neuropathies. Br Med J 1:663, 1979

186. LeQuesne PM: Neuropathy due to drugs. p. 2162. In Dyck PJ, Thomas PK, Lambert EH, Bunge R (eds): Peripheral Neuropathy. 2nd Ed. W.B. Saunders, Philadelphia, 1984

187. Wilbourn AJ: The direct effects of neoplasms on the peripheral neuromuscular system. Syllabus from Course on Neuromuscular Complications of Cancer. American Association of Electromyography and Electrodiagnosis, 1985

188. Kaufman MD, Hopkins LC, Hurwitz BJ: Progressive sensory neuropathy in patients without carcinoma: A disorder with distinctive clinical and electrophysiological findings. Ann Neurol 9:237, 1981

189. Horwich MS, Cho L, Porro RS, Posner JB: Subacute sensory neuropathy: A remote effect of carcinoma. Ann Neurol 2:7, 1977

190. Lisak RP, Mitchell M, Zweiman B, Orrechio E, Asbury AK: Guillain-Barré syndrome and Hodgkin's disease: Three cases with immunological studies. Ann Neurol 1:72, 1977

191. Johnson PC, Rolak LA, Hamilton RH, Laguna JF: Paraneoplastic vasculitis of nerve: A remote effect of cancer. Ann Neurol 5:437, 1979

192. Schold SC, Cho ES, Somasundaram M, Posner JB: Subacute motor neuronopathy: A remote effect of lymphoma. Ann Neurol 5:271, 1979

193. Kelly JJ Jr: Peripheral neuropathies associated with monoclonal proteins: A clinical review. Muscle Nerve 8:138, 1985

194. Dalakas MC, Engel WK: Polyneuropathy with monoclonal gammopathy: Studies of 11 patients. Ann Neurol 10:45, 1981

195. Kelly JJ Jr, Kyle RA, O'Brien PC, Dyck PJ: The natural history of peripheral neuropathy in primary systemic amyloidosis. Ann Neurol 6:1, 1979

196. Kelly JJ Jr, Kyle RA, Miles JM, O'Brien PC, Dyck PJ: The spectrum of peripheral neuropathy in myeloma. Neurology 31:24, 1981

197. Parry GJ, Holtz SJ, Ben-Zeev D, Drori JB: Gammopathy with proximal motor axonopathy simulating motor neuron disease. Neurology 36:273, 1986

198. Bolton CF, Gilbert JJ, Hahn AF, Sibbald WJ: Polyneuropathy in critically ill patients. J Neurol Neurosurg Psychiatry 47:1223, 1984

199. Levy RM, Bredesen DE, Rosenblum ML: Neurological manifestations of the acquired immuno-deficiency syndrome (AIDS): Experience at UCSF and review of the literature. J Neurosurg 62:475, 1985

200. Stern R, Gold J, DiCarlo EF: Myopathy complicating the acquired immune deficiency syndrome. Muscle Nerve 10:318, 1987

210. Dalakas MC, Pezeshkpour GH, Gravell M, Sever JL: Polymyositis associated with AIDS retrovirus. JAMA 256:2381, 1986

12

The Facial Nerve

The anatomy of the seventh cranial nerve is summarized in Figure 12.1. The fibers destined for it have a long, intrapontine course, hooking around the sixth nerve nucleus before emerging from the pons in the cerebellopontine angle to pass to the internal auditory meatus, and thence to the facial canal. The nerve leaves the skull through the stylomastoid foramen, and passes laterally and forward in the parotid gland, dividing behind the ramus of the mandible into branches to the muscles of facial expression. Various branches are given off within the facial canal, including the branch to the stapedius and the chorda tympani. As it exits from the stylomastoid foramen, the facial nerve gives off posterior auricular, stylohyoid, and digastric branches, and in the parotid it divides into five terminal branches—the temporal, zygomatic, buccal, mandibular, and cervical—to the muscles of facial expression.

Involvement of facial nerve fibers at any point along their course will lead to a facial paresis of lower motor neuron type. A paresis of this sort is characterized clinically by impaired voluntary and emotive movements because of flaccid weakness of the muscles in both the upper and lower parts of the face. It may result from nuclear lesions such as occur with vascular disease, tumors, motor neuron disease, poliomyelitis, or syringobulbia. Clinical evidence of more widespread brain stem involvement is then generally found, and electromyographic signs of chronic partial denervation are usually present in the facial muscles if sufficient time has elapsed after onset of the weakness.

A facial paresis may also result from more peripheral lesions of the seventh cranial nerve. When attributable to idiopathic facial nerve involvement outside the central nervous system and unaccompanied by evidence of aural or more widespread neurologic disease, the condition is designated as *Bell's palsy*. In other cases, it may be caused by tumors in the cerebellopontine angle or other areas; trauma; acute otitis media; sarcoidosis; infectious mononucleosis; viral disorders, such as geniculate herpes zoster; or bacterial infection, such as leprosy. The facial nerves may also be affected in patients with polyneuropathies or diseases, such as diabetes, in which peripheral nerve involvement is likely to occur.

In this chapter, the electrophysiologic evaluation of facial palsy is considered. The reader is referred to Chapter 6 for discussion of the findings in facial myokymia and hemifacial spasm.

257

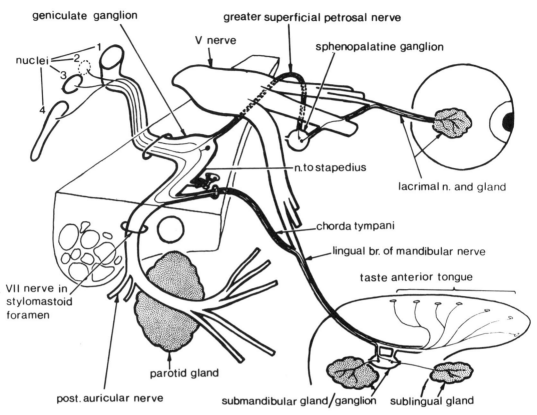

Fig. 12.1 Anatomy of the facial nerve. For simplicity, only some of the branches of the nerve are shown. Nuclei: 1, motor nucleus of the seventh cranial nerve; 2, ? special nucleus for lacrimal gland; 3, superior salivatory nucleus; 4, nucleus tractus solitarius. (Aminoff MJ: Clinical aspects of Bell's palsy. Br J Hosp Med 12:559, 1974.)

ELECTROPHYSIOLOGIC EXAMINATION OF THE FACIAL MUSCLES AND NERVE

Needle Electromyography

A fine concentric needle electrode is used to sample the facial muscles, the most convenient of which to examine are the frontalis and orbicularis oris. The mean duration of motor unit potentials is shorter in these muscles than in the limb muscles, and there is a higher incidence of polyphasic potentials. The examiner should, therefore, be familiar with the electromyographic appearance of normal facial muscles. This is important because of the ease with which the short-duration motor unit potentials can be mistaken for fibrillation potentials when the amount of voluntary activity is grossly reduced. When sampling is performed near the midline, the possibility that muscles are supplied by the contralateral facial nerve must be considered and excluded, if necessary, by stimulating the nerve on that side.

Facial Nerve Stimulation

The facial nerve can conveniently be stimulated using surface electrodes, with the cathode being placed at the angle of the jaw just in front of the mastoid process, and the anode being placed more posteriorly. A search is made on the normal side for the point at which a submaximal stimulus yields the greatest response and excites muscles supplied by all branches of the nerve. The corresponding site on the affected side is then stimulated after a similar search to confirm that this is, indeed, the most effective point. Alternatively, needle electrodes may be used for stimulation, with the cathode being placed next to the nerve as it emerges from the stylomastoid foramen by inserting it to a depth of about 2 cm at right angles to the skin and just in front of the tip of the mastoid process.[1] The anode is placed subcutaneously 2 to 3 cm posterior and inferior to the cathode.[1] The response is usually recorded from the frontalis or orbicularis oris or oculi muscles; either needle or surface electrodes are suitable for this purpose. Surface electrodes are particularly useful in children; when they are used, the reference electrode can generally be placed on the side of the nose. The ground electrode is placed between the stimulating and recording electrodes, or on the forehead (Fig. 12.2).

The normal side is examined first and the findings are then compared with those obtained on the affected side. Although some authors have reported electrophysiologic abnormalities on the nonparetic side in patients with Bell's palsy and have taken this to indicate subclinical involvement,[2,3] the study by Olsen does not support this interpretation and suggests that a comparison of the findings on the two sides is fully justified.[1] Care must be taken, however, to ensure that the distance between the stimulating cathode and recording electrode is equal on both sides.

When nerve excitability is being studied, the smallest amount of current necessary to produce a minimal visible response in the facial muscles is measured. Campbell and co-workers found that this level of current was usually 3 to 8 mA when the stimulus was of 1-msec duration.[4] Minor differences

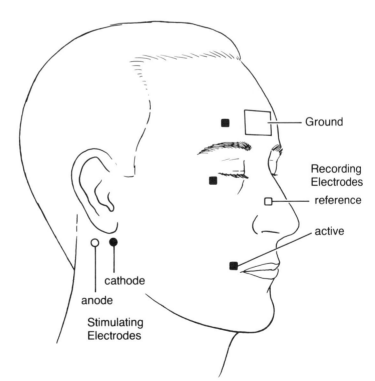

Fig. 12.2 Electrode placements for facial nerve conduction studies.

between the two sides of the face were found in normal subjects, and differences of at least 2 mA were required before these authors attributed any clinical significance to them. Even differences of this magnitude, however, may not be a reliable predictor of denervation in patients with Bell's palsy.[5]

The latency of the motor response evoked by supramaximal stimulation of the facial nerve can also be measured and compared on the two sides. When recording from the orbicularis oris, the latency is normally less than 4.0 msec, with a difference between the two sides of less than 0.5 msec. The latency may be prolonged in patients with diabetes,[6] generalized polyneuropathies,[7] or chronic renal failure.[8] It is also prolonged in some patients with Bell's palsy of more than a week's duration.[9]

When the size of the response evoked by supramaximal stimulation of the facial nerve is to be examined, the peak-to-peak amplitude or the amplitude of the initial negative phase of the action potential recorded from the frontalis, orbicularis oris, or depressor anguli oris muscle is measured. This provides an indication of the number of muscle fibers activated and thus, of the number of nerve fibers remaining excitable. Recordings are best made with surface or subcutaneous needle electrodes, the position of which is adjusted until the response obtained is of maximal amplitude and is as synchronized as possible. The reference electrode is placed on the opposite side of the face. Olsen found that recording in this "unipolar" way is more satisfactory than recording with a concentric needle electrode because there is less variability in the size of the response.[1] The results obtained on the normal and affected sides of the face are then compared, and may provide information of prognostic significance in patients with Bell's palsy.[1]

The use of supramaximal stimuli is necessary when the latency or amplitude of the motor response is being studied, but spread of the stimulating current—when of high intensity—may lead to unintended activation of the masseter muscle at its motor point. The response of this muscle may then be picked up by the recording electrode as a result of volume conduction. The contraction of the masseter should be evident on visual inspection of the face.

Stimulation of the unaffected facial nerve in patients with facial palsy may evoke action potentials from the contralateral (paralyzed) perioral muscles. These contralateral responses are probably attributable to conduction along muscle fibers crossing the midline rather than to cross-innervation, and similar responses may be evoked contralateral to the stimulated facial nerve in normal subjects.[10]

Blink Reflex

The technique of recording blink reflexes in the laboratory has already been discussed in Chapter 8.

BELL'S PALSY

The electromyographic investigation of patients with Bell's palsy exemplifies the approach to patients with facial nerve lesions of other types. In Bell's palsy, facial weakness is usually preceded or accompanied by pain in or about the ear, but this usually lasts for no more than a few days. The onset of weakness is relatively abrupt, and it may progress over the initial 2 to 3 days or, less commonly, over a somewhat longer period. Depending on the site of the lesion, it may be accompanied by impaired lacrimation, hyperacusis, or a disturbance of taste. All of the muscles supplied by the affected nerve are paralyzed when the lesion is complete, whereas the degree of weakness varies in different muscles if the lesion is incomplete. The majority of patients recover completely, without treatment, after a period of time that varies from a few days to several months.[11] In other instances, the cosmetic result is acceptable even though recovery is incomplete, and only about 10 percent of patients with Bell's palsy are "seriously dissatisfied" with the final outcome because of permanent disfigurement or other sequelae.[12] Treatment with steroids may increase the proportion of patients who recover completely, but it is generally believed that such treatment must commence within 5 days of onset of the palsy to be effective. Some means of predicting the outcome at an early stage is, therefore, required if treatment is to be offered to the minority of patients who will benefit from it.

Useful clinical indicators of a poor prognosis for complete recovery are initial pain and the presence of a complete palsy when the patient is first seen.[12,13] Electrophysiologic methods have also been used to assess prognosis, but do not permit this to be determined sufficiently early to guide the selection of patients for treatment. In considering the electrophysiologic evaluation of patients with Bell's palsy, it must be remembered that the facial nerve does not degenerate in those who completely recover, its dysfunction being caused by a reversible conduction block. In contrast, degeneration always occurs to some extent in those who have residual, long-term sequelae.

Electromyographic Sampling

Electromyographic sampling of facial muscles may reveal that some motor units survive under voluntary control in patients with clinically complete palsies, thereby indicating a more favorable prognosis than is implied by an absence of motor unit activity. Similarly, in patients with palsies secondary to other causes, such as trauma, the presence of surviving units is of prognostic significance in indicating that the nerve re-

mains in continuity. This finding must be interpreted with caution, however, because fibers of the orbicularis oris muscle cross from one side of the face to the other, so that it may be necessary to block the unaffected facial nerve with an anesthetic agent in order to establish that the palsy is, in fact, complete.[14]

The presence of fibrillation potentials and positive sharp waves in patients with Bell's palsy suggests that denervation has occurred and, therefore, that the eventual outcome may be unsatisfactory. The absence of such activity when the patient is first seen does not necessarily indicate, however, that a good outcome can be anticipated. The appearance of these signs may be delayed for about 3 weeks after onset of palsy, and incomplete recovery may occur even if fibrillation potentials are never detected.

Needle examination may indicate at an early stage whether recovery is occurring after an initially complete palsy, for volitional motor unit activity reappears at a time when movement is not yet visible on attempted contraction of the facial muscles. It also provides an ancillary method of studying the outcome in patients with Bell's palsy who have participated in trials of treatment regimens to prevent denervation. In patients with little, if any, residual deficit after recovery, electromyography may provide evidence that denervation has occurred at some stage during the course of the disorder. Slight movements occur in one part of the face when another part is moved after recovery from denervation, regardless of the extent to which power is regained,[15] and the detection of such associated movements is facilitated by simultaneous recording from the different muscles.

Facial Nerve Excitability

Campbell and co-workers compared the intensity of current required to evoke a minimal visible contraction of the facial muscles on the normal and affected sides in patients with a clinically complete Bell's palsy.[4] They found that full recovery subsequently occurred in 90 percent of patients when there was no difference on the two sides, presumably because the underlying pathophysiology was a conduction block proximal to the site of stimulation. When the affected nerve was inexcitable, it was assumed to have degenerated completely, and full recovery ultimately occurred in only 20 percent of cases. The affected nerve was excitable, but only at a higher intensity than normal, in the remaining patients, 49 percent of whom recovered completely, and this change in excitability was attributed to partial degeneration.

The prognostic implications of an inexcitable facial nerve were subsequently confirmed by others.[5,9] Groves, however, found that the nerve never became inexcitable before the fourth day.[5] He also reported that a difference between the two sides of less than 5 mA in the requisite intensity of stimulating current was an unreliable predictor of denervation, but that a difference of 5 mA or greater was followed by total inexcitability within hours. He concluded, therefore, that nerve excitability tests do not permit cases with a poor outlook to be detected sufficiently early for effective treatment to be instituted.

Motor Latency

Gilliatt and Taylor stimulated the facial nerve percutaneously after it had been divided for therapeutic purposes in three patients.[16] They found little change in latency of the muscle response recorded electromyographically until the response became unobtainable 4 to 7 days later (Fig. 12.3). Langworth and Taverner stimulated the nerve at the angle of the jaw in patients with Bell's palsy and reported that the latency of the muscle response was normal (that is, less than 4.0 msec) in patients who ulti-

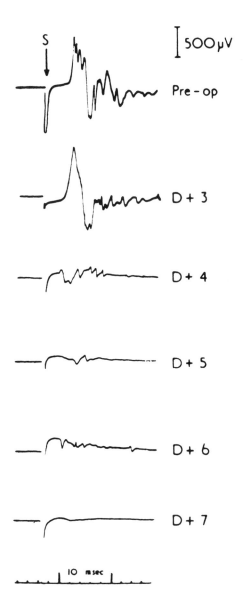

Fig. 12.3 Tracings to show muscle response to facial nerve stimulation before, and on successive days after, nerve section. The stimulus (S) is shown by artifact in each trace and is followed by muscle action potentials up to the sixth postoperative day (D + 6) but not after this time. (Gilliatt RW, Taylor JC: Electrical changes following section of the facial nerve. Proc R Soc Med 52:1080, 1959.)

mately made a complete recovery.[9] Latency sometimes became prolonged after about the first week in those who eventually developed partial denervation, but usually remained normal until the nerve became inexcitable in those who went on to develop complete denervation.

Amplitude of the Muscle Action Potential Evoked by Nerve Stimulation

Olsen found that the amplitude of the muscle action potential evoked by maximally stimulating the facial nerve was a reliable indicator of eventual outcome.[1] He studied patients after 5 or more days had elapsed from onset of the palsy and reported that a reduction in amplitude of 10 to 50 percent of that on the unaffected side was associated with only minor residual sequelae, but that a reduction to less than 10 percent was followed by poor recovery. Clearly, the amplitude of the response relates to the number of surviving axons in the nerve, and thus reflects the severity of nerve damage. Its value as a means of assessing the prognosis in Bell's palsy has since been confirmed in other studies.[17] However, in some patients, the muscle action potential continues to decline for as long as several weeks after the onset of facial weakness, suggesting that nerve degeneration is continuing over this relatively long period of time. Such a finding implies that Bell's palsy may be a heterogeneous group of disorders rather than representing a simple, acute, monophasic disturbance.

Blink Reflex

The blink reflex reflects the functional status of the seventh cranial nerve in its entirety. Abnormalities of the blink reflex have been described in patients with Bell's palsy or other lesions of the facial nerve.[18,19] The response may be delayed or absent, as described in Chapter 8, and abnormalities may progress over the first few days rather than being maximal at onset of the facial weakness. Blink reflex studies will not identify at an early stage patients with a poor prognosis. Some patients with an initial response that is markedly abnormal may do well clinically, whereas in others an initially near-normal response (that might be taken to imply a good prognosis) becomes unelicitable after several days.

If axonal degeneration occurs, it is followed to a variable extent by regeneration. Fibers originally going to the orbicularis oculi may come to supply other facial muscles if aberrant regeneration occurs. In such circumstances, a blink reflex may be elicited in these other muscles, and the demonstration of synkinetic movements by this means will obviate any uncertainty as to whether the movements have a volitional basis.

Electrogustometry

Electrogustometry tests the integrity of the chorda tympani fibers and is a reliable indicator, at an early stage, of which patients with Bell's palsy are likely to develop denervation. A detailed account of the method is beyond the scope of this book, but can be obtained elsewhere.[20,21] In brief, however, the anterior portion of the tongue is stimulated electrically on each side, at increasing strength, until a distinct acidic taste is evoked. The threshold levels on the two sides are then compared. In one study, 20 of 21 patients who were seen within 2 weeks of onset of Bell's palsy and who ultimately developed denervation exhibited an increased threshold on the affected side.[21] In nine of these patients, the threshold was raised while the facial nerve was still excitable. By contrast, in 21 other patients, there were no significant differences in the galvanic threshold on the two sides, and all of the patients subsequently made a complete recovery.

Equipment for anodal galvanic stimula-

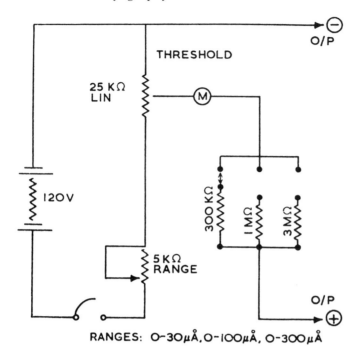

THRESHOLD

25 KΩ
LIN

O/P

120V

300 KΩ

1 MΩ

3 MΩ

5 KΩ
RANGE

O/P

RANGES: 0-30μÅ, 0-100μÅ, 0-300μÅ

Fig. 12.4 Circuit diagram of an electrogustometer. (Peiris OA, Miles DW: Galvanic stimulation of the tongue as a prognostic index in Bell's palsy. Br Med J 2:1162, 1965. By permission of the Authors and Editors of the British Medical Journal.)

tion of the tongue is easily constructed. A circuit diagram of such equipment is shown in Figure 12.4.

a reliable indication of prognosis at a sufficiently early stage for treatment to be instituted for those requiring it.

Summary

In patients with Bell's palsy, a poor prognosis for full recovery is indicated electrophysiologically by the absence of volitional motor unit activity, the presence of fibrillation potentials and positive sharp waves, an inexcitable facial nerve, and a gross reduction in amplitude of the muscle action potential evoked by nerve stimulation. Treatment is usually ineffective by the time such changes have occurred, but the changes may be used to monitor the progress of individual patients. Moreover, the high spontaneous recovery rate of patients with Bell's palsy implies that patients who are participating in therapeutic trials should be matched as far as possible for these prognostic indicators. Electrogustometry has not achieved widespread use in clinical practice, but it does seem to provide

REFERENCES

1. Olsen PZ: Prediction of recovery in Bell's palsy. Acta Neurol Scand 52:suppl. 61, 1, 1975
2. Safman BL: Bilateral pathology in Bell's palsy. Arch Otolaryngol 93:55, 1971
3. Chaco J: Subclinical peripheral nerve involvement in unilateral Bell's palsy. Am J Phys Med 52:195, 1973
4. Campbell EDR, Hickey RP, Nixon KH, Richardson AT: Value of nerve-excitability measurements in prognosis of facial palsy. Br Med J 2:7, 1962
5. Groves J: Facial palsies: Selection of cases for treatment. Proc R Soc Med 66:545, 1973
6. Johnson EW, Waylonis GW: Facial nerve conduction delay in patients with diabetes mellitus. Arch Phys Med Rehabil 45:131, 1964
7. Waylonis GW, Johnson EW: Facial nerve conduction delay. Arch Phys Med Rehabil 45:539, 1964

8. Taylor N, Jebsen RH, Tenckhoff HA: Facial nerve conduction latency in chronic renal insufficiency. Arch Phys Med Rehabil 51:259, 1970

9. Langworth EP, Taverner D: The prognosis in facial palsy. Brain 86:465, 1963

10. Trojaborg W: Does cross-innervation occur after facial palsy? J Neurol Neurosurg Psychiatry 40:712, 1977

11. Aminoff MJ: Clinical aspects of Bell's palsy. Br J Hosp Med 12:559, 1974

12. Taverner D: The prognosis and treatment of spontaneous facial palsy. Proc R Soc Med 52:1077, 1959

13. Matthews WB: Prognosis in Bell's palsy. Br Med J 2:215, 1961

14. Buchthal F: Electromyography in paralysis of the facial nerve. Arch Otolaryngol 81:463, 1965

15. Taverner D: Bell's palsy. A clinical and electromyographic study. Brain 78:209, 1955

16. Gilliatt RW, Taylor JC: Electrical changes following section of the facial nerve. Proc R Soc Med 52:1080, 1959

17. Boongird P, Vejjajiva A: Electrophysiologic findings and prognosis in Bell's palsy. Muscle Nerve 1:461, 1978

18. Kimura J, Powers JM, Van Allen MW: Reflex response of orbicularis oculi muscle to supraorbital nerve stimulation: Study in normal subjects and in peripheral facial paresis. Arch Neurol 21:193, 1969

19. Kimura J: The blink reflex as a clinical test. p. 347. In Aminoff MJ (ed): Electrodiagnosis in Clinical Neurology. 2nd Ed. Churchill Livingstone, New York, 1986

20. Krarup B: Electro-gustometry: A method for clinical taste examinations. Acta Otolaryngol (Stockh) 49:294, 1958

21. Peiris OA, Miles DW: Galvanic stimulation of the tongue as a prognostic index in Bell's palsy. Br Med J 2:1162, 1965

13

Root and Plexus Lesions

RADICULOPATHIES

Electrophysiologic techniques have an important role in the evaluation of patients with suspected radiculopathies. In the first place, the findings may confirm the presence of a radiculopathy and indicate the level of root involvement. Conversely, the findings may indicate that a lesion at some other site is responsible for the patient's symptoms and signs, and the examination must always be conducted with this possibility in mind. Second, the nature of any electromyographic abnormalities may indicate the severity of the underlying pathologic process by permitting the distinction of a localized demyelinative lesion from axonal degeneration. This is an important distinction because the former implies a good prognosis for complete and rapid recovery, whereas the latter suggests that recovery is likely to be delayed and incomplete. Axonal degeneration results from a severe focal lesion, whereas a relatively milder lesion may lead solely to conduction slowing or blocking from localized demyelination. Third, the electrophysiologic findings may help to determine whether an abnormality that is detected by myelography or computed tomography (CT) scanning is of any functional relevance. In other words, electrophysiologic techniques have an impor-

tant complementary role to radiologic imaging procedures, and one is certainly not a substitute for the other. Fourth, in patients who have undergone surgical treatment for a compressive root lesion, postoperative complaints may be hard to evaluate except by electrophysiologic means, especially if these studies can be compared with preoperative studies. It must be emphasized, however, that although the electrophysiologic evaluation of patients with a root lesion is clearly important, normal findings do not exclude the possibility of a radiculopathy if this disorder is suspected clinically.

The clinical features of root lesions are well known. Pain is common and may be accompanied by a segmental motor or sensory deficit, and there is depression of those tendon reflexes whose arc is subserved by the affected roots. In the cervical region, the sixth and seventh roots are affected most commonly by disc disease, with the fifth and eighth roots being involved somewhat less frequently. In the lumbosacral region, the fifth lumbar and first sacral roots and, to a lesser extent, the fourth lumbar root, are most commonly affected by compressive disc lesions, whereas other roots are involved infrequently.

The neurologic deficit resulting from damage to one root is often masked because of the overlap that exists with other nerve roots that remain intact. Since most muscles are supplied from several different segments, it may be difficult to demonstrate clinically any weakness when a mild lesion involves one nerve root. When weakness is found, it probably relates to conduction block or axonal degeneration rather than to conduction slowing. When it occurs in the presence of muscle atrophy, significant axonal degeneration should be suspected. The cutaneous distribution of nerve fibers is such that there is a similar overlap of, and variation in, segmental territory. For example, Inouye and Buchthal examined the segmental sensory innervation in different regions of the upper limbs by studying the potentials recorded from cervical spinal nerves following stimulation of different digits and various nerves.[1] They found that the little finger seemed to be supplied as often by C8 as by both C7 and C8, and that the cutaneous areas of the first and second digits connected as often to C7 as to C6. Dermatomal sensory changes may, therefore, be more restricted than anticipated in patients with an isolated radiculopathy.

There is wide variation in published charts delineating the anatomic distribution of single spinal roots. This is partly a result of the variation in normal anatomy, but is also partly attributable to attempts to extrapolate from experimental findings in animals to expected findings in humans.

Radiculopathies may occur for many reasons, including compression (for example, from prolapse of an intervertebral disc, or degenerative osteoarthritis), trauma, neoplastic disease, diabetes, ischemia, and infective or inflammatory pathology (for example, Guillain-Barré syndrome or zoster infection). The resulting electrophysiologic findings depend upon the nature and severity of the underlying process. For convenience, the electrophysiologic findings in patients with compressive radiculopathy secondary to compression from disc disease are considered in detail, and the findings in

other disorders are then briefly summarized.

Compressive Radiculopathies

Needle electromyography is performed to delineate the distribution of affected muscles, and to determine whether it conforms to a myotomal pattern. The findings are also important in providing a prognostic guide by indicating whether or not denervation has occurred or reinnervation is proceeding. With severe damage, there is axonal degeneration, and this leads to the presence of positive sharp waves and fibrillation potentials in a myotomal distribution, and to loss of motor units. Especially in chronic radiculopathies, complex repetitive discharges are sometimes found, but fasciculations are rare. There may also be a reduction in the size of the compound muscle action potential elicited by supramaximal stimulation of the motor nerve supply of affected muscles. With lesser degrees of damage, pathophysiologic changes may consist solely of localized conduction block or slowing. Abnormal spontaneous activity is then inconspicuous or absent in affected muscles, although there is reduced recruitment of motor units on volitional activity, and the compound muscle action potential recorded from affected muscles by stimulation distal to the lesion is normal.

Lesions may develop acutely or over a longer period of time, and the timing of the examination in relation to the onset of the lesion also affects the electrophysiologic findings. In patients with an acute root lesion, the first abnormality to be found on needle examination is impaired recruitment of motor units in affected muscle, with an increase in recruitment frequency and a reduction in the number of units activated. Although the presence of fibrillation potentials and positive sharp waves in a myotomal distribution is helpful in establishing the diagnosis of a root lesion, as well as in indicating that axonal degeneration has occurred, such abnormal spontaneous activity does not develop for 7 to 10 days or longer after the onset of the lesion, depending upon the muscle that is examined. (If found earlier, it suggests either that there has been previous pathology or that onset of the current lesion occurred earlier than originally thought.) It appears sooner in proximal than in distal muscles, and is found first in the paraspinal muscles, usually about 1 week or so after onset of the lesion. Therefore, these muscles should always be examined in patients suspected of having a root lesion unless they have had previous back surgery, in which case any paraspinal electromyographic abnormalities may be hard to interpret.

Electromyographic abnormalities in the paraspinal muscles help to localize the lesion to the nerve roots or spinal cord, and would not be expected to occur in patients with a plexus or peripheral nerve lesion. This is because the paraspinal muscles are supplied by the posterior primary rami of the spinal nerves, whereas the limb plexuses and peripheral nerves are derived from the anterior primary rami.

It is particularly important to examine the paraspinal muscles if the peripheral limb muscles are normal. Abnormal spontaneous activity may not develop until 2 to 6 weeks after onset of the lesion in different limb muscles, depending upon their location. For the examination of paraspinal muscles, the needle electrode is generally inserted about 2 to 3 cm to the side of the appropriate spinous process. It may be advanced for approximately 4 to 5 cm, or alternatively, it may be advanced until it reaches the subjacent transverse process, and then is withdrawn slightly so that its tip lies in the multifidus muscle. Although segmental representation is said to be greatest in this muscle, the findings in the paraspinal muscles should not be relied upon to determine the segmental level of the lesion because there is so much segmental overlap.

As reinnervation occurs (by collateral sprouting from surviving axons, regeneration of degenerated axons, or both), an increased incidence of polyphasic potentials, some of which may show pathologic variation in amplitude or configuration, is noted. The size and duration of motor unit potentials increases with continued reinnervation so that the needle examination may provide evidence of a long-standing root lesion even when the clinical deficit has resolved. Fibrillation potentials become less conspicuous and eventually disappear as reinnervation proceeds, first in the proximal muscles and then more distally. From the distribution of fibrillation potentials, therefore, it may be possible to gain some idea of the duration of the lesion. Reinnervation generally tends to be more complete in the proximal than in the distal muscles, and this should be considered when muscles are selected for study.

Thus, in patients who undergo electromyographic examination soon (7 to 10 days) after onset of a radiculopathy, impaired recruitment of motor units in a myotomal distribution is evident and, if axonal degeneration has occurred, fibrillation and positive sharp waves are found in the paraspinal muscles. During the following days or weeks, abnormal spontaneous activity may be noted, first in other proximal muscles and then in the distal muscles of the affected myotome. Even later, as reinnervation occurs, fibrillations and positive sharp waves are found predominantly in the distal muscles of the myotome, whereas an increasing number of large, long-duration, polyphasic motor unit potentials are found, first proximally and ultimately in a more widespread segmental distribution.

The distribution of abnormalities must conform to a myotomal pattern if an isolated root lesion is to be diagnosed on electromyographic grounds. Abnormalities are usually not found in all of the muscles of the involved myotome, but must be found in at least two separate muscles supplied by

Table 13.1. The Innervation of Selected Muscles in the Upper Limbs[a]

Spinal Segment	Dorsal Scapular Nerve	Long Thoracic Nerve	Suprascapular Nerve	Subscapular Nerve	Thoracodorsal Nerve	Pectoral Nerve	Circumflex Nerve	Musculocutaneous Nerve	Radial Nerve	Median Nerve	Ulnar Nerve
C4	(Rhomboids)										
C5	Rhomboids	Serratus anterior	Supraspinatus Infraspinatus	Subscapularis		(Pectoralis major)	Deltoid	Biceps	Brachioradialis Supinator		
C6		Serratus anterior	(Infraspinatus)	Subscapularis	Latissimus dorsi	Pectoralis major	(Deltoid)	Biceps	Brachioradialis Supinator Extensor carpi radialis longus	Pronator teres Flexor carpi radialis	
C7		Serratus anterior		(Subscapularis)	Latissimus dorsi	Pectoralis major			Extensor carpi radialis longus Triceps Extensor digitorum Extensor carpi ulnaris Extensor indicis (Extensor pollicis longus and brevis)	Pronator teres Flexor carpi radialis Palmaris longus (Flexor digitorum sublimis) (Flexor digitorum profundus I and II) (Flexor pollicis longus)	(Flexor carpi ulnaris) (Flexor digitorum profundus III and IV)
C8					Latissimus dorsi	Pectoralis major			Triceps (Extensor digitorum) Extensor carpi ulnaris Extensor indicis Extensor pollicis longus and brevis	(Flexor carpi radialis) Palmaris longus Flexor digitorum sublimis Flexor digitorum profundus I and II Flexor pollicis longus (Abductor pollicis brevis) (Opponens pollicis)	Flexor carpi ulnaris Flexor digitorum profundus III and IV Abductor digiti minimi First dorsal interosseous
T1						(Pectoralis major)				(Palmaris longus) (Flexor digitorum sublimis) (Flexor digitorum profundus I and II) (Flexor pollicis longus) Abductor pollicis brevis Opponens pollicis	(Flexor digitorum profundus III and IV) Abductor digiti minimi First dorsal interosseous

[a] Only a limited number of muscles are included, but these are conveniently accessible for electromyographic examination. The name of the muscle has been placed in parentheses when its innervation from a particular spinal segment is not of major importance. There is no general agreement on the precise segmental innervation of certain muscles, and minor discrepancies may, therefore, be found between the material presented here and that of other authors.

the involved root in the affected limb. These muscles must not be supplied by the same peripheral nerve or some common structural component of the limb plexus. Furthermore, similar abnormalities must not be present in muscles supplied by other nerve roots, and the muscles with electromyographic abnormalities must have only the one root in common. Abnormalities in the paraspinal muscles help to support the diagnosis, but are not always present. Electromyographic abnormalities would not be expected to occur in the paraspinal muscles in patients with plexus or peripheral nerve lesions.

The electromyographic examination of limb muscles is continued until it is clear that the distribution of electromyographic abnormalities is, indeed, radicular rather than conforming to a peripheral nerve distribution or to a pattern indicative of a plexus lesion. Similarly, it must be shown that muscles in other myotomes are not involved. For convenience, some of the limb muscles that can be examined electromyographically are shown in Tables 13.1 and

Table 13.2. The Innervation of Seleced Muscles in the Lower Limbs[a]

| | | | | | Sciatic Nerve | | |
Spinal Segments	Femoral Nerve	Obturator Nerve	Superior Gluteal Nerve	Inferior Gluteal Nerve		Common Peroneal Nerve or Its Branches	Tibial Nerve or Its Branches
L2	(Quadriceps femoris) Iliacus	Adductors of thigh Gracilis					
L3	Quadriceps femoris Iliacus	Adductors of thigh Gracilis					
L4	Quadriceps femoris	Adductors of thigh (Gracilis)	Gluteus medius Tensor fasciae latae		(Semimembranosus) (Semitendinosus) (Biceps femoris)	Tibialis anterior	
L5			Gluteus medius Tensor fasciae latae	Gluteus maximus	Semimembranosus Semitendinosus Biceps femoris	Tibialis anterior Peronei Extensor digitorum brevis Extensor digitorum longus Extensor hallucis longus	(Flexor digitorum longus) Tibialis posterior
S1			Gluteus medius	Gluteus maximus	Semimembranosus Semitendinosus Biceps femoris	Peronei Extensor digitorum brevis (Extensor digitorum longus) (Extensor hallucis longus)	Gastrocnemius Soleus Flexor digitorum longus (Tibialis posterior) Abductor hallucis Abductor digiti quinti pedis
S2				(Gluteus maximus)	(Semimembranosus) (Semitendinosus) (Biceps femoris)		Gastrocnemius Soleus (Flexor digitorum longus) Abductor hallucis Abductor digiti quinti pedis

[a] Only a limited number of muscles are included, but these are conveniently accessible for electromyographic examination. The name of the muscle has been placed in parentheses when its innervation from a particular spinal segment is not of major importance. There is no general agreement on the precise segmental innervation of certain muscles, and minor discrepancies may, therefore, be found between the material presented here and that of other authors.

13.2, where the details of their nerve supply are indicated. The importance of a well-planned needle examination can be illustrated by several examples. For instance, needle examination of the rhomboid muscles may help to distinguish C5 radiculopathy from a brachial plexus lesion, since the rhomboid muscles are supplied by the dorsal scapular nerve which arises directly from the C5 nerve root. In the legs, it is often difficult clinically to distinguish between an L5 radiculopathy and a peroneal nerve palsy, but needle examination of the tibialis posterior, gluteus medius, and tensor fasciae latae may be helpful since these are not supplied by the peroneal nerve.

The diagnosis of radiculopathy should not be made on electrophysiologic grounds solely because of an increased incidence of polyphasic potentials. Such potentials are nonspecific in character, may occur in both neuropathic and myopathic disorders, and may represent sequelae from a previous root lesion that has resolved and that is not responsible for the patient's complaint. Similarly, electromyographic abnormalities in just one muscle do not permit a definitive diagnosis to be made.

The presence of *paraspinal abnormalities* are by no means diagnostic of either a radiculopathy or a compressive lesion. Electromyographic abnormalities in the paraspinal muscles may be found in several different clinical contexts and provide evidence of damage to the nerve roots, spinal nerves, or spinal cord. With compressive, infiltrative, or infarctive pathology of the cord, paraspinal fibrillations are generally present bilaterally and at multiple levels.[2] Similar abnormalities may also be found in diabetes, acute or chronic inflammatory polyradiculopathy, the polyradiculopathy or polyneuropathy associated with monoclonal gammopathy, other inflammatory or infiltrative processes (such as metastatic pathology) involving the nerve roots, amyotrophic lateral sclerosis, progressive spinal muscular atrophy, porphyria, and

compressive lesions of the cauda equina. They may also accompany muscle trauma or inflammatory myopathy, and commonly occur following laminectomy.

Fasciculation potentials may be found in patients with a chronic radiculopathy, but they are uncommon. Their presence should prompt a more detailed electromyographic examination to exclude motor neuron disease (p. 85).

The main value of *standard motor and sensory nerve conduction studies* is to exclude other, more peripheral disorders that might otherwise be mistaken for a radiculopathy. These studies generally show no abnormalities in patients with isolated root lesions because the sites of stimulation and recording are located more distally than the site of damage. However, if marked axonal degeneration has occurred, the size of the compound muscle action potentials may be reduced significantly in muscles supplied by the affected nerve root when compared to the unaffected side or to the normal values obtained for that muscle in the laboratory where the study is performed. By contrast, a compound muscle action potential of normal size, when recorded 3 weeks or more after the onset of symptoms, suggests either that the lesion is attributable to demyelination (therefore carrying a favorable prognosis) or that only mild axonal loss has occurred. Because muscles are generally supplied by two or more nerve roots, mild axonal loss in one root usually has little effect on the size of the compound muscle action potential. However, a similar mild loss in two (or more) adjacent roots often leads to a marked reduction in the size of the response recorded from muscles that are supplied from both roots. If the fastest-conducting nerve fibers are preferentially affected by the lesion or if marked axonal loss has occurred, there may be slight slowing of maximal motor conduction velocity. Because the site of the lesion is proximal to the dorsal root ganglion, however, there is no change in the size or latency of the sensory nerve action potential, even in patients with clinically severe sensory disturbances. This may be helpful in distinguishing radiculopathies from plexopathies or peripheral nerve disorders.

The functional integrity of proximal segments of peripheral nerves may be evaluated by recording *F responses* or *H reflexes*. Because the H reflex can normally be elicited from just a limited number of muscles (as indicated in Chapter 8), it can only be used in evaluating patients with suspected lesions of the S1 nerve root. Unfortunately, these late responses often have a normal latency in patients with an established radiculopathy. This is because the affected length of nerve root is very short compared to the much longer segment of axons with normal conduction that is evaluated when F responses or H reflexes are recorded. Any delay at the site of the lesion is "diluted" by the long length of normally conducting axons and so is not recognized. Sensitivity is sometimes enhanced by comparing the latency of the F response or H reflex in the clinically affected limb with that found in the unaffected limb. Other parameters of these late responses, such as absence or attenuation of the H reflex or reduced persistence of the F response, may also be useful for diagnostic purposes, as discussed in Chapter 8.

Even when abnormalities of late responses are found, they may not be clinically helpful. For example, responses may have a prolonged latency because of previous disease rather than any concurrent pathology. Moreover, abnormalities in these responses do not localize the lesion to the root itself because a lesion at any point between the sites of stimulation and recording could be responsible for the abnormality.

Proximal conduction has also been assessed by the technique of *nerve root stimulation*. However, the site of stimulation is generally distal to the site of compression in patients with, for example, prolapse of an intervertebral disc.

Somatosensory evoked potential studies have recently been used to evaluate patients with suspected radiculopathies. Somewhat surprisingly, perhaps, abnormal cortical responses to stimulation of a plurisegmental, mixed, peripheral nerve have been reported in patients with an isolated root lesion. Indeed, in one study of 77 patients with lumbar disc lesions confirmed by myelogram, every patient was found to have an abnormal cortical response to peroneal nerve stimulation.[3] However, in our experience, peroneal-derived somatosensory evoked potentials are normal in patients with isolated L5 or S1 root lesions.[4]

Median- or ulnar-derived somatosensory evoked potentials have been used to study patients with cervical spondylosis. Unfortunately, patients without objective neurologic signs frequently have normal responses, and it is precisely in this group of patients that some ancillary investigative technique would be of most help. In patients who have a severe spondylotic radiculopathy causing objective neurologic signs, somatosensory evoked potentials may be abnormal as a result of loss of components of the response or an abnormally prolonged latency,[5,6] regardless of whether there is an associated myelopathy. It may be that response amplitude, rather than latency, would be more helpful in evaluating compressive root lesions,[7] but in general, this parameter is so variable that it is of relatively limited clinical utility. At the present time, then, somatosensory evoked potentials elicited by stimulation of nerve trunks in the arms are not really useful in the investigation of patients with a cervical radiculopathy. In particular, they are no more useful than careful clinical examination in determining the severity or prognosis of cervical spondylosis.

The segmental specificity of somatosensory evoked potentials may be increased by dermatomal or cutaneous nerve stimulation, and these techniques have, therefore, been used in the evaluation of patients with root lesions.[4,8–10] Using cutaneous nerve stimulation, Eisen and associates evaluated 28 patients with suspected cervical or lumbosacral root lesions and found that, in 16 patients (57 percent), the somatosensory evoked potentials were abnormal, usually in association with clinical sensory changes.[10] To evaluate cervical radiculopathies, they stimulated the musculocutaneous nerve when the C5 segment was to be evaluated, the median nerve fibers in the thumb for C6, the median nerve fibers along the adjoining surfaces of the second and third fingers for C7, and the ulnar nerve in the little finger for C8. The saphenous nerve was stimulated at the knee to evaluate L3 and at the ankle for L4, the superficial peroneal nerve was stimulated above the ankle to evaluate L5, and the sural nerve was stimulated at the ankle to assess S1. However, their subsequent experience with this technique has been more disappointing, although others remain enthusiastic. Perlik and co-workers recently examined the utility of recording somatosensory evoked responses elicited by stimulating specific cutaneous sensory nerves.[11] They found that, in 21 of 27 patients in whom the findings on CT scans were consistent with root injury, somatosensory evoked potential studies were also abnormal, and were consistent with focal root dysfunction and the radiographic abnormalities.

Dermatomal somatosensory evoked potentials (p. 155) are easy to record, and in one study of patients with surgically verified L5 or S1 root lesions, most patients (92 percent) were found to have abnormal responses, although it is not clear how the criteria for abnormality were derived.[9] However, in their more rigorous study, which incorporated a strict definition of abnormality, Aminoff and associates found that the yield was 25 percent, although in two of seven patients with abnormal responses, the other electrophysiologic studies were normal.[8] The poor diagnostic yield of somatosensory evoked potential studies probably relates to the very short segment along the somatosensory pathway in which conduction is impaired, in contrast to the very long segment in which conduction is normal. It is possible, however, that the diagnostic yield will increase when more sensitive parameters of the response—such as a quantitative definition of morphology or dispersion—are developed.

Aminoff and co-workers compared the diagnostic utility of needle electromyography, F response and H reflex studies, and peroneal and dermatomal somatosensory evoked potential studies in evaluating patients with clinically unequivocal L5 or S1 compressive root lesions.[8] They found that the single most useful electrophysiologic technique was the needle examination. Indeed, this mode of examination often provided evidence of denervation in a myotomal pattern when other electrophysiologic findings were normal. There was a disappointingly low diagnostic yield from studies of late responses, with the yield with F responses being only 18 percent, and the yield with H reflex studies being 41 percent among the patients with S1 lesions. Abnormal late responses were found in 14 of 28 patients studied (50 percent), which compares favorably with the experience of Tonzola and associates,[12] who found late response abnormalities in 15 of 57 patients (26 percent). All of the patients with abnormal late responses reported by Aminoff and colleagues also had abnormalities on needle examination.

Tonzola and associates correlated the electrophysiologic and myelographic findings in patients with a clinical diagnosis of lumbosacral root disease and found that 14 of 36 patients (39 percent) with abnormal myelograms had normal electrophysiologic studies, whereas 8 of 29 patients (28 percent) with abnormal electrophysiologic studies had a normal myelogram.[12] Such findings emphasize the complementary nature of these two investigative approaches.

In an attempt to derive guidelines for the

most cost-effective approach to evaluation, others have attempted to correlate the electromyographic findings with CT scan results in patients with low back pain. In one study of 80 consecutive patients, 42 had abnormal electromyographic findings (despite a rather limited examination) that could be explained on the basis of anatomic defects seen on CT scan, 9 had normal CT scans but abnormal electromyographic findings, and 5 had abnormal CT scans but normal electromyographic findings.[13] Of the patients who eventually underwent surgery, the abnormal CT and electromyographic findings were confirmed by surgery in most instances. However, in some patients, the abnormality was confirmed only at the level shown by electromyographic examination. An abnormal electromyogram seemed to corrrelate better with the prognosis and ultimate outcome of radiculopathy than the CT findings.[13]

Noncompressive Radiculopathies

Asymptomatic electromyographic abnormalities in the paraspinal muscles may be encountered in diabetic patients, often with a widespread distribution although sometimes the abnormalities are more restricted (but generally tend to be bilateral and symmetric).[14] Symptomatic radiculopathy is probably more common in diabetics than is generally appreciated, however, and reference to it has been made already in Chapter 11, where the different peripheral nerve complications of diabetes are considered. Diabetic radiculopathy may involve one or more of the limbs, or may be confined to, or most conspicuous in, the trunk. The presenting sign is generally pain, which often is severe in intensity, may not be clearly radicular in character, and may be associated with marked weight loss.[14] Electromyographic examination of the paraspinal muscles usually reveals bilateral abnormal-

ities that may span several segments, and there may be abnormalities in the intercostal, abdominal, or limb muscles, depending upon the level of the lesion. Intercostal nerve conduction studies have been said to help in the diagnosis of thoracic radiculopathy and in determining the level of involvement. However, pneumothorax may complicate the procedure,[15] so it is not performed routinely in most clinical neurophysiology laboratories. Electrophysiologic evidence of coexisting polyneuropathy or entrapment neuropathy may also be found.

Multisegmental, paraspinal, electromyographic abnormalities have been described in patients with occult metastatic carcinoma.[16] Further, a localized disease process, such as herniation of an intervertebral disc, sometimes leads to electromyographic changes over several paraspinal segments.[16] Reference has already been made (p. 272) to the wide variety of other disorders in which similar abnormalities may be encountered.

Muscle weakness, which is sometimes profound, may occur in patients with herpes zoster. The diagnosis is usually easily made when there is an accompanying skin rash, but herpes zoster may rarely occur without a rash,[17] and the development of a motor or sensory radiculopathy then poses a diagnostic dilemma. Thomas and Howard found that, of 1210 patients with herpes zoster seen at the Mayo Clinic over a 10-year period, 61 had zoster-induced segmental muscle weakness.[18] In their experience, the weakness always followed a cutaneous eruption and led to cranial nerve (usually facial) palsies in 28 patients, upper limb weakness in 16, lower limb weakness in 15, and weakness of the abdominal musculature in 2 patients. The motor deficit varied in severity from mild to very profound, and there was an uneven distribution of weakness within the myotome, depending on the extent to which muscles were also supplied by other, nonaffected nerve roots. Electromyography confirms the neurogenic basis of the weakness and indicates its radicular origin. Changes are found both in the paraspinal muscles and in muscles supplied by the anterior primary ramus of the spinal nerve.[18]

Cauda Equina Lesions

In patients with multiple lumbosacral radiculopathies, such as occur with a cauda equina lesion, clinical and electrophysiologic evaluation usually reveals bilateral abnormalities, although one side may be more severely affected than the other. Needle electromyography reveals abnormalities indicative of multiple root lesions, but the precise findings will, as indicated on p. 268, depend upon the severity of the underlying pathologic process and the timing of the electrophysiologic study. When axonal degeneration has occurred, supramaximal stimulation of motor nerves may reveal small compound muscle action potentials from clinically affected muscles. Motor conduction velocity and terminal latency are normal, as are the sensory nerve action potentials in the legs. If there is involvement of the S1 root on one or both sides, the H reflex is commonly absent. The clinical and electrophysiologic findings sometimes simulate amyotrophic lateral sclerosis, especially if—as is common in the elderly—the plantar responses are extensor on one or both sides. However, the presence of pain, sensory disturbances, or sphincter involvement should raise the possibility of some underlying local structural lesion, and needle electromyography of the upper limbs is normal unless there is some coexisting pathology.

PLEXUS LESIONS

Lesions of a limb plexus are often difficult to evaluate, both clinically and by electrophysiologic means, and require detailed knowledge of normal anatomy (such as is provided in most major textbooks of anatomy). The relative inaccessibility of the limb plexuses makes their electrophysiologic evaluation especially challenging. Several general points in this regard have been made by Wilbourn.[19] First, extensive electromyographic sampling is often necessary for adequate evaluation. Second, it is frequently necessary to examine both the affected and unaffected limb when nerve conduction studies are performed in patients with unilateral plexus lesions in order to detect subtle abnormalities. Third, a detailed assessment of plexopathies may necessitate conduction studies of nerves that are not studied routinely. Finally, special techniques may be required to evaluate conduction through inaccessible segments of a limb plexus. These include the recording of F responses (p. 146), H reflexes (p. 149), and somatosensory evoked potentials (p. 150), as well as the technique of nerve root stimulation.

For *nerve root stimulation*, a Teflon-coated monopolar needle with about 2 mm of insulation removed from its tip is used as a stimulating cathode.[20,21] It is inserted perpendicular to the skin, in a sagittal plane, to lie adjacent to the spinal nerve and close to the intervertebral foramen. It is placed about 1 to 2 cm to the side of the midline at the level of interest, and advanced down to the bone. A surface anode is placed proximal to the cathode, or opposite it on the front of the neck or trunk. Motor fiber conduction to different muscles can then be studied, depending upon the level of the stimulating electrodes and the placement of the recording electrodes. Normal latency values for responses recorded from the biceps, triceps, and abductor digiti minimi in the upper limbs, and the vastus medialis and abductor hallucis in the lower limbs have been published by MacLean.[20] The method is more easily applied to the evaluation of cervical rather than lumbosacral pathology. Its main limitations are discomfort to the patient; the necessity, in many instances, to examine both the symptomatic and asymptomatic sides to improve the diagnostic yield; and the fact that sensory function cannot easily be evaluated. Its main value is in demonstrating the presence of conduction block across a limb plexus.

The nature, severity, and time course of the underlying pathology will govern the electrophysiologic findings. Mild compressive or traction lesions often lead to a focal demyelinative lesion that results in conduction slowing or block. In general, the prognosis for recovery after such a lesion is excellent. Electrophysiologic evaluation may reveal no abnormalities other than reduced recruitment of motor units from affected muscles if conduction block has occurred. This is because the lesion is so proximal that conduction across it cannot easily be assessed. More severe lesions lead to axonal loss, and so to a poorer prognosis. Electromyographic evidence of denervation may be found in affected muscles (provided examination is deferred for a suffi-

cient amount of time after onset of the lesion), and there is an attenuation of sensory nerve action potentials and, to a lesser extent, compound muscle action potentials from appropriate nerves and muscles that are affected by the lesion. There is little or no change in maximal motor and sensory conduction velocity.

Brachial Plexopathies

The anatomy of the brachial plexus is illustrated in Figures 13.1 and 13.2 and is summarized in Table 13.3. In brief, the plexus is formed by the anterior primary rami of the lower four cervical nerves and the first thoracic nerve with variable contributions from C4 and T2. The C5 and C6 roots unite to form the upper trunk of the plexus, C7 continues as the middle trunk, and C8 and T1 unite to form the lower trunk. Each trunk then divides into anterior and posterior branches at about the upper border of the clavicle. The anterior divisions

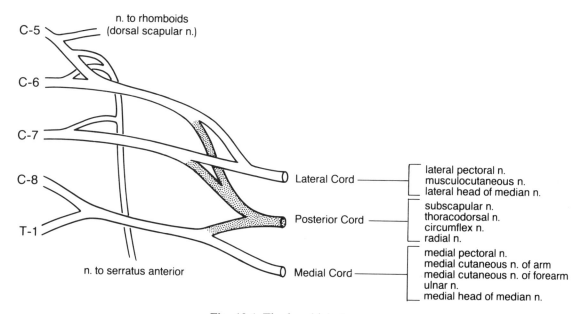

Fig. 13.1 The brachial plexus.

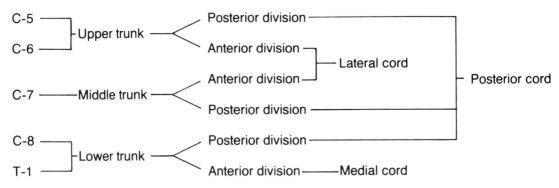

Fig. 13.2 A summary of the anatomy of the brachial plexus.

of the upper and middle trunks combine to form the lateral cord of the plexus, the anterior division of the lower trunk continues as the medial cord, and the posterior divisions of all the trunks join as the posterior cord. The various nerves that arise from the cords are shown in Table 13.3.

Brachial plexopathies may occur in a variety of different contexts and these govern the clinical and electrophysiologic findings. Their manifestations depend on the level and severity of pathologic involvement, and particularly on the components of the plexus that are affected, but they generally extend beyond the distribution of an isolated nerve root or peripheral nerve. The distribution of clinical signs and electro-

myographic abnormalities depends on the site and extent of the lesion. In a complete lesion of an entire plexus, the affected limb is paralyzed and senseless. The distribution of abnormalities in partial lesions of the brachial plexus depends on whether the plexus is affected above or below the clavicle. In supraclavicular lesions, abnormalities have a radicular distribution that depends on whether the upper (C5 and C6), middle (C7), or lower (C8 and T1) trunks of the plexus are involved. Infraclavicular lesions affect the cords of the plexus and the nerves which arise from them, and this governs the distribution of motor and sensory signs. A lesion of the lateral cord affects the musculocutaneous nerve and lateral root of the

Table 13.3. Nerves Arising from the Cords of the Brachial Plexus, with Their Root Derivation

Cord Segment	Nerve	Root Derivation
Lateral cord	Lateral pectoral nerve	C5, C6, C7
	Musculocutaneous nerve	C5, C6, C7
	Lateral head of median nerve	(C5), C6, C7
Medial cord	Medial pectoral nerve	C8, T1
	Medial cutaneous nerve of arm	C8, T1
	Medial cutaneous nerve of forearm	C8, T1
	Ulnar nerve	(C7),[b] C8, T1
	Medial head of median nerve	C8, T1
Posterior cord	Subscapular nerves	C5, C6, (C7)
	Thoracodorsal nerve	C6, C7, C8
	Circumflex nerve	C5, C6
	Radial nerve	C5, C6, C7, C8, (T1)

[a] Note: root derivations shown in parentheses are inconstant or only minor.
[b] These fibers enter the ulnar nerve through the plexus or more distally.

median; a medial cord lesion involves the ulnar nerve, the medial root of the median, and the medial cutaneous nerves of the arm and forearm; whereas posterior cord involvement affects the radial and circumflex nerves and sometimes, the nerves to subscapularis, teres major, and latissimus dorsi, as well.

Wilbourn has emphasized that lesions may be localized incorrectly when a plexopathy with only mild axonal loss leads to electromyographic abnormalities in a single peripheral nerve distribution, or when several nerves arising from the same component of the plexus are involved at the same time so that a plexopathy is simulated.[19] Radiculopathies can usually be distinguished from plexopathies by the presence of electromyographic abnormalities in the paraspinal muscles, and of preserved sensory nerve action potentials. However, it is sometimes impossible to distinguish between an isolated root lesion and a mild plexopathy if there are no paraspinal electromyographic abnormalities.

TRAUMATIC PLEXOPATHIES

Trauma is the most common cause of a brachial plexus lesion. Electrophysiologic studies are performed to localize the lesion and to determine its severity, as described on p. 277. It may be difficult clinically to distinguish between a plexopathy and root avulsion, and the electrophysiologic findings may help in this regard. When root avulsion has occurred, electromyographic sampling reveals spontaneous fibrillation and positive sharp waves in the cervical paraspinal muscles, and nerve conduction studies indicate that sensory nerve action potentials in the affected arm are preserved. By contrast, loss of the sensory nerve action potentials indicates a lesion distal to the dorsal root ganglion. In such circumstances, if needle electromyography provides evidence of denervation in the para-

spinal muscles, it can be inferred that there is a lesion involving both the plexus and the nerve roots. In contrast, the roots may be functionally intact if there are no paraspinal abnormalities found on examination performed about 10 days or so after injury. (As indicated earlier on p. 269, it may take 7 to 10 days before signs of denervation are found in the paraspinal muscles.)

Electromyographic sampling of other muscles that are supplied proximal to the plexus may also help in localizing the lesion. Examination of the rhomboid, levator scapulae, and serratus anterior muscles should, therefore, not be neglected.

Some authors have suggested that recording the somatosensory evoked potentials elicited by stimulation of nerves in the arm increases the accuracy of electrophysiologic evaluation of patients with traumatic lesions of the brachial plexus. Attenuation of N13 will reflect the total proportion of damaged nerve fibers, whereas N9 attenuation relates solely to the proportion damaged postganglionically. Jones and associates used this approach to evaluate patients with unilateral traction lesions of the brachial plexus.[22] The somatosensory evoked potentials were thought to indicate a postganglionic lesion when the N9 and N13 peaks were attenuated to a similar extent. When there was little or no attenuation of the N9 component but N13 and N20 were markedly attenuated, a preganglionic lesion was inferred. A combined lesion was suggested when, despite some attenuation of N9, the N13 component was attenuated to a greater extent or was absent. Abnormalities of the median-elicited response were thought to reflect damage to the C6 or C7 roots, or both, whereas abnormalities of the ulnar-elicited response suggested damage of the C8 or T1 nerve roots, or both. These researchers compared the preoperative electrophysiologic findings with the site of the surgically verified lesion in 16 patients, however, and found that electrophysiologic findings correctly localized the lesion in only 8. Indeed, in three patients, there was a marked discrepancy between the electrophysiologic findings and those revealed at operation.

Recently, Synek reviewed his extensive experience of median-derived somatosensory evoked potentials in patients with supraclavicular lesions of the brachial plexus.[23] First, he emphasized that, in patients with multiple root avulsions, the Erb's point (N9) potential was usually attenuated because of concomitant damage to the cords and trunks of the plexus. Moreover, he found that the median-elicited responses were always normal in injuries of the upper trunk and with root avulsions confined to one or two levels. Previously, he had stressed the relatively greater value of musculocutaneous-derived somatosensory evoked potentials in patients with brachial plexus injuries causing C5 and C6 root avulsion.[24]

Somatosensory evoked potentials, then, do not appear to offer any particular advantage in the preoperative evaluation of patients with traumatic lesions of the brachial plexus. However, intraoperative recordings across plexus lesions may be helpful in determining the continuity of individual segments of the plexus, and in guiding surgical treatment.

IDIOPATHIC BRACHIAL PLEXOPATHY

In many cases of neuralgic amyotrophy or idiopathic brachial plexopathy, there is a history of preceding viral infection, injection, injury, or surgery. The disorder usually commences acutely with pain about the shoulder or arm, with subsequent development of muscle weakness and wasting. Sensory complaints are commonly overshadowed by the motor deficit. Recovery generally occurs gradually over many months, and ultimately, there may be little or no residual deficit. Familial and recurrent cases have been described. Spontaneous at-

tacks of brachial plexopathy can also occur in patients with a hereditary susceptibility to pressure palsy (p. 225), as can plexopathies related to mild trauma.[25]

Needle electromyography is helpful in determining the distribution and severity of the disorder, which is patchy and therefore difficult to localize to any particular segment of the plexus. Typically, there is impaired recruitment or loss of motor unit potentials, as well as abnormal spontaneous activity (positive sharp waves and fibrillation potentials) in affected muscles. In some instances, the pattern of muscle involvement may suggest involvement of particular nerves, with mild or no abnormalities detected on needle examinations of other muscles supplied from the same and other levels of the plexus.[26] Such a pattern of abnormalities involves the axillary, suprascapular, or radial nerves most frequently.[26] In some instances, bilateral electromyographic abnormalities may be encountered. The electromyographic findings can be particularly confusing if abnormalities are found in the serratus anterior muscle (which is supplied from the roots rather than from the brachial plexus), especially if sensory nerve action potentials are then found to be normal when elicited from the median nerve fibers supplying the thumb.

Abnormalities of motor conduction, as determined by the latency to different muscles, may occasionally be encountered, but the findings are usually normal, even when recordings are made from severely affected muscles (as judged by the degree of weakness or wasting). However, the evoked muscle response may be attenuated, and sensory nerve action potentials are also commonly diminished in amplitude. F response latencies are sometimes abnormally prolonged.[26]

THORACIC OUTLET SYNDROME

Many patients with pain about the shoulder or vague sensory complaints in the arm or hand are said to have thoracic outlet syndrome, and it is assumed that nerves, blood vessels, or both are compressed between the neck and axilla. In most of these patients, clinical examination reveals no neurologic abnormalities whatsoever, and electrophysiologic evaluation is similarly normal. Swift and Nichols have recently defined the "droopy shoulder syndrome,"[27] which generally occurs in women with droopy shoulders and a long neck. The resulting traction on the brachial plexus produces pain about some portion of the upper limb, shoulder, or neck. Postural maneuvers often influence symptoms; traction on the shoulders may exacerbate the symptoms whereas proper posturing relieves them.

The neurogenic thoracic outlet syndrome has been well defined, especially by Gilliatt and his colleagues.[28,29] The medial cord or lower trunk of the brachial plexus, or the anterior primary rami of the C8 and T1 roots, are compressed by a cervical rib or band, and the middle trunk or anterior primary ramus of the C7 root may also be affected. In addition to pain and other sensory symptoms in the appropriate (C8 and T1) dermatomes, there is weakness and wasting of various muscles in the hand and, to a lesser extent, in the forearm, with the muscles in the lateral part of the thenar eminence being particularly affected. Careful clinical examination shows that these motor changes are more extensive than can be accounted for by a median nerve lesion, conforming instead to the distribution of muscles innervated by the T1 and C8 segments and, in a few cases, to those supplied by the C7 segment as well. In many cases, a cervical rib is visible on radiographic examination and is frequently bilateral; in other patients, there is no radiologic abnormality but surgical exploration shows the presence of a fibrous band. Surgical resection of the rib or band prevents further progression of symptoms and signs and helps to reverse the neurologic deficit.

The thoracic outlet syndrome may occur on a familial basis, although this is not common. Presentation may be with pain and paresthesias without any specific neurologic features,[30] or neurogenic atrophy.[31]

In neurogenic thoracic outlet syndrome, electromyography of the affected hand muscles reveals a reduced number of motor units under voluntary control. There may also be an increased incidence of large, long-duration, polyphasic potentials. Abnormal spontaneous activity is sometimes found but, in the experience of Gilliatt and associates, is unusual.[28] Needle examination of the paraspinal muscles is normal, thereby providing no evidence of a more proximal lesion. Maximal motor conduction velocity in the forearm may be slightly slowed in the median nerve but is normal in the ulnar nerve, and the distal motor latency of both nerves is normal. However, the size of the compound muscle action potential recorded over the thenar muscles is reduced if there has been marked axonal loss, whereas that of the hypothenar muscles is generally normal. Sensory action potentials are of normal amplitude and latency when recorded from the median nerve at the wrist after stimulation of digital sensory fibers in the index finger, but are frequently small or absent when recorded from the ulnar nerve after stimulation of the little finger. The F response recorded from hypothenar muscles with stimulation of the ulnar nerve may be prolonged.[32] Ulnar somatosensory evoked potentials may be abnormal (see p. 154). The findings thus typically indicate a lesion involving fibers from the C8 and T1 segments and located distal to the dorsal root ganglia.

NEOPLASMS

Malignant infiltration leads to a progressive brachial plexus lesion that often involves the lower trunk in particular, and that may occur in association with epidural deposits.[33] Pain is usually a conspicuous feature, and Horner's syndrome may be present.[33,34] The electrophysiologic findings may resemble those accompanying the cervical rib syndrome, but needle examination usually shows profuse, abnormal spontaneous activity in the affected myotomes, whereas, as already indicated, this is unusual in patients with a cervical rib. Although there may be local conduction slowing or block, this may be hard to demonstrate because of the inaccessibility of the lesion.

IRRADIATION

The slowly progressive plexopathy produced as a result of irradiation is usually painless, and Horner's syndrome is a rare accompaniment.[33,34] Radiation injuries seem to affect the upper plexus (C5 and C6) especially,[33] but not necessarily exclusively. On needle examination, myokymia and complex repetitive discharges are commonly found in affected muscles.[35] The findings may not otherwise differ from other plexopathies. Nerve conduction studies may show reduced response amplitudes, regardless of the site of stimulation and despite normal conduction velocities and distal latencies. Median nerve sensory action potentials elicited from the thumb are often the most severely affected.[19] Only rarely is it possible to demonstrate conduction block with stimulation at Erb's point.[34]

Lumbosacral Plexopathies

The lumbosacral plexus is divided into an upper portion (the lumbar plexus, derived from L1, L2, L3, and L4) and a lower portion (the sacral plexus, which arises mainly from L5, S1, and S2). They are connected by the furcal nerve. The main nerves that arise from the lumbar plexus are the femoral and obturator nerves, whereas the gluteal and sciatic nerves are the main nerves derived from the sacral plexus.

Lumbosacral plexopathies may occur as a result of infiltration or compression by neoplasms, radiation therapy, or trauma. In patients with bleeding disorders or in those receiving anticoagulant drugs, a compressive lumbosacral plexopathy may be secondary to hematoma within the psoas muscle; its early recognition is important if serious permanent damage is to be prevented. (A pure femoral neuropathy may also result from hematoma within the iliacus or iliopsoas muscle.)

In general, pain is an early and conspicuous feature of tumor-induced plexopathy, which typically is unilateral. Radiation-induced plexopathy, by contrast, is characterized by weakness that is frequently bilateral and often painless.[36] In both types of plexopathy, sensory loss and reflex changes are common.

A condition that is clinically similar to idiopathic brachial plexopathy may involve the lumbosacral plexus. It is characterized by the sudden onset of pain, followed by wasting and weakness of affected muscles in a patchy distribution. There may be major involvement of just the upper or lower portions of the plexus and, especially when the lower plexus is involved, the condition may be mistaken for disc disease manifesting as "sciatica."[37] As is true when the condition affects the brachial plexus, the long-term prognosis is usually good, although recovery may take many months and is not always complete.

A plexopathy may occur in patients with diabetes, sometimes in combination with a radiculopathy. The etiology is presumed to be ischemic, pain is common, and axonal degeneration usually occurs.

Electrophysiologic evaluation of patients with suspected lumbosacral plexopathies is important. Needle electromyography is the single most important technique. Electromyographic evidence of denervation in the limb muscles beyond the territory of individual peripheral nerves, and associated with normal findings in the paraspinal muscles, suggests a lesion of the plexus. For example, electromyographic abnormalities in the thigh adductor muscles and the vasti muscles would not be expected in an isolated femoral or obturator neuropathy, and the absence of lumbar paraspinal abnormalities would suggest the diagnosis of lumbar plexopathy. There may be exclusive or predominant involvement of either the upper or lower portion of the plexus, or there may be more diffuse involvement. Myokymia may be found in affected muscles in radiation-induced plexopathies, and fasciculation potentials are sometimes present.[36] In some patients with tumor- or radiation-induced plexopathy, paraspinal electromyographic abnormalities are also found,[36] presumably because of concomitant involvement more proximally.[38] Maximal motor conduction velocities are normal, but F responses may be prolonged in some cases. The compound muscle action potential of weak muscles may be low in amplitude, especially if there has been marked axonal loss, and the sural sensory action potential may be absent or attenuated.

REFERENCES

1. Inouye Y, Buchthal F: Segmental sensory innervation determined by potentials recorded from cervical spinal nerves. Brain 100:731, 1977
2. Levin KH, Daube JR: Spinal cord infarction: Another cause of "lumbosacral polyradiculopathy." Neurology 34:389, 1984
3. Feinsod M, Blau D, Findler G, Hadani M, Beller AJ: Somatosensory evoked potential to peroneal nerve stimulation in patients with herniated lumbar disc. Neurosurgery 11:506, 1982
4. Aminoff MJ, Goodin DS, Barbaro NM, Weinstein PR, Rosenblum ML: Dermatomal somatosensory evoked potentials in unilat-
eral lumbosacral radiculopathy. Ann Neurol 17:171, 1985
5. Ganes T: Somatosensory conduction times and peripheral, cervical and cortical evoked potentials in patients with cervical spondylosis. J Neurol Neurosurg Psychiatry 43:683, 1980
6. El Negamy E, Sedgwick EM: Delayed cervical somatosensory potentials in cervical spondylosis. J Neurol Neurosurg Psychiatry 42:238, 1979
7. Siivola J, Sulg I, Heiskari M: Somatosensory evoked potentials in diagnostics of cervical spondylosis and herniated disc. Electroencephalogr Clin Neurophysiol 52:276, 1981
8. Aminoff MJ, Goodin DS, Parry GJ, Barbaro NM, Weinstein PR, Rosenblum ML: Electrophysiologic evaluation of lumbosacral radiculopathies: Electromyography, late responses, and somatosensory evoked potentials. Neurology 35:1514, 1985
9. Scarff TB, Dallman DE, Toleikis JR, Bunch WH: Dermatomal somatosensory evoked potentials in the diagnosis of lumbar root entrapment. Surg Forum 32:489, 1981
10. Eisen A, Hoirch M, Moll A: Evaluation of radiculopathies by segmental stimulation and somatosensory evoked potentials. Can J Neurol Sci 10:178, 1983
11. Perlik S, Fisher MA, Patel DV, Slack C: On the usefulness of somatosensory evoked responses for the evaluation of lower back pain. Arch Neurol 43:907, 1986
12. Tonzola RF, Ackil AA, Shahani BT, Young RR: Usefulness of electrophysiological studies in the diagnosis of lumbosacral root disease. Ann Neurol 9:305, 1981
13. Khatri BO, Baruah J, McQuillen MP: Correlation of electromyography with computed tomography in evaluation of lower back pain. Arch Neurol 41:594, 1984
14. Kikta DG, Breuer AC, Wilbourn AJ: Thoracic root pain in diabetes: The spectrum of clinical and electromyographic findings. Ann Neurol 11:80, 1982
15. Johnson ER, Powell J, Caldwell J, Crane C: Intercostal nerve conduction and posterior rhizotomy in the diagnosis and treatment of thoracic radiculopathy. J Neurol Neurosurg Psychiatry 37:330, 1974
16. Watson R, Waylonis GW: Paraspinal elec-

tromyographic abnormalities as a predictor of occult metastatic carcinoma. Arch Phys Med Rehabil 56:216, 1975

17. Lewis GW: Zoster sine herpete. Br Med J 2:418, 1958
18. Thomas JE, Howard FM: Segmental zoster paresis—A disease profile. Neurology 22:459, 1972
19. Wilbourn AJ: Electrodiagnosis of plexopathies. Neurol Clin 3:511, 1985
20. MacLean IC: Nerve root stimulation to evaluate conduction across the brachial and lumbosacral plexuses. p. 51. Syllabus, Annual Continuing Education Course, American Association of Electromyography and Electrodiagnosis, 1980
21. MacLean IC: Nerve root stimulation to evaluate conduction across the lumbosacral plexus. Acta Neurol Scand 60:suppl. 73, 270, 1979
22. Jones SJ, Wynn Parry CB, Landi A: Diagnosis of brachial plexus traction lesions by sensory nerve action potentials and somatosensory evoked potentials. Injury 12:376, 1981
23. Synek VM: Validity of median nerve somatosensory evoked potentials in the diagnosis of supraclavicular brachial plexus lesions. Electroencephalogr Clin Neurophysiol 65:27, 1986
24. Synek VM: Somatosensory evoked potentials from musculocutaneous nerve in the diagnosis of brachial plexus injuries. J Neurol Sci 61:443, 1983
25. Bosch EP, Chui HC, Martin MA, Cancilla PA: Brachial plexus involvement in familial pressure-sensitive neuropathy: Electrophysiological and morphological findings. Ann Neurol 8:620, 1980
26. Flaggman PD, Kelly JJ: Brachial plexus neuropathy. An electrophysiologic evaluation. Arch Neurol 37:160, 1980
27. Swift TR, Nichols FT: The droopy shoulder syndrome. Neurology 34:212, 1984
28. Gilliatt RW, LeQuesne PM, Logue V, Sumner AJ: Wasting of the hand associated with a cervical rib or band. J Neurol Neurosurg Psychiatry 33:615, 1970
29. Gilliatt RW, Willison RG, Dietz V, Williams IR: Peripheral nerve conduction in patients with a cervical rib and band. Ann Neurol 4:124, 1978
30. Lascelles RG, Mohr PD, Neary D, Bloor K: The thoracic outlet syndrome. Brain 100:601, 1977
31. Thompson T: Familial atrophy of the hand muscles. Brain 31:286, 1908
32. Wulff CH, Gilliatt RW: F waves in patients with hand wasting caused by a cervical rib and band. Muscle Nerve 2:452, 1979
33. Kori SH, Foley KM, Posner JB: Brachial plexus lesions in patients with cancer: 100 cases. Neurology 31:45, 1981
34. Lederman RJ, Wilbourn AJ: Brachial plexopathy: Recurrent cancer or radiation? Neurology 34:1331, 1984
35. Albers JW, Allen AA, Bastron JA, Daube JR: Limb myokymia. Muscle Nerve 4:494, 1981
36. Thomas JE, Cascino TL, Earle JD: Differential diagnosis between radiation and tumor plexopathy of the pelvis. Neurology 35:1, 1985
37. Evans BA, Stevens JC, Dyck PJ: Lumbosacral plexus neuropathy. Neurology 31:1327, 1981
38. Jaeckle KA, Young DF, Foley KM: The natural history of lumbosacral plexopathy in cancer. Neurology 35:8, 1985

14

Neuromuscular Transmission and Its Disorders

The transmission of impulses from nerve to muscle occurs at the neuromuscular junctions (Fig. 14.1), which are the regions in which the terminal processes of motor neurons come into close contact with the muscle fibers that they innervate. There is normally one such neuromuscular junction on each muscle fiber, and it lies about midway along the fiber. At each junction, the terminal processes, which contain numerous mitochondria and vesicular structures, are separated from the postjunctional structures by a space, the so-called synaptic cleft, which is approximately 200 to 300 Å wide and contains ground substance. The membrane of the muscle fiber is arranged in folds in this region, so that its surface area is increased by secondary synaptic clefts that open into the primary one.

When an impulse arrives at the terminals of a motor nerve fiber, it leads to the release of acetylcholine which diffuses across the synaptic cleft to combine with receptors on the muscle membrane, thereby altering the membrane permeability to sodium and potassium. The muscle membrane is consequently depolarized in the junctional—or motor end-plate—region. When this local end-plate potential reaches a critical level, it excites the adjacent membrane of the muscle fiber, thereby producing an action potential that is propagated along the fiber, and ultimately leads to its contraction.

Acetylcholine is synthesized in the motor nerve cells and stored in the vesicles that are found in the nerve terminals. It is released in multimolecular packets or quanta. Small amounts are released spontaneously and randomly, giving rise to nonpropagated miniature end-plate potentials[1] that are below the threshold for generating propagated action potentials. Much larger quantities of acetylcholine are released with the arrival of a nerve impulse, however, because calcium enters the depolarized terminals from the extracellular fluid, increasing the rate of acetylcholine release.[2] Magnesium competes with calcium, and therefore inhibits this process. Once released, the acetylcholine is rapidly removed by diffusion or by the action of acetylcholinesterase on the muscle membrane in the junctional region, which breaks it down into choline and acetate. The choline is then taken up again by the nerve fiber for the synthesis of further acetylcholine.

The size of the end-plate potentials produced by a single nerve impulse depends on the amount of acetylcholine that is released by the nerve terminals. The potentials are

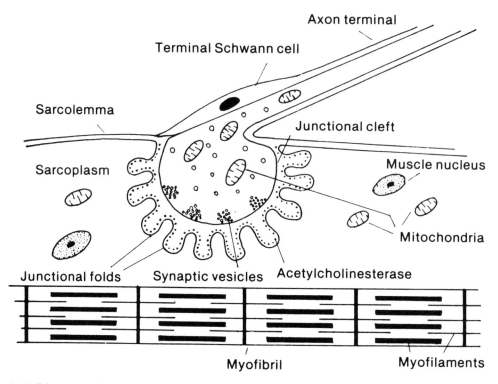

Fig. 14.1 Diagrammatic representation of the neuromuscular junction. (Slightly modified by the original authors and reproduced with permission from Bowman WC, Rand MJ, West GB: Textbook of Pharmacology. Blackwell Scientific Publications, Oxford, 1968.)

greater when evoked by an impulse that follows a preceding (that is, a conditioning) stimulus by a short interval than they are when evoked by one that does not. This is because the calcium that has accumulated within the nerve terminals as a result of the initial stimulus causes an increase in the amount of acetylcholine released by the subsequent nerve impulse.[3] As the interval between the two stimuli is increased, this facilitation becomes less prominent and is eventually succeeded by a longer lasting period of depression, during which the end-plate potentials are reduced in amplitude. This reduction has been attributed to depletion of the acetylcholine immediately available for release, and to a reduced probability of release of individual quanta.[4]

The size of the end-plate potentials evoked by a test impulse may also be al-tered by a preceding period of tetanic stimulation, being enhanced with short intervals between conditioning and test shocks, and reduced at longer ones. The extent and duration of these changes depend on the parameters of the conditioning train of shocks.

Preceding activity in the junctional regions thus influences the amount of acetylcholine released—and therefore, the size of the end-plate potentials evoked—by a test stimulus. This does not normally lead to a failure of neuromuscular transmission because more acetylcholine is released than is required to bring the end-plate potentials to the threshold for generating muscle fiber action potentials. In other words, the end-plate potentials evoked by a nerve impulse are considerably greater than is needed to generate propagated action potentials. When this normal *safety factor* is reduced, however, the effect of previous junctional activity may be sufficient to alter the number of end-plate potentials that reach the threshold for generating propagated muscle fiber action potentials in response to the stimulus, and thus may affect the number of muscle fibers that are activated.

Neuromuscular transmission will be impaired if there is a disturbance of any of the physiologic events just described. Thus, it is impaired when the synthesis of acetylcholine and its storage within nerve terminals is inhibited, as by hemicholinium, or when the normal release of acetylcholine from nerve terminals in response to the arrival of an impulse is prevented (as may occur, for example, following administration of certain antibiotics or in the presence of botulinum toxin). A deficiency of calcium ions or an excess of magnesium ions in the extracellular fluid similarly disturbs neuromuscular transmission by interfering with the release of acetylcholine. Some pharmacologic agents, such as curare, gallamine triethiodide, quinine, and certain anesthetic substances, impair neuromuscular transmission because they are competitive antagonists of acetylcholine. Others, such as physostigmine, neostigmine, and edrophonium, do so by antagonizing the acetylcholinesterase system so that acetylcholine accumulates in the junctional region and causes a prolonged depolarization and refractoriness of the muscle fibers. Yet other substances, such as decamethonium and suxamethonium, have an action which is similar to, but of longer duration than, acetylcholine, and they also cause prolonged depolarization and refractoriness of muscle fibers after an initial excitatory effect.

ELECTROPHYSIOLOGIC EVALUATION OF NEUROMUSCULAR TRANSMISSION

The amplitude of the compound muscle action potential, or M response, provides an indication of the number of muscle fibers activated by a stimulus. Neuromuscular transmission is, therefore, tested by examining the electrical response of muscle to supramaximal stimulation of its motor nerve by paired or repetitive shocks, or by single shocks delivered at selected intervals after a period of maximal voluntary activity. Neuromuscular transmission can also be evaluated by single fiber electromyography (see Chapter 8).

Normal Subjects

The amplitude of the compound action potential recorded from muscle by surface or subcutaneous electrodes after a single supramaximal stimulus to its motor nerve varies among different subjects, and depends on the muscle examined and the precise recording arrangements. Measurements are usually made of the amplitude of the negative spike. Lambert and colleagues found that this amplitude normally ranged between 5.6 and 20.8 mV (with a mean of 11.4 mV) for the hypothenar muscles.[5]

The responses to repetitive stimulation depend upon the rate at which the stimuli are applied. At a rate of 10 or less per second in normal subjects, there is usually no change in the size of the compound muscle action potential, but sometimes a small decrement does occur. Desmedt and Borenstein reported that, if a decrement occurs with a stimulation rate of 3 per second, the fifth potential is reduced by less than 7 percent of the first.[6] When the rate of stimulation is between 10 and 50 per second, the amplitude of the potential usually remains steady for a variable period of time, depending upon the frequency of stimulation. It may, however, increase with the first few stimuli because an increase in conduction velocity of the muscle fibers leads to improved synchronization of the individual potentials contributing to the compound muscle action potential.[7] This increment is usually on the order of 10 to 15 percent, but occasionally may be as much as 20 to 30 percent of the size of the initial response. At rates of 50 or more per second, the M responses decrease as a result of the refractory period of the muscle fibers.

If a pair of stimuli is applied to the motor nerve, the amplitude of the second M response depends on the interval between the two stimuli. If this interval is less than 20 msec, the second M response is smaller than the first because some of the muscle fibers are still in the refractory period that follows the initial stimulus when the subsequent one is delivered. If the interval between stimuli is more than 20 msec, the second M response is usually the same size as the first, although when the interval is 20 to 100 msec, it may be slightly larger because of improved synchronization in the responses of individual muscle fibers.

The response to a single stimulus delivered after tetanic stimulation or maximal voluntary activity is studied by recording the compound muscle action potential evoked by a single stimulus before, and at selected intervals after, such conditioning. For clinical purposes, a 10-second period of voluntary contraction is convenient, with the muscle responses to single stimuli being recorded 3, 10, and 30 seconds later and after 1, 2, 3, 4, 5, and 10 minutes. The size of the M response of the rested muscle relates to activation of all the fibers in that muscle. Accordingly, although the amount of acetylcholine released by the test stimulus is increased for a short time after maximal voluntary activity of the muscle in normal subjects, the number of fibers activated cannot increase, and the size of the M response therefore remains unchanged. In the period that follows, the end-plate potentials produced by the test stimulus are reduced in amplitude, but the number of muscle fibers activated—and thus, the size of the M response—remains unaltered because of the normal safety factor governing transmission.

Single fiber electromyography is an important method of investigating the functional integrity of neuromuscular junctions, but is currently being used in only a limited number of medical centers. A special electrode is used to record the action potentials of single muscle fibers, as described in Chapter 8. Using this technique, Ekstedt recorded the action potentials from two fibers belonging to the same motor unit at the same time and found the interval between the two potentials differed slightly with consecutive discharges.[8] This variability—the jitter—is usually between 10 and 30 μsec, and in normal subjects, is attributable mainly to variability in the synaptic delays of the two neuromuscular junctions involved. The jitter is increased in patients with defective neuromuscular transmission, even when all the muscle fibers may still be activated and the response to repetitive stimulation is normal.

CLINICAL DISORDERS OF NEUROMUSCULAR TRANSMISSION

Myasthenia Gravis

Myasthenia gravis is an autoimmune disease that may occur at any age, is more common in females than males, may be associated with a thymic tumor or thyrotoxicosis, and is characterized by weakness and easy fatiguability of affected muscles. Muscle activity cannot be maintained, and movements which initially are powerful fatigue readily. The external ocular muscles are often the first to be involved, but the masticatory, facial, pharyngeal, laryngeal, respiratory, and limb muscles may also be affected. The distribution of affected muscles varies in different patients, and severity of weakness varies both between patients and in the same patient at different times. There appears to be a reduced number of functioning acetylcholine receptors, and antibodies to these receptors have been found in the serum of 70 to 90 percent of patients.[9] Indeed, measurement of acetyl-choline receptor antibodies is an important means of confirming the diagnosis, although the assay is currently only performed at a limited number of medical centers. Symptomatic benefit often follows treatment with anticholinesterases, such as physostigmine or neostigmine. Thymectomy may lead to remission and should be considered in all patients, especially those who are young and have weakness that is not restricted to the extraocular muscles. Patients who have responded poorly to anticholinesterases and who have already undergone thymectomy may benefit from steroids, azathioprine, or plasmapheresis.

Infants born to women with myasthenia gravis may develop a transient neonatal form of the disorder that is manifested by a weak cry and suck. Transplacental transfer of maternal acetylcholine receptor antibodies is responsible. Drug treatment may be necessary in severe cases, but the disorder resolves in 6 to 8 weeks.

Myasthenia gravis that is similar in all respects to the variety just described may occur in patients who are taking D-penicillamine, especially for the treatment of rheumatoid arthritis. Fortunately, remission frequently occurs when the drug is discontinued.[10–12] Other drugs may also influence neuromuscular transmission, and these are considered on p. 298.

ELECTROPHYSIOLOGIC EVALUATION OF MYASTHENIA GRAVIS

Needle electromyography of affected muscles only rarely reveals any abnormal spontaneous activity. Motor unit potentials are usually normal in appearance, but their amplitude may vary considerably, often declining with activity as a result of progressive failure of neuromuscular transmission. In some cases, an increased incidence of polyphasic or short-duration units, or both, is found. This presumably relates to a reduction in the number of functional muscle fibers per unit, caused either by the transmission defect itself or by the development of a secondary myopathy. The interference pattern is generally full, but becomes reduced in amplitude if voluntary activity is maintained. Furthermore, active units then develop a tendency to fire in synchronized bursts, the number of active units declines, and it sometimes becomes possible to recognize the potentials of individual motor units which may be seen to suddenly stop firing despite continued effort.[13]

Nerve conduction studies generally reveal no abnormality. The electrical response of muscle to motor nerve stimulation is occasionally abnormal, but the amplitude of the M response evoked from rested muscle by a single supramaximal stimulus is usually within the normal range. In a group of patients with myasthenia gravis, the mean amplitude of the M response is slightly reduced, however, compared to that of normal subjects, suggesting that some impairment of neuromuscular transmission occurs even in rested muscle.

The electrical responses of muscle to paired or repetitive stimulation of its motor nerve, or to stimulation after a period of maximal voluntary activity, may be abnormal in patients with myasthenia gravis, especially if proximal or clinically affected muscles are examined. It is important, however, that muscles be warm when tested because the safety factor for neuromuscular transmission declines with increasing temperature, and abnormalities may then be found that were not evident in cold muscles (Fig. 14.2). Unfortunately, it is not uncommon for normal responses to be obtained, even in warm muscles, and the clinical diagnosis is not excluded by such findings. Attempts have been made to increase the diagnostic yield to repetitive stimulation of distal hand muscles by inducing ischemia or by regional infusion of curare. The role of ischemia is considered below, but the curare test is potentially hazardous and should not be employed routinely.

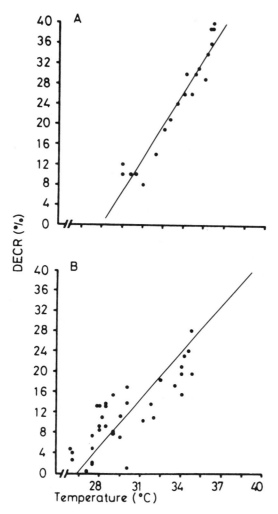

Fig. 14.2 Effect of temperature on the decrement (first:fourth response) in two patients with myasthenia gravis. (**A**) From deltoid muscle. (**B**) From abductor digiti minimi muscle. The temperature is slowly changed with a heating lamp and icebags, and is measured with an intramuscular thermocouple. (Stalberg E: Clinical electrophysiology in myasthenia gravis. J Neurol Neurosurg Psychiatry 43:622, 1980. Reproduced by permission of the Authors and Editors of the Journal of Neurology, Neurosurgery and Psychiatry.)

Repetitive stimulation at either low (1 to 10 Hz, but usually between 2 and 5 Hz) or high (10 to 50 Hz) rates may lead to a depression of neuromuscular transmission in patients with myasthenia gravis. When abnormalities occur, the findings vary considerably in different patients, and in different muscles from the same patient. There may be a rapid decline in amplitude of the compound muscle action potential, as shown in Fig. 14.3, but in most cases, the decline levels off after about four to eight stimuli so that the potentials remain at a steady but reduced amplitude. In other instances, the initial decrement is followed by a temporary increase in size of the potentials for 2 to 3 seconds, after which further decrement occurs. A progressive increment occurs very occasionally during repetitive stimulation at high rates,[14] but is more characteristic of the myasthenic syndrome.

When paired stimuli, separated by an interval of 4 to 20 msec, are applied to the motor nerve, the second M response may be similar in size to the first, or even slightly greater. At intervals longer than this (but less than about 10 seconds), the second response is commonly smaller, with this depression being maximal when the interstimulus interval is 200 to 1000 msec (which corresponds to a stimulation rate of 1 to 5 per second).

In myasthenia gravis, the amplitude of the M response to a single stimulus delivered after a 10-second period of maximal voluntary activity may be slightly increased 3 seconds after the period of activity, but declines to its pre-exercise level within about 30 seconds. The increase indicates that more muscle fibers are responding to the stimulus, thereby implying that prior to exercise, not all of the muscle fibers were responding to it.[15] This postactivation facilitation of neuromuscular transmission is followed by a longer period of depression, which is maximal 2 to 4 minutes after the

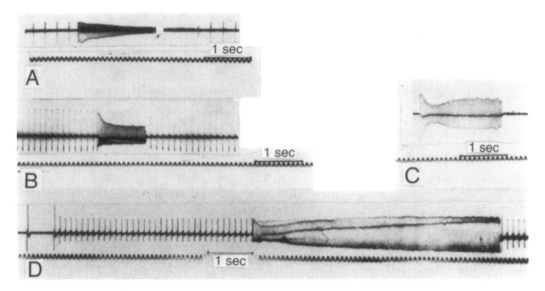

Fig. 14.3 Muscle response to repetitive, supramaximal nerve stimulation in myasthenia gravis. **(A)** Classical response. **(B)** Immediate decrement followed by a leveling off of the response. **(C)** Decrement followed by a temporary increment. **(D)** Decrement during stimulation at a rate of 8 per second, and progressive increment with stimulation at 50 per second. (Simpson JA: Disorders of neuromuscular transmission. Proc R Soc Med 59:993, 1966.)

conditioning period, but which may last for about 10 minutes. During this time, the M response may be reduced in amplitude, sometimes to less than 50 percent of its pre-exercise size, because of the reduced safety factor governing transmission.

A train of five or six shocks, delivered at a rate of 2 to 3 per second, can be used instead of a single stimulus to assess the manner in which neuromuscular transmission has been influenced by preceding activity. Compared with the findings in rested muscle, the decrement in size of successive responses is commonly reduced or even abolished during the period of postactivation facilitation, and is increased during the subsequent period of depression (Fig. 14.4).

The double-step test described by Desmedt and Borenstein[16] may increase the diagnostic yield in patients with mild or localized myasthenia gravis. It involves the combined use of both preceding activity and ischemia to challenge apparently normal muscles. The first step involves 3-Hz supramaximal ulnar nerve stimulation for 4 minutes while the electrical responses of the muscles of the hand and forearm are recorded to detect abnormal decrements. Following this, the procedure is repeated with the circulation of blood arrested by a cuff which is inflated to 25 cm Hg and placed proximal to the site of stimulation around the arm. This permits abnormal decrements to be elicited from subclinically involved muscles that reacted normally to the first step (Fig. 14.5).

Single fiber electromyography is even more valuable in investigating patients with suspected myasthenia gravis. The diagnostic yield is very high, and the procedure is especially helpful in patients with mild disease or ocular myasthenia. The jitter is typically increased, and impulse blocking may occur.[17] There is, however, considerable variation in the extent to which the different

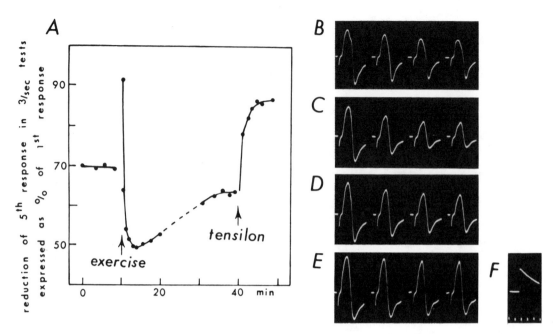

Fig. 14.4 Electrical responses of flexor carpi radialis to trains of supramaximal stimuli delivered at 3 per second to the median nerve. (**A**) The variation that occurs in the degree of neuromuscular block after a 10-second period of maximal voluntary contraction of the muscle (*first arrow*), and after administration of edrophonium (Tensilon, 20 mg; *second arrow*). (**B–E**) Samples of the responses obtained during the experiment: (**B**) before; (**C**) 4 minutes after; and (**D**) 24 minutes after maximal voluntary activity. The decrement in size of successive responses is greater in **C** than in **B** because of the depression in neuromuscular transmission that follows activity. (**E**) Responses 6 minutes after administration of edrophonium (Tensilon). (**F**) 10 mV calibration signal, and 200-per-second time marker. (Desmedt JE: Identification and titration of myasthenic defect by nerve stimulation. Electroencephalogr Clin Neurophysiol Suppl. 22:63, 1962.)

neuromuscular junctions are affected. The jitter between some potentials may be increased, whereas between others, it may remain in the normal range (Fig. 14.6). Furthermore, increased jitter may result from causes other than defective neuromuscular transmission.[18] However, if the jitter in a weak muscle is always within the normal range, the diagnosis of myasthenia gravis is extremely unlikely.[19,20]

The mechanical responses to nerve stimulation have also been used to differentiate between normal and myasthenic subjects; the technical details of this approach are provided elsewhere.[21] There is no unanimity concerning the nature and frequency of the findings in myasthenia gravis, however, and this approach is of no clinical utility at the present time.

Congenital Myasthenic Syndromes

Several different hereditary disorders of neuromuscular transmission have been recognized. Unlike transient neonatal myasthenia (referred to above), congenital myasthenic syndromes occur in infants born to nonmyasthenic mothers, and are not transient. Unlike classical myasthenia gravis, these syndromes are not associated with the

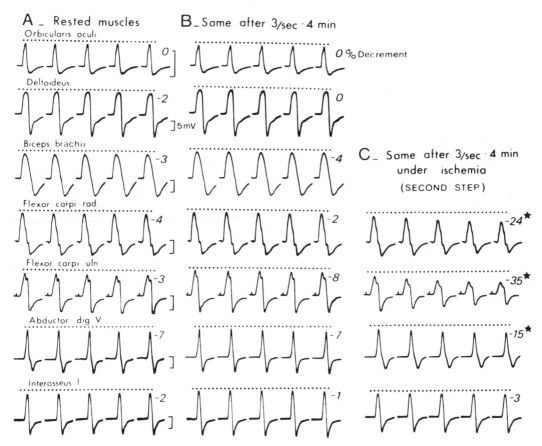

Fig. 14.5 A 53-year-old male patient with ocular myasthenia and preserved muscle force in face and limbs. Electrical responses to supramaximal nerve stimulation at 3 Hz in various muscles (from above downward): orbicular, deltoid, biceps, radial, ulnar, abductor of the fifth finger, and first interosseus. Intramuscular temperatures, 35° to 36.3°C. (**A**) Rested muscles. (**B**) Fifteen seconds after a series of 3-Hz stimulations for 4 minutes (first step). (**C**) Fifteen seconds after a similar stimulation under ischemia (second step). The decrement of the fifth response, expressed as a percentage, is indicated at the right of each record. The three stars indicate a significant decrement in the subclinically involved muscles. The first step is negative in all of the tested muscles. Vertical calibration, 5 mV. (Desmedt JE, Borenstein S: Double-step nerve stimulation test for myasthenic block: Sensitization of postactivation exhaustion by ischemia. Ann Neurol 1:55, 1977.)

presence of serum antibodies to the acetylcholine receptors. Difficulty in feeding and ptosis are the most common presenting features in infancy or early childhood, but weakness in the limbs may also occur and sometimes has a characteristic distribution. In mild cases, the disorder may not become evident clinically until later life.

Several different varieties of this disorder

have been described. These include the recessively inherited types that occur with either end-plate acetylcholinesterase deficiency, a defect in acetylcholine synthesis or mobilization, or an abnormality of acetylcholine receptor synthesis, and the dominantly inherited, slow-channel syndrome, in which slow closure of the acetylcholine receptor ion channel permits excessive cal-

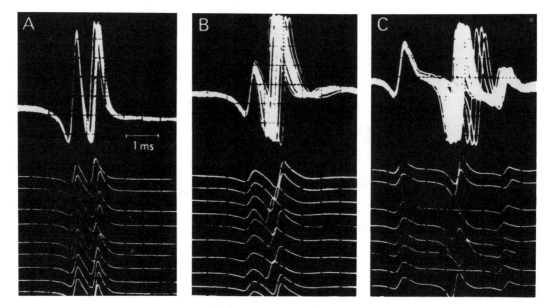

Fig. 14.6 Single fiber electromyography of the extensor digitorum communis muscle of a patient with myasthenia gravis. The oscilloscope sweep is triggered by the first action potential, delayed by 1 to 2 msec. The jitter is seen as a variable position of the second and, in **C**, a third action potential. Upper tracings: 20 superimposed sweeps. Lower tracings: sweeps moved downward. Within the same muscle, one can see normal jitter (**A**), increased jitter but no blocking (**B**), and increased jitter and intermittent blocking (second potential in **C**). In (**C**), different degrees of abnormality among motor end-plates in the same motor unit are demonstrated. Jitter in **A** is 29 μsec, in **B** is 65 μsec, and in **C** is 81 μsec and 49 μsec. (Stalberg E: Clinical electrophysiology in myasthenia gravis. J Neurol Neurosurg Psychiatry 43:622, 1980. Reproduced by permission of the Authors and Editors of the Journal of Neurology, Neurosurgery and Psychiatry.)

cium influx into the junctional region. Other varieties have also been described.[22,23]

In the four types described above, decremental responses to 2-Hz repetitive stimulation, as well as abnormalities in single fiber electromyography, are reported to occur, although in the type characterized by defective acetylcholine synthesis or mobilization, this may not be apparent unless tested after 10-Hz stimulation for 5 to 10 minutes. In some varieties, a repetitive compound muscle action potential is elicited by a single supramaximal stimulus to the motor nerve (Fig. 14.7). Further details of these disorders are provided elsewhere.[22]

The Lambert-Eaton Myasthenic Syndrome

The Lambert-Eaton myasthenic syndrome is a disorder of neuromuscular transmission in which the release of acetylcholine in response to a nerve impulse is defective.[24] It is more common in men than in women. It may occur in association with malignant disease, usually a bronchogenic carcinoma of oat cell type, but in some cases (about 30 percent) no neoplastic lesion is evident. It is occasionally associated with autoimmune disorders. The syndrome is characterized clinically by weakness and easy fatigability of muscles, especially the proximal muscles of the limbs. Other symp-

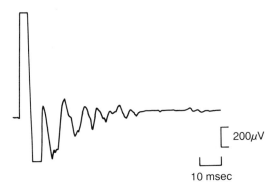

Fig. 14.7 Repetitive compound muscle action potential elicited by a single stimulus.

toms include dryness of the mouth, constipation, impotence, and bladder disturbances. Examination shows that voluntary contraction is weak initially, but power often increases if the contraction is briefly maintained.[25] The tendon reflexes are usually depressed, but may be increased after activity. Marked but temporary clinical deterioration may follow administration of neuromuscular blocking drugs. Clinical benefit may be derived from treatment of the underlying neoplasm or from administration of guanidine, which increases the calcium-mediated release of acetylcholine from nerve terminals. Immunosuppressant drug therapy or plasmapheresis may also be helpful,[26] but the response to anticholinesterase treatment is generally disappointing.

An autoimmune basis for the disorder has been suggested. The disorder has been induced in mice by passive transfer of the IgG component of plasma from patients with the syndrome.[27]

ELECTROPHYSIOLOGIC EVALUATION

Needle electromyography during voluntary activity reveals that the amplitude of individual motor unit potentials varies considerably from moment to moment, but tends to increase with time. This presumably relates to a variation in the number of muscle fibers responding to each nerve impulse, with the number tending to increase with activity. An increased incidence of polyphasic or short-duration units, or both, may also be found, particularly when a weak muscle is first contracted, suggesting a myopathic disorder. Abnormal spontaneous activity is not present.

Motor and sensory conduction velocity is normal in the peripheral nerves unless there is a coexisting peripheral neuropathy. However, the compound action potential of rested muscle is greatly reduced in amplitude in patients with the myasthenic syndrome. For example, Lambert and co-workers[5] found that the M response of the hypothenar muscles was smaller than 6 mV in all of 15 patients with this disorder, with the mean value being 1.9 mV. This reduced size reflects the reduced number of muscle fibers that are activated by the stimulus as a result of the defective release of acetylcholine.

The M response to a single stimulus is much smaller than normal and, with repetitive stimulation at a rate of 1 to 10 per second, the first four to eight responses show a progressive decrement in size. However, subsequent responses show an increment, and may eventually reach a size several times larger than the initial response. At rates of stimulation of 10 to 50 per second, a progressive increment usually occurs from the start of stimulation. Thus, whereas repetitive stimulation at low rates initially depresses neuromuscular transmission, stimulation at higher rates usually leads to an immediate facilitation.

When paired stimuli are used, facilitation of the second response occurs when the interstimulus interval is between about 4 and 100 msec; it is maximal at an interval of 4 to 10 msec. When the interval is lengthened so that it is between 100 msec and 10 seconds, there is usually some depression of the second response.

The changes that occur in the response

to single stimuli delivered at selected intervals after a 10-second period of maximal voluntary activity are similar qualitatively, but not quantitatively, to those occurring in patients with myasthenia gravis. Within a few seconds of the period of maximal voluntary activity, the M response increases markedly in amplitude (Fig. 14.8), sometimes reaching a size that is more than 10 times that of the pre-exercise response.

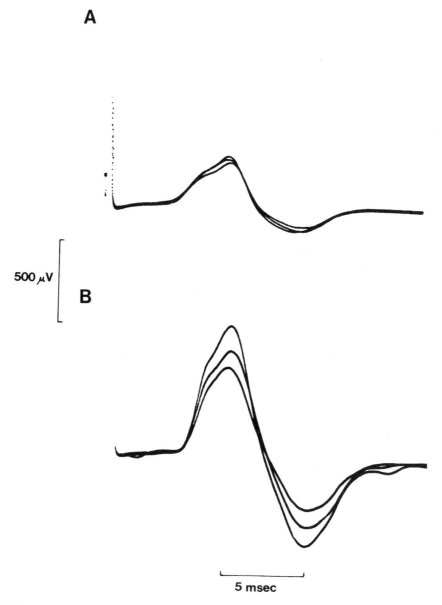

A

500 μV

B

5 msec

Fig. 14.8 The compound action potentials evoked in the hypothenar muscles of a patient with the Lambert-Eaton myasthenic syndrome by three supramaximal stimuli delivered to the ulnar nerve at the wrist at a rate of 2 per second. (**A**) Responses of the rested muscle. (**B**) Responses evoked in the muscle 3 seconds after a 10-second period of maximal voluntary contraction.

After about 60 seconds, however, this period of facilitated neuromuscular transmission is followed by a longer-lasting period of depression, just as occurs in myasthenia gravis.

Single fiber electromyography reveals an increased jitter. This finding is similar to that which occurs in myasthenia gravis except that, with an increase in firing rate, the jitter and degree of blocking increase in myasthenia gravis but decrease in Lambert-Eaton syndrome.[20]

OTHER DISORDERS WITH ABNORMAL RESPONSES TO REPETITIVE STIMULATION

Botulism

The weakness that occurs in patients with botulism results from the defective release of acetylcholine from nerve terminals. This may relate to a reduction in calcium sensitivity of the transmitter release mechanism in the nerve terminals.[28] Symptoms generally begin within 48 hours of eating contaminated food and are usually the result of the presence of type A, B, or E toxin in the food. Rarely, wound infection with *Clostridium botulinum*, an anaerobic soil bacillus, is followed by local production of the toxin with subsequent hematogenous dissemination. Extraocular and bulbar weakness is followed by weakness of the respiratory and limb muscles. Accompanying autonomic disturbances, such as blurred vision, dilated pupils, constipation, and urinary retention, are important in suggesting the correct diagnosis.

In infants, presentation may be with constipation, hypotonia, weakness, poor suck, loss of head control, and other symptoms. There is enteric infection with the offending organism, with local production of toxin.[29] This "spontaneous" form of botulism is now recognized as a common and very important cause of rapidly progressive weakness in the first 9 months of life.[30]

The diagnosis of botulism depends on epidemiologic factors and the clinical findings, and may be confirmed by electrophysiologic studies and by the discovery of the toxin or organism in the patient or a food source. Treatment of food-borne or wound botulism involves administration of trivalent antitoxin. Wound infection also requires appropriate local therapy. Penicillin is usually given routinely. Neither antitoxin nor antibiotic therapy is advised for infant botulism.[30] The role of guanidine in treating botulism is unclear. There is little response to anticholinesterases. Ventilatory support may be necessary, and appropriate facilities should therefore be available.

On electrophysiologic examination, the muscle responses to supramaximal nerve stimulation may resemble those occurring in the Lambert-Eaton myasthenic syndrome, although the findings are more variable and not all muscles are affected. It is, therefore, important to evaluate the responses of several different muscles if the initial findings are unremarkable or inconclusive. The M response to a single supramaximal nerve stimulus is usually low in amplitude if the tested limb is clinically affected, and a small decrement sometimes occurs in the size of the responses evoked by repetitive stimulation at low rates.[31,32] An increment (Fig. 14.9) may occur at high rates of stimulation[33] or after a 10-second period of voluntary activity.[31] Although this post-tetanic facilitation is not as great as that occurring in the Lambert-Eaton myasthenic syndrome, it may persist for several minutes, which is much longer than in myasthenia gravis or the Lambert-Eaton syndrome.[34] Distal motor latency and motor and sensory conduction velocity are normal.

In infants, the response to motor nerve stimulation may be recorded most conveniently using subcutaneous needle electrodes, while stimuli are delivered at the

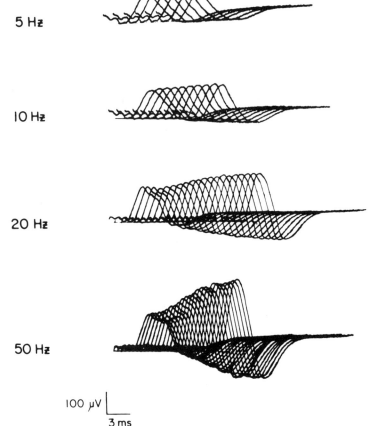

5 Hz

10 Hz

20 Hz

50 Hz

100 μV

3 ms

Fig. 14.9 Repetitive stimulation of the left median innervated abductor pollicis brevis in infantile botulism. On the left are listed the rates of stimulation. At 5 Hz, a mild decrement is seen (8%). At 10 Hz, an increment is seen (25%) that increases with higher rates of stimulation (20 Hz, 38%; 50 Hz, 94%). (Cornblath DR, Sladky JT, Sumner AJ: Clinical electrophysiology of infantile botulism. Muscle Nerve 6:448, 1983. Copyright © 1983 John Wiley & Sons, Inc. Reprinted by permission.)

elbow or knee (rather than more distally) to reduce the likelihood of artifacts.[35] Approximately half of infants with botulism show a decrement in the M response to low-frequency (2 to 5 Hz) stimulation, one quarter show no change and one fifth have an increment.[35] High-frequency (20 to 50 Hz) repetitive stimulation produces an incremental response in most infants.[35]

Needle examination of clinically involved muscles may also be abnormal in patients of all ages, with an increased incidence of short, low-amplitude, polyphasic motor unit potentials that are recruited rapidly, causing an excessive number of potentials during mild contractions. Abnormal spontaneous activity, consisting of fibrillations and positive sharp waves, is also a common finding in affected muscles. Increased jitter

and impulse blocking, which often diminish as the firing rate increases, may be found on single fiber electromyography.[36]

Drug-Induced Weakness

Myasthenia gravis may occur in patients taking D-penicillamine, as described earlier (p. 289). Neuromuscular transmission can also be impaired by certain antibiotics, especially neomycin, streptomycin, kanamycin, gentamicin, amikacin, and tobramycin. Clinical dysfunction is more likely to occur if there is hepatic or renal disease, or a preexisting disturbance of neuromuscular transmission. Affected patients may develop respiratory difficulty, weakness of the limb and bulbar muscles, and dilated pupils. The M response of affected muscles to a single supramaximal nerve stimulus is reduced, and progressive decrement occurs with repetitive stimulation at rates of up to 50 per second.[37] Post-tetanic facilitation is inconstant and insignificant.[38] The disorder is usually attributed to defective release of acetylcholine and to a reduced effect of acetylcholine on the postsynaptic membrane.

Other antibiotics and drugs that may affect neuromuscular transmission include tetracyclines, polymixin, colistin, phenytoin, quinine, quinidine, procainamide, β-adrenergic blockers, adrenocorticotropic hormone (ACTH), corticosteroids, lithium, phenothiazines, magnesium-containing cathartics, and chloroquine. A detailed account of these and other drugs influencing junctional mechanisms is provided by Swift[12] and Layzer.[11]

Other Neuromuscular Disorders

An abnormal decrement in size of the muscle responses to repetitive stimulation may occur in the myotonic disorders,[39] in polymyositis and dermatomyositis,[14] in certain of the muscular dystrophies,[40] and in disorders affecting the anterior horn cells[41,42] or peripheral nerves.[12,41] Such a decrement has even been described in multiple sclerosis[43] and in patients with upper motor neuron disorders or parkinsonism.[44] In motor neuron disease, such a response has been held to indicate active disease and a poor prognosis.[45]

PRACTICAL CONSIDERATIONS

Tests of neuromuscular transmission are performed most commonly in patients with suspected myasthenia gravis and will be discussed with this in mind. There is no general agreement about the manner in which these tests are best performed, and many individual modifications have been described.

The response to stimulation of the motor fibers of any accessible peripheral nerve can be studied, provided that movements of the stimulating and recording electrodes can be prevented by mechanical fixation of the extremity. It is usually most convenient to immobilize the hand and record the response of the abductor digiti minimi muscle to stimulation of the ulnar nerve at the wrist. When recordings from a more proximal muscle in the upper limb are desired, however, the deltoid or biceps muscle may be used, with the arm being held to the side while the brachial plexus or musculocutaneous nerve is stimulated. In the lower extremity, satisfactory recordings can be made from the extensor digitorum brevis muscle while the peroneal nerve is stimulated at the ankle, or from the tibialis anterior muscle while the peroneal nerve is stimulated more proximally.

The stimulating cathode is placed distal to the anode and as close to the nerve as possible, with its optimal position being determined by finding the point at which the muscle response evoked by a submaximal stimulus is greatest in size. Stimulus intensity is then increased so that, for subsequent test procedures, it is at least 50 percent greater than that required to elicit a maximal response.

Surface or subcutaneous electrodes are used for recording, with the active one being placed in the end-plate region of the muscle and the reference one being positioned over its tendon. The ground electrode is positioned between the stimulating and recording sites. All electrodes are securely attached to the patient to prevent their movement during subsequent test procedures.

The safety factor for neuromuscular transmission declines as the muscle temperature increases within the physiologic range.[46] Therefore, is important to ensure that muscles are warm (35° to 37°C) prior to conducting the test.

The extent of the examination depends

upon the nature of the diagnostic problem. In myasthenia gravis, abnormal responses are found more often in muscles that are involved clinically than in those that are not, but normal responses are frequently obtained even in the former. Accordingly, the responses of several muscles, including the facial muscles, may have to be examined before the diagnosis can be confirmed. If the examination is to be restricted to one muscle, however, the selection of a proximal rather than a distal one may improve the diagnostic yield.[47] Single fiber electromyography may be rewarding if conventional studies fail to reveal any abnormality. If this technique is not available, the diagnostic yield to repetitive stimulation of the distal hand muscles may be increased either by inducing ischemia or by regional infusion of curare, following which initially normal responses to repetitive stimulation may be replaced by an abnormal decrement. Ischemia is produced by inflating a cuff around the upper arm to a level exceeding systolic pressure (25 cm Hg), but this may be uncomfortable for the patient. Administration of curare, especially to patients with a suspected disorder of neuromuscular transmission, involves some risk and should not be used routinely. Since the electrophysiologic findings are influenced by anticholinesterases, administration of these substances should be discontinued for at least 6 hours, and preferably for 24 hours, prior to the examination (when this is clinically feasible). Once abnormalities have been found, however, an attempt can be made to determine whether they may be corrected by intravenous edrophonium.

In patients with the Lambert-Eaton myasthenic syndrome, electrophysiologic abnormalities indicative of impaired neuromuscular transmission are found in all muscles. Therefore, only one muscle needs to be examined.

After the size of the M response to a single supramaximal nerve stimulus has been measured, the response to repetitive stimulation at a rate of 2 to 3 per second is examined. With a repetition rate of 2 per second, the interval between the stimuli is 500 msec, at which time the depression of neuromuscular transmission that occurs after a stimulus is most marked. Stimulation can either be discontinued after five or six stimuli, with the amplitude of the fifth response being compared to that of the first, or it may be continued for 10 seconds. A decrement of 10 percent or more is generally regarded as indicative of defective neuromuscular transmission.

The responses to repetitive stimulation at higher rates can also be examined. The findings are sometimes abnormal even when the response to stimulation at 2 to 3 per second is unremarkable. Rates of 10 and 30 per second are commonly used, and stimulation is continued for 10 seconds. The prominent increase in size of the M response that occurs in the Lambert-Eaton myasthenic syndrome serves to distinguish it from myasthenia gravis.

Defective neuromuscular transmission may also be revealed by the responses elicited by a single stimulus delivered at selected intervals (for example, at 3, 10, and 30 seconds and at 1, 2, 3, 4, 5, and 10 minutes) after a 10-second period during which the patient either maintains a maximal muscle contraction or contracts the muscle repetitively. A train of five or six shocks at a rate of 2 or 3 per second may be used instead of the single stimulus. This approach may help to reveal a latent defect of transmission in patients with myasthenia gravis.

As the technique of single fiber electromyography is discussed briefly in Chapter 8, recapitulation here is unnecessary.

In reporting the results of electrophysiologic examination, full details are given of the muscles that were studied, the procedures that were used, and the findings that were obtained. The physiologic implications of the findings are then related to the clinical problem under investigation. In this regard, particular care must be exercised when the electrophysiologic findings are normal in a patient with suspected myasthenia gravis, since this does not exclude the diagnosis.

REFERENCES

1. Katz B: Microphysiology of the neuro-muscular junction. A physiological 'quantum of action' at the myoneural junction. Bull Johns Hopkins Hosp 102:275, 1958
2. Katz B, Miledi R: The timing of calcium action during neuromuscular transmission. J Physiol 189:535, 1967
3. Katz B, Miledi R: The role of calcium in neuromuscular facilitation. J Physiol 195:481, 1968
4. Betz WJ: Depression of transmitter release at the neuromuscular junction of the frog. J Physiol 206:629, 1970
5. Lambert EH, Rooke ED, Eaton LM, Hodgson CH: Myasthenic syndrome occasionally associated with bronchial neoplasm: Neurophysiologic studies. p. 362. In Viets HR (ed): Myasthenia Gravis. Charles C Thomas, Springfield, Illinois, 1961
6. Desmedt JE, Borenstein S: The testing of neuromuscular transmission. p. 104. In Vinken PJ, Bruyn GW (eds): Handbook of Clinical Neurology. Vol. 7. North-Holland, Amsterdam, 1970
7. Stalberg E: Propagation velocity in human muscle fibers in situ. Acta Physiol Scand, 70:suppl. 287, 1, 1966
8. Ekstedt J: Human single muscle fiber action potentials. Acta Physiol Scand, 61:suppl. 226, 1, 1964
9. Lindstrom JM, Seybold ME, Lennon VA, Whittingham S, Duane DE: Antibody to acetylcholine receptor in myasthenia gravis. Neurology 26:1054, 1976
10. Albers JW, Hodach RJ, Kimmel DW, Treacy WL: Penicillamine-associated myasthenia gravis. Neurology 30:1246, 1980
11. Layzer RB: Neuromuscular Manifestations of Systemic Disease. F.A. Davis, Philadelphia, 1985
12. Swift TR: Disorders of neuromuscular transmission other than myasthenia gravis. Muscle Nerve 4:334, 1981
13. Lundervold A: Myasthenia gravis. An electromyographic investigation. Acta Psychiatr Neurol Scand 29:151, 1954
14. Simpson JA: Disorders of neuromuscular transmission. Proc R Soc Med 59:993, 1966
15. Johns RJ, Grob D, Harvey AM: Studies in neuromuscular function. II. Effects of nerve stimulation in normal subjects and in patients with myasthenia gravis. Bull Johns Hopkins Hosp 99:125, 1956
16. Desmedt JE, Borenstein S: Double-step nerve stimulation test for myasthenic block: Sensitization of postactivation exhaustion by ischemia. Ann Neurol 1:55, 1977
17. Ekstedt J, Stalberg E: The diagnostic use of single muscle fiber recording and the neuromuscular jitter in myasthenia gravis. p. 669. In Proceedings of the 6th International Congress of Electroencephalography and Clinical Neurophysiology, 1965
18. Stalberg E, Ekstedt J: Single fibre EMG and microphysiology of the motor unit in normal and diseased human muscle. p. 113. In Desmedt JE (ed): New Developments in Electromyography and Clinical Neurophysiology, Vol. 1. S. Karger AG, Basel, 1973
19. Stalberg E, Ekstedt J, Broman A: Neuromuscular transmission in myasthenia gravis studied with single fibre electromyography. J Neurol Neurosurg Psychiatry 37:540, 1974
20. Stalberg E: Clinical electrophysiology in myasthenia gravis. J Neurol Neurosurg Psychiatry 43:622, 1980
21. Slomic A, Rosenfalck A, Buchthal F: Electrical and mechanical responses of normal and myasthenic muscle with particular reference to the staircase phenomenon. Brain Res 10:1, 1968
22. Sanders DB: Electrophysiologic study of disorders of neuromuscular transmission. p. 307. In Aminoff MJ (ed): Electrodiagnosis in Clinical Neurology, 2nd Ed. Churchill Livingstone, New York, 1986
23. Engel AG: Myasthenia gravis and myasthenic syndromes. Ann Neurol 16:519, 1984
24. Elmqvist D, Lambert EH: Detailed analysis of neuromuscular transmission in a patient with the myasthenic syndrome sometimes associated with bronchogenic carcinoma. Mayo Clin Proc 43:689, 1968
25. Eaton LM, Lambert EH: Electromyography and electrical stimulation of nerves in

diseases of motor unit. Observations on myasthenic syndrome associated with malignant tumors. JAMA 163:1117, 1957

26. Newsom-Davis J, Murray NMF: Plasma exchange and immunosuppressive drug treatment in the Lambert-Eaton myasthenic syndrome. Neurology 34:480, 1984

27. Newsom-Davis J, Murray N, Wray D, Lang B, Prior C, Gwilt M, Vincent A: Lambert-Eaton myasthenic syndrome: Electrophysiological evidence for a humoral factor. Muscle Nerve 5:S17, 1982

28. Cull-Candy SG, Lundh H, Thesleff S: Effects of botulinum toxin on neuromuscular transmission in the rat. J Physiol 260:177, 1976

29. Pickett J, Berg B, Chaplin E, Brunstetter-Shafer MA: Syndrome of botulism in infancy: Clinical and electrophysiologic study. N Engl J Med 295:770, 1976

30. Arnon SS: Infant botulism. Ann Rev Med 31:541, 1980

31. Cherington M, Ryan DW: Botulism and guanidine. N Engl J Med 278:931, 1968

32. Cherington M: Electrophysiologic methods as an aid in diagnosis of botulism: A review. Muscle Nerve 5:S28, 1982

33. Mayer RF: The neuro-muscular defect in human botulism. Electroencephalogr Clin Neurophysiol 25:397, 1968

34. Gutmann L, Pratt L: Pathophysiologic aspects of human botulism. Arch Neurol 33:175, 1976

35. Cornblath DR, Sladky JT, Sumner AJ: Clinical electrophysiology of infantile botulism. Muscle Nerve 6:448, 1983

36. Schiller HH, Stalberg E: Human botulism studied with single-fiber electromyography. Arch Neurol 35:346, 1978

37. McQuillen MP, Cantor HE, O'Rourke JR: Myasthenic syndrome associated with antibiotics. Arch Neurol 18:402, 1968

38. Wright EA, McQuillen MP: Antibiotic-induced neuromuscular blockade. Ann NY Acad Sci 183:358, 1971

39. Aminoff MJ, Layzer RB, Satya-Murti S, Faden AI: The declining electrical response of muscle to repetitive nerve stimulation in myotonia. Neurology 27:812, 1977

40. Sica REP, McComas AJ: An electrophysiological investigation of limb-girdle and facioscapulohumeral dystrophy. J Neurol Neurosurg Psychiatry 34:469, 1971

41. Simpson JA, Lenman JAR: The effect of frequency of stimulation in neuromuscular disease. Electroencephalogr Clin Neurophysiol 111:604, 1959

42. Mulder DW, Lambert EH, Eaton LM: Myasthenic syndrome in patients with amyotrophic lateral sclerosis. Neurology 9:627, 1959

43. Patten BM, Hart A, Lovelace R: Multiple sclerosis associated with defects in neuromuscular transmission. J Neurol Neurosurg Psychiatry 35:385, 1972

44. Brown JC: Repetitive stimulation and neuromuscular transmission studies. p. 958. In Walton JN (ed): Disorders of Voluntary Muscle. 3rd Ed. Churchill Livingstone, Edinburgh, 1974

45. Bernstein LP, Antel JP: Motor neuron disease: Decremental responses to repetitive nerve stimulation. Neurology 31:204, 1981

46. Barrett EP, Barrett JN, Botz D, Chang DB, Mahaffey D: Temperature-sensitive aspects of evoked and spontaneous transmitter release at the frog neuromuscular junction. J Physiol 279:253, 1978

47. Ozdemir C, Young RR: Electrical testing in myasthenia gravis. Ann NY Acad Sci 183:287, 1971

15

Electrophysiologic Evaluation of Selected Aspects of the Central and Autonomic Nervous Systems

There has been increasing interest in recent years in the application of conventional electrophysiologic techniques to the evaluation of patients with abnormal movements. In these disorders, there is generally no evidence of peripheral neuromuscular disease, but rather, the peripheral neuromuscular apparatus comes to be activated inappropriately. Electrophysiologic techniques may help to characterize the abnormal movements and to provide some quantitative guide to their severity. They are particularly important when the pattern of muscular activation must be determined, especially with regard to the sequence in which muscles are activated and the relationship between activity in agonist muscles and that in antagonist muscles. The relationship of motor activity to specific stimuli may also be determined more easily if electrophysiologic recording techniques are used. Such techniques may involve recording the electromyographic activity from a number of different muscles, the velocity of movement about different joints in the

limbs, and the displacement of the limbs that occurs about these joints.

Tremor

Tremor is defined clinically as a rhythmic oscillatory movement about a joint. Tremors are traditionally divided into different categories depending upon their relationship to activity.

Rest tremor is typically seen in patients with parkinsonism and is characterized by a tremor that is often most conspicuous when the affected limb is at rest or under only slight postural activation. *Postural tremor* is most conspicuous when the affected limb is maintained in a posture against gravity, and *intention tremor* is a tremor that is most conspicuous during movement.

Tremor may occur in a number of different clinical circumstances, and its electrophysiologic characterization may then be helpful in suggesting the underlying cause.

When a tremor is to be studied by electrophysiologic means, it is convenient to record the muscle activity using surface electrodes from agonist and antagonist muscles involved in the rhythmic motor activity. In addition, movement about a joint can be measured using accelerometers. These can be used to monitor movement along a single axis or—if more sophisticated, triaxial accelerometers are available—along three orthogonal axes. The recordings from the accelerometer allow the frequency and amplitude of movements to be determined, whereas the electromyographic recording permits the relationship of activity in apparently antagonistic muscles to be recognized. When electrophysiologic studies are performed as a means of following changes in the frequency or amplitude of tremor over time, it is important that the recording situation be standardized. Many factors will influence the amplitude of the tremor, such as the level of arousal of the patient.

Tremor occurring in healthy subjects and associated with continuous (rather than periodic bursts of) electromyographic activity in agonist and antagonist muscles is referred to as *physiologic tremor*. Its frequency is between 7 and 12 Hz. Such tremor can be enhanced in amplitude, without alteration in frequency, in a variety of circumstances as a result of synchronization of the discharges of the voluntarily firing motor neuron pool at the segmental level. This enhancement occurs through the operation of the segmental stretch reflex,[1,2] with the motor outflow producing rhythmic contractions that reinforce the mechanical resonant properties of the moving parts. Bursts of activity from agonist and antagonist muscles are then evident on electromyography.

In *essential* or *familial tremor*, which has a frequency of 4 to 8 Hz in most instances, electromyographic recordings show bursts of synchronous activity from agonist and antagonist muscles (Fig. 15.1), although in up to about 10 percent of patients, there may be alternating bursts of activity (Fig.

15.1) that are more suggestive of the tremor seen in patients with parkinsonism.[3] Whether these latter patients are at greater risk of developing Parkinson's disease is unclear.

Analysis of single motor unit discharges during essential tremor bursts has shown that the discharges tend to be grouped or synchronized at the rate of the tremor, that the pattern of recruitment does not follow the "size" principle during the tremor burst, and that newly recruited single motor units often fire with abnormally high instantaneous firing frequencies during the tremor.[4–6]

Among patients with *alcoholism*, electromyographic studies have shown that tremor may be characterized by a pattern suggestive of enhanced physiologic tremor or a slower frequency pattern characteristic of essential tremor.[7]

Tremor may occur in patients with *peripheral neuropathies* and has been attributed to imbalance of the sensory input to the motor neuron pool.[3] Electrophysiologically, it is characterized by a mixed electromyographic pattern, with activity occurring either synchronously or with an alternating pattern in agonist and antagonist muscles, usually at a frequency of 6 to 8 Hz.

In so-called *primary writing tremor*, tremor occurs only in relation to a specific skilled task, such as handwriting. This type of tremor is generally regarded as a variant of essential tremor, although in some patients, electrophysiologic recordings show alternating activity in agonist and antagonist muscles.[8]

The rest tremor of *parkinsonism* is characterized by a 3- to 7-Hz tremor in which there is alternating electromyographic activity evident in agonist and antagonist muscles (Fig. 15.1). This activity may vary spontaneously in amplitude over time, may be obscured during volitional activity, and typically disappears during sleep. This typical pattern of alternating electromy-

A

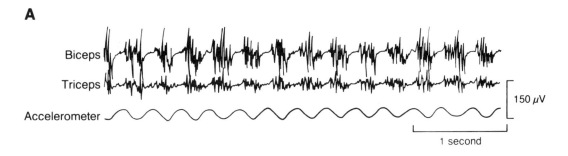

B

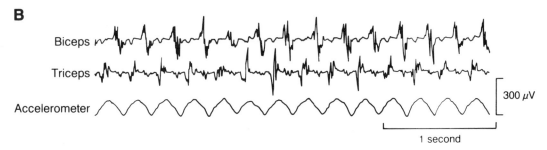

Fig. 15.1 Tremor recorded by surface electrodes over the biceps and triceps muscles, and by an accelerometer. (**A**) Bursts of synchronous activity from the two muscles. (**B**) Alternating bursts of electromyographic activity. Vertical calibration marker refers to electromyographic traces.

ographic activity may be replaced at times by coactivation of agonist and antagonist muscles. The physiologic mechanism generating the tremor is unknown; it does not relate to oscillations in the segmental stretch reflex,[9] but probably is attributable to some central generator mechanism. Analysis of the electromyographic activity by recordings of single motor unit activity has shown that some units may be active in each tremor burst, with instantaneous firing frequencies of up to 50 Hz, whereas others—of a higher threshold—have the same firing frequency as the tremor itself.[4]

Electromyographic studies have shown that some parkinsonian patients also have a tremor of the essential or familial variety. This fact may be important in determining the need for treatment with other medication.

More sophisticated studies have been performed by Findley and associates, who used spectral analysis to separate the various forms of tremor found in patients with Parkinson's disease.[10] They reported a rest tremor with a frequency of 4 to 5.3 Hz, a postural tremor at 6 Hz, and a physiologic tremor at 8 to 10 Hz. Most parkinsonian patients had tremors at both 4 to 5 Hz and 6 Hz.

Electrophysiologic techniques can be helpful in distinguishing tremor from other disorders simulating it. Cerebellar ataxia is characterized by irregular, coarse oscillations that occur in different planes, and electromyography does not show the distinctive features of essential tremor.

Asterixis is the term used when an intermittent difficulty in maintaining a sustained posture leads to a so-called "flapping tremor." Electromyographically, there is a brief lapse or interruption in the activity of tonically contracting muscles (Fig. 15.2), during which electrical silence for periods of up to about 200 msec occurs synchronously in agonist and antagonist muscles.[11] This is sometimes referred to as "negative" myoclonus. Other myoclonic phenomena

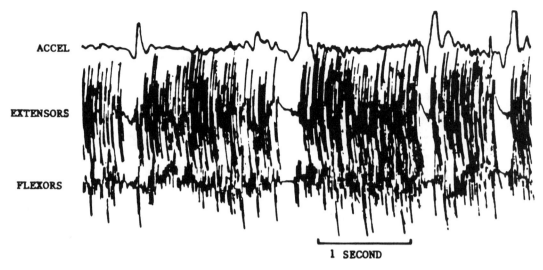

ACCEL

EXTENSORS

FLEXORS

1 SECOND

Fig. 15.2 Electromyographic and accelerometric recording of asterixis. Electromyographic recording is from flexors and extensors of the wrist and accelerometer was on the dorsum of the hand. (Hallett M: Electrophysiologic evaluation of tremor and central disorders of movement. p. 385. In Aminoff MJ (ed): Electrodiagnosis in Clinical Neurology. 2nd Ed. Churchill Livingstone, New York, 1986.)

are discussed in detail below, but apparently rhythmic myoclonus (with which tremor is most likely to be confused) is usually characterized by intermittent co-contraction of agonist and antagonist muscles that typically continues during sleep.

Myoclonus

The designation *myoclonus* refers to a quick muscle jerk that relates to dysfunction of the central nervous system. The modern classification of myoclonus depends on the presumed site of origin or physiologic basis of the abnormal activity.[12] In evaluating patients with myoclonus, it is helpful to record from a number of muscles supplied from different levels of the neuraxis while the patient is resting quietly, as well as after cutaneous stimulation, voluntary activity, and sudden startle or arousal. In many types of myoclonus, there are characteristic, repetitive patterns of muscle

jerking in terms of the muscle groups involved and the order in which they are activated. The recording of the electroencephalogram and of somatosensory evoked potentials may also be helpful, as may the demonstration of a C response (discussed below). Prospective studies suggest that these neurophysiologic studies, though time-consuming and complex, are helpful both in establishing an accurate diagnosis and in predicting responses to therapy.[12,13]

CORTICAL MYOCLONUS

Cortical myoclonus is generated by a discharge arising in the cerebral cortex, either spontaneously or in response to some triggering stimulus (cortical reflex myoclonus), and typically involves localized parts of the body. In cortical reflex myoclonus, jerks are triggered by peripheral stimuli, such as touch, muscle stretch, or voluntary activity.[14] When a number of muscles are involved, these are activated sequentially in a rostrocaudal direction, passing down the brain stem and spinal cord (Fig. 15.3). Electromyographic recordings from affected muscles show a brief discharge, often less than 30 msec in duration. Other electrophysiologic studies permit further characterization of the myoclonus. Scalp-recorded electroencephalograms may show that a focal event precedes each myoclonic jerk, especially if the cerebral activity is back-averaged from the myoclonic jerk, and somatosensory evoked potentials may be abnormally large.[15,16] Furthermore, electrical stimulation of a mixed nerve produces, in addition to an M wave and F response in the muscles innervated by that nerve, a third response—known as the C response—after a latency suggesting a transcortical pathway.[17] This response is thought to represent a myoclonic movement occur-ring as a manifestation of neural excitability.[17]

RETICULAR MYOCLONUS

Reticular myoclonus is similarly characterized by a brief (10 to 30 msec) electromyographic discharge in affected muscles that occurs either spontaneously or in response to some triggering stimulus (reticular reflex myoclonus). The myoclonus is generalized and bilateral, and if recordings are made from a number of muscles, it may be possible to show sequential activation of muscles in both a rostral and caudal direction (Fig. 15.4) starting from a particular level of the brain stem.[18] Electroencephalography fails to show any consistent preceding cerebral events that are time-locked to the jerks.

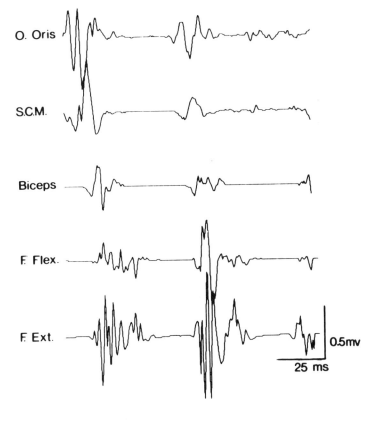

Fig. 15.3 Surface-recorded electromyographic correlate of myoclonic jerking induced by simultaneous, voluntary, tonic contraction of facial and right arm muscles. Two jerks are shown. (Hallett M, Chadwick D, Marsden CD: Cortical reflex myoclonus. Neurology 29:1107, 1979.)

O. Oris

S.C.M.

Biceps

F. Flex.

F. Ext.

0.5mv

25 ms

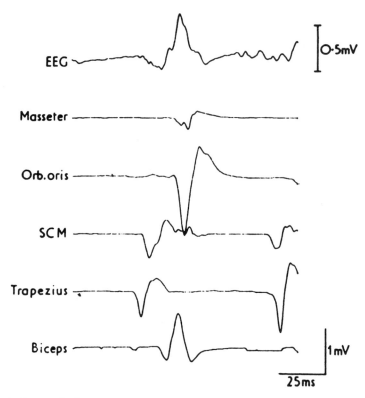

Fig. 15.4 Electrical record of spontaneous myoclonic jerk including activity in cranial nerve muscles. The electroencephalographic recording (EEG) is from a point 1 cm to the left and 2 cm behind the vertex referred to a midfrontal electrode (a positive deflection is downward). Other records are from the right masseter, left orbicular oris (Orb. oris), left sternocleidomastoid (SCM), right trapezius, and right biceps. Note the activation of the cranial nerves up the brain stem, and the onset of activity in the trapezius before that in the electroencephalogram. The upper voltage calibration refers to the electroencephalogram and the lower voltage calibration to all the electromyographic records. (Hallett M, Chadwick D, Adam J, Marsden CD: Reticular reflex myoclonus: A physiological type of human post-hypoxic myoclonus. J Neurol Neurosurg Psychiatry 40:253, 1977. Reproduced by permission of the Authors and Editors of the Journal of Neurology, Neurosurgery and Psychiatry.)

OTHER FORMS OF MYOCLONUS OF CEREBRAL ORIGIN

The two forms of myoclonus already described may coexist in the same patient. Other forms of myoclonus—for example, that associated with subacute sclerosing panencephalitis or familial essential myoclonus—may also arise in the brain subcortically, although their precise site of origin is unclear. The electromyographic discharges often last longer (50 to about 500 msec) than those that occur with the preceding cortical or reticular varieties. In one form of essential myoclonus, Hallett and associates found that voluntary activity provoked the myoclonus.[19] The volitional act elicited the typical electromyographic features of a ballistic movement[20] (activity first in the agonist, then in the antagonist, and finally in the agonist again), but inappropriate—often remote—muscles were also activated. Hence, the designation *ballistic movement overflow myoclonus* was applied.

Recent studies of *primary generalized epileptic myoclonus* suggest that it is a fragment of primary generalized epilepsy and a frequent manifestation of minipolymyoclonus of central origin. These studies indicate that a hyperexcitable cortex is driven by ascending impulses from a subcortical source.[21] The muscle jerks, which are less than 50 msec in duration, are preceded by a bilaterally synchronous, predominantly frontocentral, negative potential in the electroencephalogram when back-averaging techniques are used.[21]

The pathophysiologic basis of *palatal myoclonus*, which appears to arise in the brain stem, is unknown.

SPINAL MYOCLONUS

Spinal myoclonus is characterized by brief electromyographic bursts that are often exquisitely localized, are stable and usually rhythmic, are typically unaffected by peripheral stimulation or sleep, and can be recorded from both agonist and antagonist muscles. There are no preceding changes noted in the electroencephalogram with this form of myoclonus, which may relate to such diverse pathologic conditions as injury, infection, neoplasms, inflammatory or demyelinative lesions, or degenerative disorders.

Other Types of Abnormal Movement

Chorea is characterized electromyographically by irregular and unpredictable bursts of electromyographic activity occurring at inappropriate times in different muscles. Agonist and antagonist muscles may be activated synchronously or asynchronously, and bursts of activity may be brief

or last for several hundred milliseconds. Bursts of abnormal activity are sometimes initiated when the patient attempts a voluntary contraction.

In patients with *athetosis* or *dystonia*, there is a reduction in the maximal velocity and acceleration of voluntary movements of the affected limbs, and the latency of a motor response to a given stimulus may be increased markedly compared to that in normal subjects.[22] Prolonged electromyographic bursts may occur in agonist and antagonistic muscles synchronously, and cannot be controlled voluntarily. Such bursts of activity may last for 20 to 30 seconds, and sometimes are triggered by attempted voluntary movements. Further, electromyographic activity can often be recorded in muscles that seem clinically to be at rest.

The flexed, dystonic posture of parkinsonian patients, as well as the freezing-up phenomena that they sometimes experience, appears to result from a co-contraction of agonist and antagonist muscles.

Tics are brief, repetitive, irregularly occurring movements that can be controlled by the patient for short periods of time. Simple tics involve one or a few muscles and are characterized electromyographically by motor unit discharges that may occur synchronously or asynchronously in agonist and antagonist muscles. Discharges usually last for less than 200 msec.

Obeso and associates studied the negative premovement "readiness potential" of the electroencephalogram in patients with tics.[23] This potential usually begins about 500 to 1,500 msec before a voluntary movement and is easily recorded from the scalp. In patients with chronic multiple tics (Gilles de la Tourette's syndrome), Obeso and colleagues simultaneously recorded the electroencephalogram and electromyographic activity from those muscles showing the most frequent tics, and they used the electromyographic activity to trigger an analysis of the electrocerebral events preceding and following the tics. They found no readiness potential preceding the tics (Fig. 15.5). However, this potential was present when patients were asked to mimic their tics, usually commencing about 500 msec before the electromyographic discharge. They therefore concluded that the tics were not generated by the neural process governing normal voluntary activity.

Upper Motor Neuron Lesions

In patients with upper motor neuron syndromes, a loss of normal motor activity occurs, and a variety of abnormal reflex responses may also be found. Attempts have been made to study these responses electrophysiologically in order to gain insight into their pathophysiologic basis, as well as to provide a means of monitoring patients

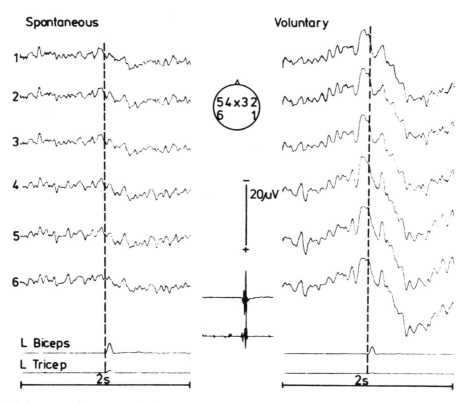

Fig. 15.5 Average electroencephalographic recordings from six sites (1–6 referred to a linked mastoid reference) in 100 spontaneous tics consisting of elbow flexion secondary to brief biceps contraction, with some co-contraction of the triceps (the electromyographic bursts producing a single such tic are seen in the middle insert), and in 128 voluntary, self-paced, willed biceps contractions mimicking the same tic, in a patient with Gilles de la Tourette's syndrome. The bottom two traces show the rectified electromyogram from biceps (used to trigger the back-averaging program) and triceps. The dotted line refers to the onset of activity in biceps. It can be seen that a negative premovement ''readiness potential'' precedes the voluntary movement but not the spontaneous tic. (Obeso JA, Rothwell JC, Marsden CD: Simple tics in Gilles de la Tourette's syndrome are not prefaced by a normal premovement EEG potential. J Neurol Neurosurg Psychiatry 44:735, 1981. Reproduced by permission of the Authors and Editors of the Journal of Neurology, Neurosurgery and Psychiatry.)

with so-called pyramidal syndromes for clinical, therapeutic, or experimental purposes.

Needle electromyography of weak muscles in patients with upper motor neuron lesions shows a reduced interference pattern on maximal voluntary effort. In some instances, fibrillation potentials and positive sharp waves have been found in limbs that are weak as a result of an upper motor neuron deficit.[24-26] Such abnormal spontaneous activity is usually not encountered for at least one week, or often longer, after onset of the weakness, and may disappear over the following weeks or months. It is sometimes attributable to an entrapment neuropathy, such as may follow prolonged bedrest, during which excessive pressure is placed on the ulnar nerve at the elbow. However, in other instances, a peripheral cause is less clear and the possibility cannot be excluded that it relates more directly to the central lesion.

In patients with spasticity, H reflexes can be elicited from muscles that, in normal adults, they would not easily be obtained from. For example, H reflexes can be elicited from the tibialis anterior muscle, and their amplitude is increased by stretching of this muscle. By contrast, although an H reflex may still be elicited in the gastrocnemius-soleus muscle, as in normal subjects, static stretch of this muscle group reduces the size of the H reflex recorded from it.[27] H reflex excitability curves following paired stimulation of the tibial nerve have been used to investigate patients with spasticity.[28-30] However, the changes found in spastic patients are of uncertain pathophysiologic significance, and the technique is of little practical relevance at the present time.

The amplitude of the F response has been taken to reflect the excitability of motor neurons. In chronic spasticity, the F response amplitude is increased on the affected side compared to that on the normal side, but in hemiplegia of recent onset the F response is reduced on the spastic side.[31] Similarly, the ratio between the maximal size of the H reflex and that of the direct motor (M) response can be taken to reflect the proportion of motor neurons activated by the reflex, and thus the excitability of the motor neuron pool.[32] In determining this ratio, the tibial nerve is stimulated at gradually increasing intensity to determine the maximal size of the H reflex; the stimulus intensity is then increased further until a maximal motor response is obtained.

The tonic vibration reflex has also been used to investigate central lesions. A vibratory stimulus to a muscle activates the primary and secondary muscle spindle endings repetitively, and an electromyographic discharge in the muscle results from the continuous bombardment of the spinal cord by impulses in group Ia and group II afferent fibers. This reflex response depends not only on motor neuron excitability, however, but also upon interneuronal interactions. Changes in the response are, therefore, hard to interpret because the reflex is influenced by so many different factors.[32]

Reflex responses with a latency greater than about 50 msec, occurring when certain voluntary movements are suddenly interrupted, have been attributed to transcortical pathways. Changes in these long-latency responses have been described in hemiplegic patients and in patients with lesions involving the ascending sensory pathways,[33,34] but such studies are currently of greater academic interest than clinical relevance.

Transcranial stimulation of motor pathways, using electrical or magnetic stimulation techniques, may provide important, clinically relevant information in patients with upper motor neuron lesions. However, such approaches are only beginning to be applied to the investigation of patients with various neurologic disorders.

In conclusion, then, electrophysiologic techniques have little clinical relevance at present to the evaluation of patients with upper motor neuron lesions.

EVALUATION OF AUTONOMIC FUNCTION

Autonomic dysfunction may complicate certain general medical disorders such as diabetes; it is a major cause of death in certain neurologic disorders, such as the Guillain-Barré syndrome or the Shy-Drager syndrome; and it is sometimes the sole manifestation of disease, as in idiopathic orthostatic hypotension. Because patients with dysautonomia are commonly referred to a clinical neurophysiologist for investigation, some discussion of the approach to their evaluation is warranted.

Symptoms of dysautonomia include paroxysmal hypertension, postprandial syncope, facial flushing, nasal congestion, declining night vision, constipation, diarrhea, vomiting, dysphagia, abdominal distention, disturbances of micturition, impaired thermoregulatory sweating, hyperhidrosis, impotence, apneic episodes, and a persistent tachycardia without any other cause. The most common and disabling symptom, however, is postural hypotension.

A variety of physiologic changes normally maintain blood pressure upon standing. An initial slight drop in systolic pressure influences the function of baroreceptors in the carotid sinus, aortic arch, and elsewhere, producing a reflex tachycardia and vasoconstriction. Other changes that occur include an immediate release of catecholamines from sympathetic ganglia, activation of the renin-angiotensin-aldosterone system, and release of vasopressin from the neurohypophysis. A slight drop in blood pressure occurs upon standing in about 10 percent of normal subjects, especially those who are elderly, and after prolonged bedrest. However, a drop of more than 25 mm Hg in systolic pressure or 10 mm Hg in diastolic pressure is abnormal.

Pathologic but non-neurologic causes of postural hypotension include disturbances of cardiac rhythm or contractility, cardiac valvular disease, a reduced blood volume, and an inadequate peripheral resistance (such as occurs with administration of phenothiazines, adrenergic blockers, and barbiturates). Neurologic causes include lesions that disrupt the reflex arc maintaining the blood pressure. This may occur because of involvement of afferent or efferent fibers in the peripheral nerves or nerve roots, such as occurs in the Guillain-Barré syndrome; in diabetic, alcoholic, amyloid, or certain toxic neuropathies; and in tabes dorsalis. In the Riley-Day syndrome of familial dysautonomia, postural hypotension is accompanied by impaired lacrimation, hyperhidrosis, defective temperature control, dysphagia, recurrent infections, indifference to pain, and depressed tendon reflexes. An acute acquired pure pandysautonomia is rare, often has a peripheral (postganglionic) basis, and is sometimes attributable to an autoimmune disturbance.

Central neurologic lesions may disrupt ascending or descending pathways, or may affect cell masses related to vasomotor regulation. In the Shy-Drager syndrome and in idiopathic orthostatic hypotension, there is degeneration of the preganglionic sympathetic efferent cells in the intermediolateral cell columns, but in the former the postural hypotension is accompanied by a variety of other neurologic symptoms and signs. Lesions in the brain stem or hypothalamus may also cause postural hypotension.

Hyperhidrosis, especially in the axillary, palmar, and plantar regions, may be idiopathic or psychogenic, whereas more widespread hyperhidrosis may be a manifestation of an underlying dysautonomia, a disturbance in thermoregulation, or certain metabolic or systemic disorders. Anhidrosis or hypohidrosis may be localized or diffuse, and is sometimes congenital. Thermoregulatory sweating is lost below a complete spinal lesion, but sweating may still occur as a spinal reflex. Sweating may be impaired in the sensory distribution of an injured peripheral nerve, leading to localized hyperhidrosis (with partial injuries) or anhidrosis, and sweating is often impaired distally in the extremities of patients with polyneuropathies. In the Ross-Adie syndrome, generalized or segmental anhidrosis is associated with tonic pupils and absent ankle jerks, and appears to relate to a peripheral neuronal deficit. Sympathectomy and various drugs also impair or block sweating.

Other autonomic symptoms result from abnormal gastrointestinal motility as well as from impaired control of micturition, defecation, and sexual function. A variety of neuro-ophthalmologic abnormalities may also occur, but these are beyond the scope of this review.

Clinical evaluation of patients with dysautonomia requires the exclusion of potentially reversible, non-neurologic causes. A detailed history of drug intake should be obtained. Hypovolemia, cardiac disease, and adrenal insufficiency must be excluded, and screening for diabetes mellitus, porphyria, and amyloidosis should also be undertaken. Neurologic examination may suggest the cause of the dysautonomia. For example, there may be signs of a polyneuropathy, evidence of a localized structural central lesion, or a combination of signs suggesting a degenerative disorder, such as the Shy-Drager syndrome.

Tests of Cardiovascular Control

The blood pressure and heart rate responses to Valsalva's maneuver and postural tilt reflect the integrity of baroreceptor reflexes, but the use of an intra-arterial needle may be necessary to record them. Valsalva's maneuver, which consists of a forced expiration against a closed glottis, is best performed by requiring patients to blow into a mouthpiece connected to a ma-

nometer so as to maintain an expiratory pressure of 40 mm Hg for about 10 seconds. The cardiovascular response has four distinct stages (Fig. 15.6). Stage 1 is characterized by a rise in blood pressure secondary to an increase in intrathoracic pressure. The reduction in venous return then leads (in stage 2) to a progressive decline in systolic and diastolic pressures, as well as in pulse pressure, accompanied by a tachycardia. Reflex vasoconstriction arrests the decline in blood pressure after about 5 to 7 seconds. When the forced expiration is discontinued in stage 3, the mean arterial pressure declines transiently as a result of the release of intrathoracic pressure. A rebound in blood pressure to above the resting level then occurs as a result of peripheral vasoconstriction, and is accompanied by a compensatory bradycardia (stage 4). Abnormalities in the response in patients with dysautonomia include loss of the tachycardia in stage 2 or bradycardia in stage 4 (or a lower heart rate in stage 2 than in stage 4), a decline in mean blood pressure in stage 2 to less than 50 percent of the previous resting mean pressure, or loss of the overshoot in systolic pressure in stage 4. In patients with autonomic insufficiency, there is often a progressive decline of intra-arterial pressure during the forced expiration, and after release of the expiration the pressure gradually returns to pre-existing levels within about a minute, without the marked overshoot and bradycardia that are normally found.

In patients with an abnormal response, it may be possible to localize the causal lesion. Central or afferent vasomotor pathways may be tested, for example, by recording the pressor or forearm blood flow response to loud noise or mental stress induced by performing mental arithmetic under harassment (or the change in blood flow through the hand with whole body heating). If no response is elicited, the lesion is probably central or efferent. There is no simple way of testing afferent pathways if an efferent lesion is present also.

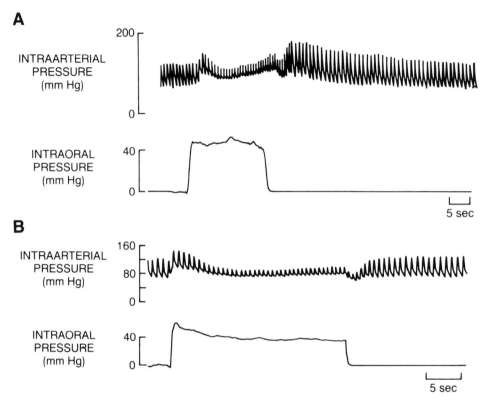

A

INTRAARTERIAL PRESSURE (mm Hg)

200

0

INTRAORAL PRESSURE (mm Hg)

40

0

5 sec

B

INTRAARTERIAL PRESSURE (mm Hg)

160

80

0

INTRAORAL PRESSURE (mm Hg)

40

0

5 sec

Fig. 15.6 Cardiovascular responses to Valsalva's maneuver, as recorded with an intra-arterial needle. (**A**) Normal response. (**B**) Abnormal response in a patient with autonomic insufficiency.

Postural changes in pulse and blood pressure are best recorded with the patient lying on a tilt table. Blood pressure and pulse are monitored with the patient lying supine until consistent values are obtained for 5 minutes; the patient is then tilted to a 60° head-up position while further measurements are made. Significant postural hypotension is commonly associated with an abnormal response to Valsalva's maneuver, but discrepancies occasionally occur that may relate to functional baroreceptors elsewhere than in the carotid sinus.

Recently developed simple tests of vagal function involve the *recording of heart rate changes* in a variety of settings, using a heart rate monitor or electrocardiogram (EKG).[35–38] Quantitative data can thereby be obtained noninvasively. The normal variation in heart rate at rest and after various stimuli is impaired or lost in dysautonomic patients. The normal tachycardia that occurs with change in position from lying to standing has been quantified by determining the ratio of the R-R interval of the thirtieth to fifteenth beat after standing. This cardiovascular response to standing has also been monitored using the peak heart rate acceleration, or the rate after 15 seconds. The beat-to-beat variation in heart rate during deep breathing has also been used as a test of autonomic function and depends on the rate and depth of respiration, as well as on an intact vagus nerve (Fig. 15.7). The response to Valsalva's maneuver can also be studied noninvasively by comparing the shortest R-R interval during forced expiration with the longest one

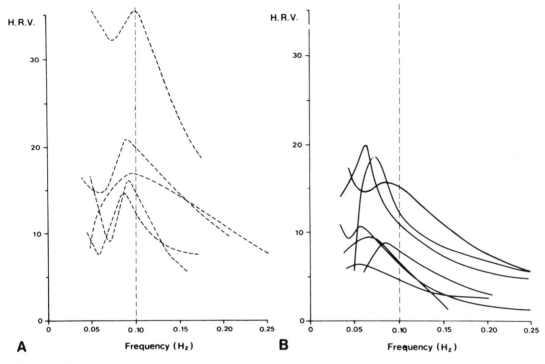

Fig. 15.7 Relation of respiration rate to heart rate variation (*H.R.V.*) in (**A**) normal subjects and (**B**) diabetic patients with peripheral and autonomic neuropathy. Frequency in Hertz is defined as the reciprocal of the time in seconds for one breath. Thus, six breaths per minute is equal to 0.1 Hz. (Reproduced, with permission from: Watkins PJ, Mackay JD: Cardiac denervation in diabetic neuropathy. Ann Intern Med 92(part 2):304, 1980.)

immediately afterward. The normal range of values depends on the duration of the forced expiration, the extent to which intrathoracic pressure is increased, and the age of the subject. These noninvasive tests of heart rate seem sensitive. For example, patients with symptoms of diabetic autonomic neuropathy almost always show some abnormality on these tests, and the results are often abnormal in patients with peripheral neuropathy who have no autonomic symptoms,[38] as shown in Figure 15.8.

The nature and extent of an autonomic deficit may be further clarified by biochemical or pharmacologic tests, but these are usually beyond the province of the clinical neurophysiologist and merit no further dis-

cussion here. In any event, the only real importance of these tests is to determine whether the sympathetic lesion is preganglionic or postganglionic, or both, because this affects the anticipated response to pressor drugs.

Tests of Sudomotor Function

Central and efferent sympathetic sudomotor fibers are tested by warming the patient with a radiant heat cradle until the body temperature has risen by 1°C. The area to be tested is then covered with a starch-iodide powder or a powder, containing alizarin or quinizarin, that changes color when wet. Alternatively, these fibers may

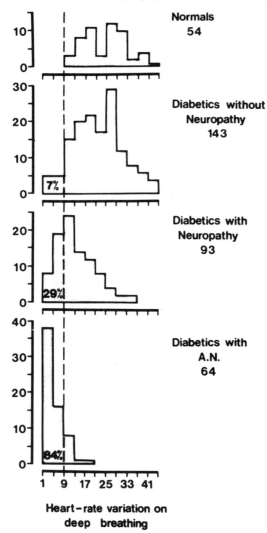

Normals
54

Diabetics without
Neuropathy
143

Diabetics with
Neuropathy
93

Diabetics with
A.N.
64

Heart-rate variation on
deep breathing

Fig. 15.8 Heart rate variation scores during deep breathing in normal subjects and diabetic patients without neuropathy, with peripheral neuropathy but no autonomic symptoms, and those with autonomic symptoms (A.N.). Heart rate variation score is calculated by measuring the difference between the minimum heart rate on inspiration and the maximum heart rate on expiration, taking the average from 10 inspirations and 10 expirations. The lower limit of normal (mean − 2 SD) is indicated by the vertical interrupted line. (Reproduced, with permission, from: Watkins PJ, Mackay JD: Cardiac denervation in diabetic neuropathy. Ann Intern Med 92(part 2):304, 1980.)

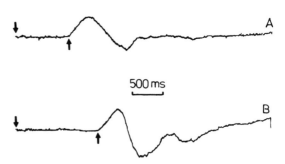

Fig. 15.9 Sympathetic skin response recorded in the proximal arm (**A**) and in the hand (**B**) of the same limb, following an electrical stimulus to the skin at the wrist. Downward pointing arrows indicate the stimulus, and upward pointing arrows demonstrate the onset of the response. (Shahani BT, Halperin JJ, Boulu P, Cohen J: Sympathetic skin response—A method of assessing unmyelinated axon dysfunction in peripheral neuropathies. J Neurol Neurosurg Psychiatry 47:536, 1984. Reproduced by permission of the Authors and Editors of the Journal of Neurology, Neurosurgery and Psychiatry.)

be tested indirectly by measuring changes in skin resistance, the so-called galvanic skin response. With sweating, there is a reduction of skin resistance that can be recorded as a voltage or current change between the region to be evaluated and an indifferent area.

Shahani and associates studied sudomotor function in patients with polyneuropathies by recording the sympathetic skin response—that is, the change in voltage (measured from the surface of the skin) following deep inspiration or a single 5- to 20-µA electrical stimulus (Fig. 15.9).[39] For recording purposes, a pair of electrodes was placed on the palm and dorsum of the hand, or the sole and dorsum of the foot. The response measured had a long latency, reflecting the slow (approximately 1 m/sec) conduction velocity of postganglionic sympathetic C fibers. Patients with predominantly demyelinative neuropathies had intact responses, whereas these responses were absent in some patients with axonal neuropathies. Abnormalities did not correlate well with clinical evidence of dysautonomia, but were thought to be a reliable indicator of disorders affecting umyelinated axons.

Other Studies

Aminoff used the technique of digital plethysmography to show that sympathetic vasomotor fibers were involved in patients with entrapment neuropathy, such as carpal tunnel syndrome, and in patients with polyneuropathies.[40,41] He studied the digital vasoconstrictor response to inspiration and found that this normal reflex response was abolished in the index finger but preserved in the little finger of the affected hand in some patients with carpal tunnel syndrome (Fig. 15.10). The reflex response was also abnormal in a number of patients with suspected polyneuropathy, most of whom had no clinical evidence of autonomic involvement. He therefore suggested that assessment of peripheral vasomotor function in patients with entrapment neuropathy or polyneuropathy may be helpful in identifying the spectrum of nerve fibers that are involved and thus in characterizing the disorder more fully. The plethysmographic technique is inconvenient and time-con-

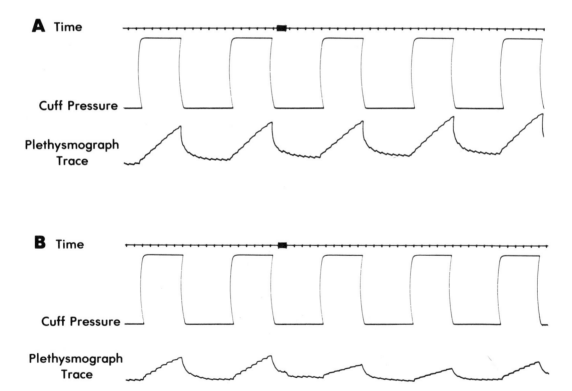

Fig. 15.10 Effect of a sudden deep inspiration (at the time shown by the marker) on blood flow to the index (**A**) and little (**B**) fingers of a patient with carpal tunnel syndrome, as recorded plethysmographically. Time in seconds. Following the deep inspiration, there is a change in blood flow to the little finger but not to the index finger, indicating dysfunction of sympathetic efferent fibers destined for the median-innervated digit. (Aminoff MJ: Involvement of peripheral vasomotor fibres in carpal tunnel syndrome. J Neurol Neurosurg Psychiatry 42:649, 1979. Reproduced by permission of the Authors and Editors of the Journal of Neurology, Neurosurgery and Psychiatry.)

suming, however, and similar information can be obtained more easily by evaluating peripheral sudomotor function, as outlined above.

The autonomic nervous system has been studied in a variety of other ways—for example, by examination of the response to intravenous lobeline (which induces a cough) to test the integrity of the glossopharyngeal nerve. Intradermally injected acetylcholine (0.1 ml of 1-percent solution) normally produces a piloerector response via an axon reflex in postganglionic sympathetic nerve fibers; loss of this response may be helpful in distinguishing ganglionic or postganglionic lesions from more proximal lesions of the sympathetic nervous system.

Metabolic studies show that, in some dysautonomic patients, plasma renin activity fails to increase upon standing, and there may also be low aldosterone levels with salt depletion, as well as an inability to conserve sodium when recumbent. The pupillary responses to different pharmacologic agents may be helpful in localizing an autonomic disturbance affecting the eyes. Radiologic studies sometimes show delayed emptying of the stomach and intestine. Bladder function may be evaluated by cystometrogram. Cystometry using gas, rather than water, as a filling medium and detrusor reflex activation procedures (with the patient being re-examined when sitting, standing, and walking in place) may be an improvement on the standard procedure. Other techniques for evaluating bladder function include uroflowmetry and urethral pressure profiles with measurement of intraurethral resistance. Absence of, or abnormal reduction in, noctural penile tumescence, as monitored with a strain gauge placed just behind the glans penis, suggests a significant organic component associated with impotence. The role and technique of sphincteric electromyography has been considered earlier in Chapter 6 (p. 93).

More invasive electrophysiologic studies have provided insight into the functioning of the sympathetic nervous system. In the technique known as microneurography, tungsten microelectrodes are inserted into nerve trunks in order to impale individual nerve fascicles. Recordings are then made of impulse traffic occurring in different types of myelinated and unmyelinated nerve fibers within the nerve fascicles. Recordings have been made from efferent postganglionic sympathetic C fibers.[42] The sympathetic fibers in a nerve fascicle tend to fire together, often with a cardiac or respiratory rhythm. The fibers conduct with a velocity of about 1 m/sec.

In nerve fascicles supplying skeletal muscles, microneurography shows bursts of impulses in sympathetic fibers that are synchronous with the pulse, and the pattern of activity recorded from nerve fascicles in different extremities is remarkably similar. Recordings from nerve fascicles to the skin indicate a greater variability in the grouped discharges in sympathetic fibers, although again, the impulse traffic recorded from two nerves in different limbs remains very similar.[43] Impulse traffic in sympathetic (sudomotor and vasomotor) nerves to the skin is influenced by a number of factors, including emotional excitement, stress, and mental activity.

Microneurography has had only limited clinical application. Nevertheless, Fagius and Wallin have used it to show that, in patients with polyneuropathies, there is impaired function of C fibers.[44] Many patients with diabetic polyneuropathy showed an absence of activity in peripheral sympathetic fibers when studied by microneurographic techniques, and this correlated with an impairment of the electrodermal and plethysmographic responses to arousal stimuli.

REFERENCES

1. Hagbarth K-E, Young RR: Participation of the stretch reflex in human physiological tremor. Brain 102:509, 1979

2. Young RR, Hagbarth K-E: Physiological tremor enhanced by manoeuvres affecting the segmental stretch reflex. J Neurol Neurosurg Psychiatry 43:248, 1980
3. Shahani BT, Young RR: Action tremors: A clinical neurophysiological review. p. 129. In Desmedt JE (ed): Physiological Tremor, Pathological Tremors and Clonus. Progress in Clinical Neurophysiology. Vol. 5. S. Karger AG, Basel, 1978
4. Shahani BT, Young RR: Specific abnormalities of single motor unit discharge patterns in tremor. Neurology 27:354, 1977
5. Young RR, Shahani BT: Analysis of single motor unit discharge patterns in different types of tremor. p. 527. In Cobb WA, Van Duijn H (eds): Contemporary Clinical Neurophysiology (Electroencephalogr Clin Neurophysiol Suppl 34). Elsevier, Amsterdam, 1978
6. Young RR, Shahani BT: Single unit behavior in human muscle afferent and efferent systems. p. 175. In Poirer LJ, Sourkes TL, Bedard PJ (eds): The Extrapyramidal System and Its Disorders. Advances in Neurology. Vol. 24. Raven Press, New York, 1979
7. Lefebvre-D'Amour M, Shahani BT, Young RR: Tremor in alcoholic patients. p. 160. In Desmedt JE (ed): Physiological Tremor, Pathological Tremors and Clonus. Progress in Clinical Neurophysiology. Vol. 5. S. Karger AG, Basel, 1978
8. Ravits J, Hallett M, Baker M, Wilkins D: Primary writing tremor and myoclonic writer's cramp. Neurology 35:1387, 1985
9. Hagbarth K-E, Wallin G, Lofstedt L, Aquilonius S-M: Muscle spindle activity in alternating tremor of Parkinsonism and in clonus. J Neurol Neurosurg Psychiatry 38:636, 1975
10. Findley LJ, Gresty MA, Halmagyi GM: Tremor, the cogwheel phenomenon and clonus in Parkinson's disease. J Neurol Neurosurg Psychiatry 44:534, 1981
11. Shahani BT, Young RR: Asterixis—A disorder of the neural mechanisms underlying sustained muscle contraction. p. 301. In Shahani M (ed): The Motor System: Neurophysiology and Muscle Mechanisms. Proceedings of a Satellite Symposium to the XXVIth International Congress of Physiology. Elsevier, Amsterdam, 1976

12. Marsden CD, Hallett M, Fahn S: The nosology and pathophysiology of myoclonus. p. 196. In Marsden CD, Fahn S (eds): Movement Disorders. Butterworths International Medical Reviews, Neurology 2. Butterworths, London, 1982
13. Kelly JJ, Sharbrough FW, Daube JR: A clinical and electrophysiological evaluation of myoclonus. Neurology 31:581, 1981
14. Hallett M, Chadwick D, Marsden CD: Cortical reflex myoclonus. Neurology 29:1107, 1979
15. Chadwick D, Hallett M, Harris R, Jenner P, Reynolds EH, Marsden CD: Clinical, biochemical, and physiological features distinguishing myoclonus responsive to 5-hydroxytryptophan, tryptophan with a monoamine oxidase inhibitor, and clonazepam. Brain 100:455, 1977
16. Shibasaki H, Yamashita Y, Kuroiwa Y: Electroencephalographic studies of myoclonus: Myoclonus-related cortical spikes and high amplitude somatosensory evoked potentials. Brain 101:447, 1978
17. Sutton GG, Mayer RF: Focal reflex myoclonus. J Neurol Neurosurg Psychiatry 37:207, 1974
18. Hallett M, Chadwick D, Adam J, Marsden CD: Reticular reflex myoclonus: A physiological type of human posthypoxic myoclonus. J Neurol Neurosurg Psychiatry 40:253, 1977
19. Hallett M, Chadwick D, Marsden CD: Ballistic movement overflow myoclonus. A form of essential myoclonus. Brain 100:299, 1977
20. Hallett M, Shahani BT, Young RR: EMG analysis of stereotyped voluntary movements in man. J Neurol Neurosurg Psychiatry 38:1154, 1975
21. Wilkins DE, Hallett M, Erba G: Primary generalised epileptic myoclonus: A frequent manifestation of minipolymyoclonus of central origin. J Neurol Neurosurg Psychiatry 48:506, 1985
22. Neilson PD: Voluntary control of arm movement in athetotic patients. J Neurol Neurosurg Psychiatry 37:162, 1974
23. Obeso JA, Rothwell JC, Marsden CD: Simple tics in Gilles de la Tourette's syndrome are not prefaced by a normal premovement EEG potential. J Neurol Neurosurg Psychiatry 44:735, 1981

24. Goldkamp O: Electromyography and nerve conduction studies in 116 patients with hemiplegia. Arch Phys Med Rehabil 48:59, 1967

25. Krueger KC, Waylonis GW: Hemiplegia: Lower motor neuron electromyographic findings. Arch Phys Med Rehabil 54:360, 1973

26. Johnson EW, Denny ST, Kelley JP: Sequence of electromyographic abnormalities in stroke syndrome. Arch Phys Med Rehabil 56:468, 1975

27. Burke D, Andrews C, Ashby P: Autogenic effects of static muscle stretch in spastic man. Arch Neurol 25:367, 1971

28. Yap CB: Spinal segmental and long-loop reflexes on spinal motoneurone excitability in spasticity and rigidity. Brain 90:887, 1967

29. Zander Olsen P, Diamantopoulos E: Excitability of spinal motor neurones in normal subjects and patients with spasticity, Parkinsonian rigidity, and cerebellar hypotonia. J Neurol Neurosurg Psychiatry 30:325, 1967

30. Masland WS: Facilitation during the H-reflex recovery cycle. Arch Neurol 26:313, 1972

31. Fisher MA, Shahani BT, Young RR: Assessing segmental excitability after acute rostral lesions. I. The F response. Neurology 28:1265, 1979

32. Delwaide PJ: EMG studies of involuntary movements. p. 89. Syllabus. Clinical EMG Course. American Academy of Neurology, 1986

33. Marsden CD, Merton PA, Morton HB, Adam J: The effect of lesions of the central nervous system on long-latency stretch reflexes in the human thumb. p. 334. In Desmedt JE (ed): Cerebral Motor Control in Man: Long Loop Mechanisms. Progress in Clinical Neurophysiology. Vol. 4. S. Karger AG, Basel, 1978

34. Lee RG, Tatton WG: Long loop reflexes in man: Clinical applications. p. 320. In Desmedt JE (ed): Cerebral Motor Control in Man: Long Loop Mechanisms. Progress in Clinical Neurophysiology. Vol. 4. S. Karger AG, Basel, 1978

35. Ewing DJ, Campbell IW, Burt AA, Clarke BF: Vascular reflexes in diabetic autonomic neuropathy. Lancet 2:1354, 1973

36. Ewing DJ, Campbell IW, Murray A, Neilson JMM, Clarke BF: Immediate heart-rate response to standing: Simple test for autonomic neuropathy in diabetes. Br Med J 1:145, 1978

37. Ewing DJ, Campbell IW, Clarke BF: Assessment of cardiovascular effects in diabetic autonomic neuropathy and prognostic implications. Ann Intern Med 92(part 2):308, 1980

38. Watkins PJ, Mackay JD: Cardiac denervation in diabetic neuropathy. Ann Intern Med 92(part 2):304, 1980

39. Shahani BT, Halperin JJ, Boulu P, Cohen J: Sympathetic skin response—A method of assessing unmyelinated axon dysfunction in peripheral neuropathies. J Neurol Neurosurg Psychiatry 47:536, 1984

40. Aminoff MJ: Involvement of peripheral vasomotor fibres in carpal tunnel syndrome. J Neurol Neurosurg Psychiatry 42:649, 1979

41. Aminoff MJ: Peripheral sympathetic function in patients with a polyneuropathy. J Neurol Sci 44:213, 1980

42. Wallin BG: New aspects of sympathetic function in man. p. 145. In Stalberg E, Young RR (eds): Butterworths International Medical Reviews. Neurology 1. Clinical Neurophysiology. Butterworths, London, 1981

43. Bini G, Hagbarth K-E, Hynninen P, Wallin BG: Regional similarities and differences in thermoregulatory vaso- and sudomotor tone. J Physiol 306:553, 1980

44. Fagius J, Wallin BG. Sympathetic reflex latencies and conduction velocities in patients with polyneuropathy. J Neurol Sci 47:449, 1980

Appendix

A Glossary of Terms Used in Clinical Electromyography*

A wave A compound action potential evoked consistently from a muscle by submaximal electrical stimuli to the nerve and frequently abolished by supramaximal stimuli. The amplitude of the A wave is similar to that of the F wave, but the latency is more constant. The A wave usually occurs before the F wave, but may occur afterwards. The A wave is due to normal or pathological axonal branching. Compare *F wave*.

Absolute refractory period See *refractory period*.

Accommodation True accommodation in neuronal physiology is a rise in the threshold transmembrane depolarization required to initiate a spike when depolarization is slow or a subthreshold depolarization is maintained. In the older literature, accommodation described the observation that the final intensity of current applied in a slowly rising fashion to stimulate a nerve was greater than the intensity of a pulse of current required to stimulate the same nerve. The latter may largely be an artifact of the nerve sheath and bears little relation to true accommodation as measured intracellularly.

Accommodation curve See *strength-duration curve*.

Action current The electrical currents associated with an *action potential*.

Action potential The brief, regenerative, all-or-nothing electrical potential that propagates along a single axon or muscle fiber membrane. See also *compound action potential*.

Active electrode Synonymous with *exploring electrode*. See *recording electrode*.

* Compiled by the Nomenclature Committee of the American Association of Electromyography and Electrodiagnosis (2nd Edition, 1987): Charles K. Jablecki, Chairman; Charles F. Bolton; Walter G. Bradley; William F. Brown; Fritz Buchthal; Roger Q. Cracco; Ernest W. Johnson; George H. Kraft; Edward H. Lamberg; Hans O. Lueders; Dong M. Ma; John A. Simpson; Erik V. Stålberg. Reprinted with permission of the American Association of Electromyography and Electrodiagnosis, © Copyright, 1987.

Adaptation A decline in the frequency of the spike discharge as typically recorded from sensory axons in response to a maintained stimulus.

After discharge The continuation of an impulse train in a neuron, axon, or muscle fiber following the termination of an applied stimulus. The number of extra impulses and their periodicity in the train may vary depending on the circumstances.

Afterpotential The membrane potential between the end of the spike and the time when the membrane potential is restored to its resting value. The membrane during this period may be depolarized or hyperpolarized.

Amplitude With reference to an *action potential*, the maximum voltage difference between two points, usually baseline to peak or peak to peak. By convention, the amplitude of the *compound muscle action potential* is measured from the baseline to the most negative peak. In contrast, the amplitude of a *compound sensory nerve action potential, motor unit potential, fibrillation potential, positive sharp wave, fasciculation potential,* and most other *action potentials* is measured from the most positive to the most negative peak.

Anodal block A local block of nerve conduction caused by *hyperpolarization* of the nerve cell membrane by an electrical stimulus. See *stimulating electrode.*

Anode The positive terminal of a source of electrical current.

Antidromic Propagation of an impulse in the direction opposite to physiologic conduction, e.g., conduction along motor nerve fibers away from the muscle and conduction along sensory fibers away from the spinal cord. Contrast with *orthodromic.*

Artifact A voltage change generated by a biological or nonbiological source other than the ones of interest. The *stimulus artifact* is the potential recorded at the time the stimulus is applied and includes the *electrical* or *shock artifact,* which represents cutaneous spread of stimulating current to the recording electrode. The stimulus and shock artifacts usually precede the activity of interest. A *movement artifact* refers to a change in the recorded activity caused by movement of the recording electrodes.

Auditory evoked potentials (Abbr. AEP). Electrical waveforms of biological origin elicited in response to sound stimuli. AEPs are classified by their latency into short-latency brainstem AEPs (Abbr. BAEP) with latency up to 10 msec, middle-latency brainstem AEPs with latency 10 to 50 msec, and long-latency AEPs with latency over 50 msec. See *brainstem auditory evoked potential.*

Axon reflex Use of term is discouraged as it is incorrect. No reflex is considered to be involved. See *A wave.*

Axon response See *A wave.*

Axon wave See *A wave.*

Axonotmesis Nerve injury characterized by disruption of the axon and myelin sheath but with preservation of the supporting connective tissue, resulting in axonal degeneration distal to the injury site.

Backfiring Discharge of an antidromically activated motor neuron.

Baseline The potential recorded from a biological system while the system is at rest.

Benign fasciculation Use of term to describe a firing pattern of fasciculation potentials is discouraged. The term has been used to describe a clinical syndrome and/or the presence of fasciculations in nonprogressive neuromuscular disorders. See *fasciculation potential.*

Bifilar (bipolar) needle electrode A *recording electrode* that measures variations in voltage between the bare tips of two insulated wires cemented side by side in a steel cannula. The bare tips of the electrodes are flush with the level of the cannula. The latter may be grounded.

Biphasic action potential An *action potential* with two phases.

Bizarre high-frequency discharge See *complex repetitive discharge.*

Bizarre repetitive discharge See *complex repetitive discharge.*

Bizarre repetitive potential See *complex repetitive discharge.*

Blink response Strictly defined, one of the *blink responses.* See *blink responses.*

Blink responses *Compound muscle action potentials* evoked from orbicularis oculi muscles as a result of brief electrical or mechanical stimuli to the cutaneous area innervated by the supraorbital (or less commonly the infraorbital) branch of the trigeminal nerve. Typically, there is an early compound muscle action potential (*R1 wave*) ipsilateral to the stimulation site with a latency of about 10 msec and a bilateral late compound muscle action potential (*R2 wave*) with a latency of approximately 30 msec. Generally, only the *R2 wave* is associated with a visible twitch of the orbicularis oculi. The configuration, amplitude, duration, and latency of the two components, along with the sites of recording and the sites of stimulation, should be specified. *R1* and *R2 waves* are probably oligosynaptic and polysynaptic brainstem reflexes, re-

spectively, together called the *blink reflex*, with the afferent arc provided by the sensory branches of the trigeminal nerve and the efferent arc provided by the facial nerve motor fibers.

Blink reflex See *blink responses.*

Brainstem auditory evoked potential (Abbr. BAEP). Electrical waveforms of biological origin elicited in response to sound stimuli. The normal BAEP consists of a sequence of up to seven waves, named I and VII, which occur during the first 10 msec after the onset of the stimulus and have positive polarity at the vertex of the head.

Brainstem auditory evoked response (Abbr. BAER, BER). See preferred term *brainstem auditory evoked potential.*

BSAP Abbreviation for "brief, small, abundant potentials." Use of term is discouraged. It is used to describe a recruitment pattern of brief-duration, small-amplitude, overly abundant motor unit action potentials. Quantitative measurements of motor unit potential duration, amplitude, numbers of phases, and recruitment frequency are to be preferred to qualitative descriptions such as this. See *motor unit action potential.*

BSAPP Abbreviation for "brief, small, abundant, polyphasic potentials." Use of term is discouraged. It is used to describe a recruitment pattern of brief-duration, small-amplitude, overly abundant, polyphasic motor unit action potentials. Quantitative measurements of motor unit potential duration, amplitude, numbers of phases, and recruitment frequency are to be preferred to qualitative descriptions such as this. See *motor unit action potential.*

Cathode The negative terminal of a source of electrical current.

Central electromyography (Abbr. central EMG). Use of electromyographic recording techniques to study the control of movement and reflexes by the spinal cord and brain.

Chronaxie See *strength-duration curve.*

Clinical electromyography Used to refer to all electrodiagnostic studies of human peripheral nerves and muscle. See *electromyography.*

Coaxial needle electrode See synonym *concentric needle electrode.*

Common peroneal nerve—short latency SEP—(Abbr. CPN-SSEP). *Short latency somatosensory evoked potentials* elicited by stimulation of the common peroneal nerve at the knee occur within 40 ms of the stimulus in normal subjects. It is suggested that individual response components be designated as follows: (1) spine components: L3 and T12 spine potentials; (2) scalp components: P27 and N35.

Complex motor unit potential A motor unit potential that is *polyphasic* or *serrated.*

Complex repetitive discharge Polyphasic or serrated action potentials that may begin spontaneously or after a needle movement. They have a uniform frequency, shape, and amplitude, with abrupt onset, cessation, or change in configuration. Amplitude ranges from 100 V to 1 mV and frequency of discharge from 5 to 100 Hz. This term is preferred to *bizarre high frequency discharge, bizarre repetitive discharge, bizarre repetitive potential, near constant frequency trains, pseudomyotonic discharge,* and *synchronized fibrillation.*

Compound action potential See *com-*

pound mixed nerve action potential, compound motor nerve action potential, compound nerve action potential, compound sensory nerve action potential, and *compound muscle action potential.*

Compound mixed nerve action potential A compound nerve action potential is considered to have been evoked from afferent and efferent fibers if the recording electrodes detect activity on a mixed nerve with the electrical stimulus applied to a segment of the nerve that contains both afferent and efferent fibers. The amplitude, latency, duration, and phases should be noted.

Compound motor nerve action potential A compound nerve action potential is considered to have been evoked from efferent fibers to a muscle if the recording electrodes detect activity only in a motor nerve or a motor branch of a mixed nerve, or if the electrical stimulus is applied only to such a nerve or a ventral root. The amplitude, latency, duration, and phases should be noted. See *compound nerve action potential.*

Compound muscle action potential The summation of nearly synchronous muscle fiber action potentials recorded from a muscle commonly produced by stimulation of the nerve supplying the muscle either directly or indirectly. Baseline-to-peak amplitude, duration, and latency of the negative phase should be noted, along with details of the method of stimulation and recording. Use of specific named potentials is recommended, e.g., *M wave, F wave, H wave, T wave, A wave,* and *R1 wave* or *R2 wave (blink responses).*

Compound nerve action potential The summation of nearly synchronous nerve fiber action potentials recorded from a nerve trunk, commonly produced by stimulation of the nerve directly or indirectly. Details of the method of stimulation and recording should be specified, together with the fiber type (sensory, motor, or mixed).

Compound sensory nerve action potential

A compound nerve action potential is considered to have been evoked from afferent fibers if the recording electrodes detect activity only in a sensory nerve or in a sensory branch of a mixed nerve, or if the electrical stimulus is applied to a sensory nerve or a dorsal nerve root, or an adequate stimulus is applied synchronously to sensory receptors. The amplitude, latency, duration, and configuration should be noted. Generally, the amplitude is measured as the maximum peak-to-peak voltage, the latency as either the *latency* to the initial deflection or the *peak latency* to the negative peak, and the duration as the interval from the first deflection of the waveform from the baseline to its final return to the baseline. The compound sensory nerve action potential has been referred to as the *sensory response* or *sensory potential.*

Concentric needle electrode

A *recording electrode* that measures an electrical potential difference between the bare tip of an insulated wire, usually stainless steel, silver, or platinum, and the bare shaft of a steel cannula through which it is inserted. The bare tip of the central wire (exploring electrode) is flush with the level of the cannula (reference electrode).

Conditioning stimulus

See *paired stimuli.*

Conduction block

Failure of an action potential to be conducted past a particular point in the nervous system, whereas conduction is possible below the point of the block. Conduction block is documented by demonstration of a reduction in the area of an evoked potential greater than that nor-

mally seen with electrical stimulation at two different points on a nerve trunk; anatomical variations of nerve pathways and technical factors related to nerve stimulation must be excluded as the cause of the reduction in area.

Conduction distance

See *conduction velocity.*

Conduction time.

See *conduction velocity.*

Conduction velocity

Speed of propagation of an *action potential* along a nerve or muscle fiber. The nerve fibers studied (motor, sensory, autonomic, or mixed) should be specified. For a nerve trunk, the maximum conduction velocity is calculated from the *latency* of the evoked potential (muscle or nerve) at maximal or supramaximal intensity of stimulation at two different points. The distance between the two points (*conduction distance*) is divided by the difference between the corresponding latencies (*conduction time*). The calculated velocity represents the conduction velocity of the fastest fibers and is expressed as meters per second (m/sec). As commonly used, the term *conduction velocity* refers to the *maximum conduction velocity.* By specialized techniques, the conduction velocity of other fibers can be determined as well and should be specified, e.g., minimum conduction velocity.

Contraction

A voluntary or involuntary reversible muscle shortening that may or may not be accompanied by *action potentials* from muscle. This term is to be contrasted with the term *contracture*, which refers to a condition of fixed muscle shortening.

Contraction fasciculation

Rhythmic, visible twitching of a muscle with weak voluntary or postural contraction. The phenomenon occurs in neuromuscular disorders in which the motor unit territory is enlarged and the tissue covering the muscle is thin.

Contracture The term is used to refer to immobility of a joint due to fixed muscle shortening. Contrast *contraction*. The term has also been used to refer to an electrically silent, involuntary state of maintained muscle contraction, as seen in phosphorylase deficiency. See preferred term, *muscle cramp*.

Coupled discharge See preferred term, *satellite potential*.

Cramp discharge Involuntary repetitive firing of *motor unit action potentials* at a high frequency (up to 150 Hz) in a large area of muscles, usually associated with painful muscle contraction. Both the discharge frequency and the number of *motor unit action potentials* firing increase gradually during development and both subside gradually with cessation. See *muscle cramp*.

Cycles per second (Abbr. cps or c/sec). Unit of frequency. See also *hertz* (Abbr. Hz).

Decremental response See preferred term, *decrementing response*.

Decrementing response A reproducible decline in the amplitude and/or area of the *M wave* of successive responses to *repetitive nerve stimulation*. The rate of stimulation and the total number of stimuli should be specified. Decrementing responses with disorders of neuromuscular transmission are most reliably seen with slow rates (2 to 5 Hz) of nerve stimulation. A decrementing response with repetitive nerve stimulation commonly occurs in disorders of neuromuscular transmission, but can also be seen in some neuropathies, myopathies, and motor neuron disease. An ar-

tifact resembling a decrementing response can result from movement of the stimulating or recording electrodes during repetitive nerve stimulation. Contrast with *incrementing response*.

Delay *Delay* as originally used in clinical electromyography referred to the time between the beginning of the horizontal sweep of the oscilloscope and the onset of an applied stimulus. The term is also used to refer to an information storage device (delay line) used to display events occurring before a trigger signal.

Denervation potential This term has been used to describe a *fibrillation potential*. The use of this term is discouraged because fibrillation potentials may occur in settings where transient muscle membrane instability occurs in the absence of denervation, e.g., hyperkalemia periodic paralysis. See *fibrillation potential*.

Depolarization See *polarization*.

Depolarization block Failure of an excitable cell to respond to a stimulus because of *depolarization* of the cell membrane.

Discharge Refers to the firing of one or more excitable element (neurons, axons, or muscle fibers) and as conventionally applied refers to the all-or-none potentials only.

Discharge frequency The rate of repetition of potentials. When potentials occur in groups, the rate of recurrence of the group and the rate of repetition of the individual components in the groups should be specified. See *firing rate*.

Discrete activity See *interference pattern*.

Distal latency See *motor latency* and *sensory latency*.

Double discharge Two action potentials (*motor unit action potential, fibrillation potential*) of the same form and nearly the same amplitude, occurring consistently in the same relationship to one another at intervals of 2 to 20 msec.

Doublet Synonymous with *double discharge*.

Duration The time during which something exists or acts. (1) The total duration of individual potential *waveforms* is defined as the interval from the beginning of the first deflection from the baseline to its final return to the baseline, unless otherwise specified. If only part of the waveform duration is measured, the points of measurement should be specified. For example, the duration of the *M wave* may refer to the interval from the deflection of the first negative phase from the baseline to its return to the baseline. (2) The duration of a single electrical stimulus refers to the interval of the applied current or voltage. (3) The duration of recurring stimuli or action potentials refers to the interval from the beginning to the end of the series.

Earth electrode Synonymous with *ground electrode*.

Electrical artifact See *artifact*.

Electrical inactivity Absence of identifiable electrical activity in a structure or organ under investigation. See preferred term *electrical silence*.

Electrical silence The absence of measurable electrical activity due to biological or nonbiological sources. The sensitivity and signal-to-noise level of the recording system should be specified.

Electrode A conducting device used to record an electrical potential (*recording electrode*) or to apply an electrical current (*stimulating electrode*). Two electrodes are always required. Depending on the relative size and location of the electrodes, however, the stimulating or recording condition may be referred to as *monopolar* or *unipolar*. See *ground electrode, recording electrode*, and *stimulating electrode*. Also see specific needle electrode configurations: *monopolar, unipolar, concentric, bipolar, multilead, single fiber,* and *macro needle electrodes*.

Electrodiagnosis The recording and analysis of responses of nerves and muscles to electrical stimulation and the identification of patterns of insertion, spontaneous, involuntary, and voluntary action potentials in muscle and nerve tissue.

Electrodiagnostic medicine A specific area of medical practice in which a physician uses information from the clinical history, observations from the physical examination, and the techniques of *electrodiagnosis* to diagnose and treat neuromuscular disorders. See *electrodiagnosis*.

Electromyelography The recording and study of electrical activity from the spinal cord and/or from the cauda equina.

Electromyogram The record obtained by *electromyography*.

Electromyograph Equipment used to activate, record, process, and display nerve and muscle action potentials for the purpose of evaluating nerve and muscle function.

Electromyography (Abbr. EMG). Strictly defined, the recording and study of insertion, spontaneous, and voluntary electrical activity of muscle. It is commonly used to refer to nerve conduction studies as well. See *clinical electromyography*.

Electroneurography (Abbr. ENG). The recording and study of the action potentials of peripheral nerves. See *nerve conduction studies*.

Electroneuromyography (Abbr. ENMG). The combined studies of *electromyography* and *electroneurography*.

End-plate activity Spontaneous electrical activity recorded with a needle electrode close to muscle end-plates. May be either of two forms:
1. **Monophasic** Low-amplitude (10 to 20 μV), short-duration (0.5 to 1 msec), monophasic (negative) potentials that occur in a dense, steady pattern and are restricted to a localized area of the muscle. Because of the multitude of different potentials occurring, the exact frequency, although appearing to be high, cannot be defined. These nonpropagated potentials are miniature end-plate potentials recorded extracellularly. This form of end-plate activity has been referred to as *end-plate noise* or *sea shell sound*.
2. **Biphasic** Moderate-amplitude (100 to 300 μV), short-duration (2 to 4 msec), biphasic (negative-positive) spike potentials that occur irregularly in short bursts with a high frequency (50 to 100 Hz), restricted to a localized area within the muscle. These propagated potentials are generated by muscle fibers excited by activity in nerve terminals. These potentials have been referred to as *biphasic spike potentials, end-plate spikes,* and, incorrectly, *nerve potentials*.

End-plate noise See *end-plate activity, monophasic*.

End-plate potential (EPP) The graded nonpropagated membrane potential induced in the postsynaptic membrane of the muscle fiber by the action of acetylcholine released in response to an action potential in the presynaptic axon terminal.

End-plate spike See *end-plate activity, biphasic*.

End-plate zone The region in a muscle where the neuromuscular junctions of the skeletal muscle fibers are concentrated.

Evoked compound muscle action potential See *compound muscle action potential*.

Evoked potential Electrical waveform elicited by and temporally related to a stimulus, most commonly an electrical stimulus delivered to a sensory receptor or nerve, or applied directly to a discrete area of the brain, spinal cord, or muscle. See *auditory evoked potential, brain stem auditory evoked potential, spinal evoked potential, somatosensory evoked potential, visual evoked potential, compound muscle action potential*, and *compound sensory nerve action potential*.

Evoked potential studies Recording and analysis of electrical waveforms of biological origin elicited in response to electrical or physiological stimuli. Generally used to refer to studies of waveforms generated in the peripheral and central nervous system, whereas *never conduction studies* refer to studies of waveforms generated in the peripheral nervous system. There are two systems for naming complex waveforms in which multiple components can be distinguished. In the first system, the different components are labeled PI or NI for the initial positive and negative potentials, respectively, and PII, PIII, NIIII, etc., for subsequent positive and negative potentials. In the second system, the components are specified by polarity and average peak latency in normal subjects to the nearest millisecond. The first nomenclature principle has been used in an abbreviated form to identify the seven positive components (I to VII) of the normal *brainstem auditory evoked potential*. The second nomenclature principle has been used to identify the positive and negative components of *visual evoked potentials* (N$\overline{75}$, P$\overline{100}$) and *somatosensory evoked potentials* (P$\overline{9}$, P$\overline{11}$, P$\overline{13}$, P$\overline{14}$, N$\overline{20}$, P$\overline{23}$). Regardless of the nomenclature system, it is possible under standardized conditions to establish normal ranges of amplitude, duration, and latency of the individual components of these *evoked potentials*. The difficulty with the second system is that the latencies of components of evoked potentials depend upon the length of the pathways in the neural tissues. Thus the components of an SEP recorded in a child have different average latencies from the same components of an SEP recorded in an adult. Despite this problem, there is no better system available for naming these components at this time. See *auditory evoked potentials, brainstem auditory evoked potential, visual evoked potential, somatosensory evoked potential, somatosensory evoked potential, median nerve—short latency SEP, common peroneal nerve—short latency SEP.*

Excitability Capacity to be activated by or react to a stimulus.

Excitatory postsynaptic potential (Abbr. EPSP). A local, graded depolarization of a neuron in response to activation by a nerve terminal of a synapse. Contrast with *inhibitory postsynaptic potential.*

Exploring electrode Synonymous with *active electrode.* See *recording electrode.*

F response Synonymous with *F wave.* See *F wave.*

F wave A compound action potential evoked intermittently from a muscle by a supramaximal electrical stimulus to the nerve. Compared with the maximal amplitude *M wave* of the same muscle, the F wave has a smaller amplitude (1 to 5 percent

of the M wave)), a variable configuration, and a longer, more variable latency. The F wave can be found in many muscles of the upper and lower extremities, and the latency is longer with more distal sites of stimulation. The F wave is due to antidromic activation of motor neurons. It was named by Magladery and McDougal in 1950. Compare the *H wave* and the *A wave.*

Facilitation Improvement of neuromuscular transmission which results in the activation of previously inactive muscle fibers. *Facilitation* may be identified in several ways:

1. *Incrementing response*—A reproducible increase in the amplitude associated with an increase in the area of successive electrical responses (M waves) during *repetitive nerve stimulation.*

2. *Postactivation* or *post-tetanic facilitation*—Nerve stimulation studies performed within a few seconds after a brief period (2 to 15 sec) of nerve stimulation producing *tetanus* or after a strong voluntary contraction may show changes in the configuration of the M wave(s) compared to the results of identical studies of the rested neuromuscular junction as follows:

   a. *Repair of the decrement*—A diminution of the decrementing response seen with slow rates (2 to 5 Hz) of *repetitive nerve stimulation.*

   b. *Increment after exercise*—An increase in the amplitude associated with an increase in the area of the M wave elicited by a single supramaximal stimulus.

Facilitation should be distinguished from *pseudofacilitation. Pseudofacilitation* occurs in normal subjects with *repetitive nerve stimulation* at high (20 to 50 Hz) rates or after strong volitional contraction, and probably reflects a reduction in the temporal dispersion of the summation of a constant number of muscle fiber action potentials. *Pseudofacilitation* produces a response characterized by an increase in the amplitude of the successive M waves with a corresponding decrease in the duration of the M wave resulting in no change in the area of the negative phase of the successive M waves.

Far-field potential Electrical activity of biological origin generated at a considerable distance from the recording electrodes. Use of the terms *near-field potential* and *far-field potential* is discouraged because all potentials in clinical neurophysiology are recorded at some distance from the generator and there is no consistent distinction between the two terms.

Fasciculation The random, spontaneous twitching of a group of muscle fibers or a motor unit. This twitch may produce movement of the overlying skin (limb), mucous membrane (tongue), or digits. The electrical activity associated with the spontaneous contraction is called the *fasciculation potential*. See also *myokymia* and *fasciculation contraction*. Historically the term *fibrillation* has been used to describe fine twitching of muscle fibers visible through the skin or mucous membrane, but this usage is no longer acceptable.

Fasciculation potential The electrical potential often associated with a visible *fasciculation* which has the configuration of a *motor unit action potential* but which occurs spontaneously. Most commonly these potentials occur sporadically and are termed ''single fasciculation potentials.'' Occasionally, the potentials occur as a grouped discharge and are termed a ''brief repetitive discharge.'' The occurrence of repetitive firing of adjacent fasciculation potentials, when numerous, may produce an undulating movement of muscle (see *myokymia*). Use of the terms *benign fasciculation* and *malignant fasciculation* is discouraged. Instead, the configuration of the

potentials, peak-to-peak amplitude, duration, number of phases, and stability of configuration, in addition to frequency of occurrence, should be specified.

Fatigue Generally, a state of depressed responsiveness resulting from protracted activity and requiring an appreciable recovery time. Muscle fatigue is a reduction in the force of contraction of muscle fibers and follows repeated voluntary contraction or direct electrical stimulation of the muscle.

Fiber density (1) Anatomically, fiber density is a measure of the number of muscle or nerve fibers per unit area. (2) In *single fiber electromyography*, the fiber density is the mean number of *muscle fiber action potentials* fulfilling amplitude and rise time criteria and belonging to one motor unit within the recording area of the *single fiber needle electrode* encountered during a systematic search in the weakly, voluntarily condtracted muscle. See *single fiber electromyography, single fiber needle electrode*.

Fibrillation The spontaneous contractions of individual muscle fibers which are not visible through the skin. This term has been used loosely in electromyography for the preferred term, *fibrillation potential*.

Fibrillation potential The electrical activity associated with a spontaneously contracting (fibrillating) muscle fiber. It is the action potential of a single muscle fiber. The action potentials may occur spontaneously or after movement of the needle electrode. The potentials usually fire at a constant rate, although a small proportion fire irregularly. Classically, the potentials are biphasic spikes of short duration (usually less than 5 msec) with an initial positive phase and a peak-to-peak amplitude of less than 1 mV. When recorded with concentric or monopolar needle electrode, the firing rate has a wide range (1 to 50 Hz) and often decreases just before cessation of an individual discharge. A high-pitched regular sound is associated with the discharge of fibrillation potentials and has been described in the old literature as "rain on a tin roof." In addition to this classic form of fibrillation potentials, *positive sharp waves* may also be recorded from fibrillating muscle fibers.

Firing pattern Qualitative and quantitative descriptions of the sequence of discharge of potential waveforms recorded from muscle or nerve.

Firing rate Frequency of repetition of a potential. The relationship of the frequency to the occurrence of other potentials and the force of muscle contraction may be described. See *discharge frequency*.

Frequency Number of complete cycles of a repetitive waveform in one second. Measured in *hertz* (Hz) or *cycles per second* (cps or c/sec).

Frequency analysis Determination of the range of frequencies composing a potential waveform, with a measurement of the absolute or relative amplitude of each component frequency.

Full interference pattern See *interference pattern*.

Functional refractory period See *refractory period*.

G1, G2 Synonymous with grid 1, grid 2. See *recording electrodes*.

"Giant" motor unit action potential Use of term is discouraged. It refers to a *motor unit action potential* with a peak-to-peak amplitude and duration much greater than the range recorded in corresponding muscles in normal subjects of sim-

ilar age. Quantitative measurements of amplitude and duration are preferable.

Ground electrode An electrode connected to the patient and to a large conducting body (such as the earth) used as a common return for an electrical circuit and as an arbitrary zero potential reference point.

Grouped discharge The term has been used historically to describe three phenomena: (1) irregular, voluntary grouping of *motor unit action potentials* as seen in a tremulous muscular contraction, (2) involuntary grouping of *motor unit action potentials* as seen in *myokymia*, (3) as a general term to describe repeated firing of *motor unit action potentials* (see preferred term *repetitive discharge*).

H reflex Abbreviation for Hoffmann reflex. See *H wave*.

H response Synonymous with *H wave*.

H wave A compound muscle action potential having a consistent latency evoked regularly, when present, from a muscle by an electrical stimulus to the nerve. It is regularly found only in a limited group of physiologic extensors, particularly the calf muscles. The reflex is most easily obtained with the cathode positioned proximal to the anode. Compared with the maximum amplitude *M wave* of the same muscle, the H wave has a smaller amplitude, a longer latency, and a lower optimal stimulus intensity; its configuration is constant. The latency is longer with more distal sites of stimulation. A stimulus intensity sufficient to elicit a maximal amplitude M wave reduces or abolishes the H wave. The H wave is thought to be due to a spinal reflex—the Hoffmann reflex—with electrical stimulation of afferent fibers in the mixed nerve to the muscle and activation of motor neurons to the muscle through a monosynaptic connection in the spinal cord. The reflex and wave are named in honor of Hoffmann's description (1918). Compare the *F wave*.

Habituation Decrease in size of a reflex motor response to an afferent stimulus when the latter is repeated, especially at regular and recurring short intervals.

Hertz (Abbr. Hz). Unit of frequency equal to *cycles per second*.

Hoffmann reflex See *H wave*.

Hyperpolarization See *polarization*.

Increased insertion activity See *insertion activity*.

Increment after exercise See *facilitation*.

Incremental response See preferred term *incrementing response*.

Incrementing response A reproducible increase in amplitude and/or area of successive responses (M wave) to *repetitive nerve stimulation*. The rate of stimulation and the number of stimuli should be specified. An incrementing response is commonly seen in two situations. First, in normal subjects the configuration of the M wave may change with repetitive nerve stimulation so that the amplitude progressively increases as the duration decreases, but the area of the M wave remains the same. This phenomenon is termed *pseudofacilitation*. Second, in disorders of neuromuscular transmission, the configuration of the M wave may change with repetitive nerve stimulation so that the amplitude progressively increases as the duration remains the same or increases, and the area of the M wave increases. This phenomenon is termed *facilitation*. Contrast with *decrementing response*.

Indifferent electrode Synonymous with *reference electrode*. Use of term is discouraged. See *recording electrode*.

Inhibitory postsynaptic potential (Abbr. IPSP). A local graded hyperpolarization of a neuron in response to activation at a synapse by a nerve terminal. Contrast with *excitatory postsynaptic potential*.

Injury potential The potential difference between a normal region of the surface of a nerve or muscle and a region that has been injured; also called a demarcation potential. The injury potential approximates the potential across the membrane because the injured surface is almost at the potential of the inside of the cell.

Input terminal 1 The input terminal of the differential amplifier at which negativity, relative to the other input terminal, produces an upward deflection on the graphic display.

Input terminal 2 The input terminal of the differential amplifier at which negativity, relative to the other input terminal, produces a downward deflection on the graphic display.

Insertion activity Electrical activity caused by insertion or movement of a needle electrode. The amount of the activity may be described as normal, reduced, increased (prolonged), with a description of the waveform and repetitive rate.

Interdischarge interval Time between consecutive discharges of the same potential. Measurements should be made between the corresponding points on each waveform.

Interference Unwanted electrical activity arising outside the system being studied.

Interference pattern Electrical activity

recorded from a muscle with a needle electrode during maximal voluntary effort. A *full interference pattern* implies that no individual *motor unit action potentials* (MUAPs) can be clearly identified. A *reduced interference pattern (intermediate pattern)* is one in which some of the individual MUAPs may be identified while other individual MUAPs cannot be identified because of overlapping. The term *discrete activity* is used to describe the electrical activity recorded when each of several different MUAPs can be identified. The term *single unit pattern* is used to describe a single MUAP, firing at rapid rate (should be specified) during maximum voluntary effort. The force of contraction associated with the interference pattern should be specified. See also *recruitment pattern*.

Intermediate interference pattern   See *interference pattern*.

International 10-20 system   A system of electrode placement on the scalp in which electrodes are placed either 10 percent or 20 percent of the total distance between the nasion and inion in the sagittal plane, and between right and left preauricular points in the coronal plane.

Interpeak interval   Difference between the peak latencies of two components of a waveform.

Interpotential interval   Time between two different potentials. Measurement should be made between the corresponding parts of each waveform.

Involuntary activity   *Motor unit potentials* that are not under voluntary control. The condition under which they occur should be described, e.g., spontaneous or reflex potentials, or, if elicited by a stimulus, the nature of the stimulus. Contrast with *spontaneous activity*.

Irregular potential   See preferred term *serrated potential*.

Iterative discharge   See preferred term *repetitive discharge*.

Jitter   Synonymous with single fiber electromyographic jitter. Jitter is the variability with consecutive discharges of the *interpotential interval* between two muscle fiber action potentials belonging to the same motor unit. It is usually expressed quantitatively as the mean value of the difference between the interpotential intervals of successive discharges (the mean consecutive difference, abbr. MCD). Under certain conditions, jitter is expressed as the mean value of the difference between interpotential intervals arranged in the order of decreasing interdischarge intervals (the mean sorted difference, abbr. MSD).

Jolly test   A technique described by Jolly (1895), who applied an electric current to excite a motor nerve while recording the force of muscle contraction. Harvey and Masland (1941) refined the technique by recording the M wave evoked by repetitive, supramaximal nerve stimulation to detect a defect of neuromuscular transmission. Use of the term is discouraged. See preferred term *repetitive nerve stimulation*.

Late component (of a motor unit action potential)   See synonymous term *satellite potential*. Also called *parasite potential*, *linked potential*, and *coupled discharge*.

Late response   A general term used to describe an evoked potential having a longer latency than the *M wave*. See *A wave*, *F wave*, *H wave*, *T wave*.

Latency   Interval between the onset of a stimulus and the onset of a response. Thus the term *onset latency* is a tautology and should not be used. The *peak latency* is the interval between the onset of a stimulus and a specific peak of the evoked potential.

Latency of activation   The time required for an electrical stimulus to depolarize a nerve fiber (or bundle of fibers as in a nerve trunk) beyond threshold and to initiate a regenerative action potential in the fiber(s). This time is usually of the order of 0.1 msec or less. An equivalent term now rarely used in the literature is the *utilization time*.

Latent period   See synonym *latency*.

Linked potential   See preferred term *satellite potential*.

Long latency SEP   That portion of a *somatosensory evoked potential* normally occurring at a time greater than 100 msec after stimulation of a nerve in the upper extremity at the wrist, or the lower extremity at the knee or ankle.

M response   See synonym *M wave*.

M wave   A *compound action potential* evoked from a muscle by a single electrical stimulus to its motor nerve. By convention, the M wave elicited by supramaximal stimulation is used for motor nerve conduction studies. Ideally, the recording electrodes should be placed so that the initial deflection of the evoked potential is negative. The *latency*, commonly called the *motor latency*, is the latency (msec) to the onset of the first phase (positive or negative) of the M wave. The amplitude (mV) is the baseline-to-peak amplitude of the first negative phase, unless otherwise specified. The *duration* (msec) refers to the duration of the first negative phase, unless otherwise specified. Normally, the configuration of the M wave (usually biphasic) is quite stable with repeated stimuli at slow rates (1 to 5 Hz). See *repetitive nerve stimulation*.

Macro motor unit action potential   (Abbr. macro MUAP). The average electrical activity of that part of an anatomical motor unit that is within the recording range of a *macro EMG electrode*. The potential is characterized by its consistent appearance when the small recording surface of the macro EMG electrode is positioned to record action potentials from one muscle fiber. The following parameters can be specified quantitatively: (1) maximal peak-to-peak amplitude, (2) area contained under the waveform, (3) number of phases.

Macro MUAP   See *macro motor unit action potential*.

Macroelectromyography   (Abbr. Macro EMG). General term referring to the technique and conditions that approximate recording of all *muscle fiber action potentials* arising from the same motor unit.

Macro EMG   See *macroelectromyography*.

Macro EMG needle electrode   A modified *single fiber electromyography* electrode insulated to within 15 mm from the tip and with a small recording surface (25 μm in diameter) 7.5 mm from the tip.

Malignant fasciculation   Use of term to describe a firing pattern of fasciculation potentials is discouraged. Historically, the term was used to describe large, polyphasic fasciculation potentials firing at a slow rate. This pattern has been seen in progressive motor neuron disease, but the relationship is not exclusive. See *fasciculation potential*.

Maximal stimulus   See *stimulus*.

Maximum nerve conduction velocity   See *conduction velocity*.

MCD   See *jitter*.

Median nerve—short latency SEP (Abbr. MN-SSEP). *Short-latency somatosensory evoked potentials* elicited by electrical stimulation of the median nerve at the wrist occur within 25 msec of the stimulus in normal subjects. Normal short-latency response components to median nerve stimulation are designated $P\overline{9}$, $P\overline{11}$, $P\overline{13}$, $P\overline{14}$, $N\overline{20}$, and $P\overline{23}$ in records taken between scalp and noncephalic reference electrodes, and $N\overline{9}$, $N\overline{11}$, $N\overline{13}$, and $N\overline{14}$ in cervical spine-scalp derivation. It should be emphasized that potentials having opposite polarity but similar latency in spine-scalp and scalp-noncephalic reference derivations do not necessarily have identical generator sources.

Membrane instability Tendency of a cell membrane to depolarize spontaneously upon mechanical irritation or after voluntary activation.

Microneurography The technique of recording peripheral nerve action potentials in man by means of intraneural microelectrodes.

Mid-latency SEP That portion of the waveforms of a *somatosensory evoked potential* normally occurring within 25 to 100 msec after stimulation of a nerve in the upper extremity at the wrist, within 40 to 100 msec after stimulation of a nerve in the lower extremity at the knee, and within 50 to 100 msec after stimulation of a nerve in the lower extremity at the ankle.

Miniature end-plate potential The postsynaptic muscle fiber potentials produced through the spontaneous release of individual quanta of acetylcholine from the presynaptic axon terminals. As recorded with conventional concentric needle electrodes inserted in the end-plate zone, such potentials are characteristically monophasic, negative, of relatively short dura-

tion (less than 5 msec) and generally less than 20 μV in amplitude.

Monophasic action potential An *action potential* with one phase.

Monopolar needle electrode A solid wire, usually stainless steel, usually coated, except at its tip, with an insulating material. Variations in voltage between the tip of the needle (active or exploring electrode) positioned in a muscle and a conductive plate on the skin surface or a bare needle in subcutaneous tissue (reference electrode) are measured. By convention, this recording condition is referred to as a monopolar needle electrode recording. It should be emphasized, however, that potential differences are always recorded between two electrodes.

Motor latency Interval between the onset of a stimulus and the onset of the resultant *compound muscle action potential (M wave)*. The term may be qualified as *proximal motor latency* or *distal motor latency*, depending on the relative position of the stimulus.

Motor nerve conduction velocity (Abbr. MNCV). See *conduction velocity*.

Motor point The point over a muscle where a contraction of a muscle may be elicited by a minimal-intensity, short-duration electrical stimulus. The motor point corresponds anatomically to the location of the terminal portion of the motor nerve fibers (end-plate zone).

Motor response (1) The compound muscle action potential (*M wave*) recorded over a muscle with stimulation of the nerve to the muscle, (2) the muscle twitch or contraction elicited by stimulation of the nerve to a muscle, (3) the muscle twitch elicited by the muscle stretch reflex.

Motor unit   The anatomical unit of an anterior horn cell, its axon, the neuromuscular junctions, and all of the muscle fibers innervated by the axon.

Motor unit action potential   (Abbr. MUAP). Action potential reflecting the electrical activity of a single anatomical motor unit. It is the compound action potential of those muscle fibers within the recording range of an electrode. With voluntary muscle contraction, the action potential is characterized by its consistent appearance with, and relationship to, the force of contraction. The following parameters should be specified, quantitatively if possible, after the recording electrode is placed so as to minimize the *rise time* (which by convention should be less than 0.5 msec):
  I.   Configuration
      A.   *Amplitude*, peak-to-peak (μV or mV)
      B.   *Duration*, total (msec)
      C.   Number of *phases (monophasic, biphasic, triphasic, tetraphasic, polyphasic)*
      D.   Sign of each *phase* (negative, positive)
      E.   Number of *turns*.
      F.   Variation of shape, if any, with consecutive discharges
      G.   Presence of *satellite (linked) potentials*, if any
  II.   *Recruitment* characteristics
      A.   Threshold of activation (first recruited, low threshold, high threshold)
      B.   *Onset frequency* (Hz)
      C.   *Recruitment frequency* (Hz) or *Recruitment interval* (msec) of individual potentials
Descriptive terms imply diagnostic significance are not recommended, e.g., *myopathic, neuropathic, regeneration, nascent, giant, BSAP,* and *BSAPP.*

Motor unit fraction   See *scanning EMG.*

Motor unit potential   (Abbr. MUP). See synonym *motor unit action potential.*

Motor unit territory   The area in a muscle over which the muscle fibers belonging to an individual motor unit are distributed.

Movement artifact   See *artifact.*

MSD   See *jitter.*

MUAP   Abbreviation for *motor unit action potential.*

Multielectrode   See *multilead electrode.*

Multilead electrode   Three or more insulated wires inserted through a common metal cannula with their bared tips at an aperture in the cannula and flush with the outer circumference of the cannula. The arrangement of the bare tips relative to the axis of the cannula and the distance between each tip should be specified.

Multiple discharge   Four or more *motor unit action potentials* of the same form and nearly the same amplitude occurring consistently in the same relationship to one another and generated by this same axon or muscle fiber. See *double* and *triple discharge.*

Multiplet   See *multiple discharge.*

MUP   Abbreviation for *motor unit potential*. See synonym *motor unit action potential.*

Muscle action potential   Term commonly used to refer to a *compound muscle action potential.*

Muscle cramp   Most commonly, an involuntary, painful muscle *contraction* associated with electrical activity (See *cramp discharge*). Muscle cramps may be accompanied by other types of *repetitive dis-*

charges, and in some metabolic myopathies (McArdle's disease), the painful, contracted muscle may show *electrical silence*.

Muscle fiber action potential Action potential recorded from a single muscle fiber.

Muscle fiber conduction velocity The speec of propagation of a single *muscle fiber action potential*, usually expressed as meters per second. The muscle fiber conduction velocity is usually less than most nerve conduction velocities, varies with the rate of discharge of the muscle fiber, and requires special techniques for measurement.

Muscle stretch reflex Activation of a muscle which follows stretch of the muscle, e.g., by percussion of a muscle tendon.

Myoedema Focal muscle contraction produced by muscle percussion and not associated with propagated electrical activity; may be seen in hypothyroidism (myxedema) and chronic malnutrition.

Myokymia Continuous quivering or undulating movement of surface and overlying skin and mucous membrane associated with spontaneous, repetitive discharge of *motor unit potentials*. See *myokymic discharges, fasciculation,* and *fasciculation potential*.

Myokymic discharge *Motor unit action potentials* that fire repetitively and may be associated with clinical myokymia. Two firing patterns have been described. Commonly, the discharge is a brief, repetitive firing of single units for a short period (up to a few seconds) at a uniform rate (2 to 60 Hz) followed by a short period (up to a few seconds) of silence, with repetition of the same sequence for a particular potential. Less commonly, the potential recurs continuously at a fairly uniform firing rate (1 to 5 Hz). Myokymic discharges are a subclass

of *grouped discharges* and *repetitive discharges*.

Myopathic motor unit potential Use of term is discouraged. It was used to refer to low-amplitude, short-duration, polyphasic *motor unit action potentials*. The term incorrectly implies specific diagnostic significance of a motor unit potential configuration. See *motor unit action potential*.

Myopathic recruitment Use of term is discouraged. It is used to describe an increase in the number of and firing rate of *motor unit action potentials* compared with normal for the strength of muscle contraction.

Myotonia The clinical observation of delayed relaxation of muscle after voluntary contraction or percussion. The delayed relaxation may be electrically silent, or accompanied by propagated electrical activity such as *myotonic discharge, complex repetitive discharge,* or *neuromyotonic discharge*.

Myotonic discharge Repetitive discharge at rates of 20 to 80 Hz are of two types: (1) biphasic (positive-negative) spike potentials less than 5 msec in duration resembling *fibrillation potentials*, and (2) positive waves 5 to 20 msec in duration resembling *positive sharp waves*. Both potential forms are recorded after needle insertion, after voluntary muscle contraction, or after muscle percussion, and are due to independent, repetitive discharges of single muscle fibers. The amplitude and frequency of the potentials must both wax and wane to be identified as myotonic discharges. This change produces a characteristic musical sound in the audio display of the electromyograph due to the corresponding change in pitch, which has been likened to the sound of a ''dive bomber.'' Contrast with *waning discharge*.

Myotonic potential See preferred term *myotonic discharge*.

Nascent motor unit potential From the Latin *nascens*, to be born. Use of term is discouraged as it incorrectly implies diagnostic significance of a motor unit potential configuration. Term has been used to refer to very low-amplitude, long-duration, highly polyphasic motor unit potentials observed during early states of reinnervation of muscle. See *motor unit action potential*.

Near constant frequency trains See *complex repetitive discharge*.

Near-field potential Electrical activity of biological origin generated near the recording electrodes. Use of the terms *near-field potential* and *far-field potential* is discouraged because all potentials in clinical neurophysiology are recorded at some distance from the generator and there is no consistent distinction between the two terms.

Needle electrode An electrode for recording or stimulating, shaped like a needle. See specific electrodes: *bipolar needle electrode, concentric needle electrode, monopolar needle electrode, single fiber needle electrode, macro needle electrode, multilead electrode*.

Nerve action potential Strictly defined, refers to an action potential recorded from a single nerve fiber. The term is commonly used to refer to the compound nerve action potential. See *compound nerve action potential*.

Nerve conduction studies Recording and analysis of electrical *waveforms* of biological origin elicited in response to electrical or physiological *stimuli*. Generally *nerve conduction studies* refers to studies of waveforms generated in the peripheral nervous system, whereas *evoked potential studies* refers to studies of waveforms generated in both the peripheral and central nervous system. The waveforms recorded in *nerve conduction studies* are *compound sensory nerve action potentials* and *compound muscle action potentials*. The *compound sensory nerve action potentials* are generally referred to as *sensory nerve action potentials*. The *compound muscle action potentials* are generally referred to by letters which have historical origins: *M wave, F wave, H wave, T wave, A wave, R1 wave,* and *R2 wave*. It is possible under standardized conditions to establish normal ranges of amplitude, duration, and latencies of these *evoked potentials* and to calculate the *maximum condition velocity* of sensory and motor nerves.

Nerve conduction velocity (Abbr. NCV). Loosely used to refer to the maximum nerve conduction velocity. See *conduction velocity*.

Nerve fiber action potential Action potential recorded from a single nerve fiber.

Nerve potential Equivalent to *nerve action potential*. Also commonly, but inaccurately, used to refer to the biphasic form of *end-plate activity*. The latter use is incorrect because muscle fibers, not nerve fibers, are the source of these potentials.

Nerve trunk action potential See preferred term *compound nerve action potential*.

Neurapraxia Failure of nerve conduction, usually reversible, due to metabolic or microstructural abnormalities without disruption of the axon. See preferred electrodiagnostic term *conduction block*.

Neuromyotonia Clinical syndrome of continuous muscle fiber activity manifested as continuous muscle rippling and stiffness. The accompanying electrical activity may be intermittent or continuous. Terms used to describe related clinical syndromes are continuous muscle fiber activity, Isaac syndrome, Isaac-Merton syndrome, quantal squander syndrome, generalized myokymia, pseudomyotonia, normocalcemic tetany, and neurotonia.

Neuromyotonic discharge Bursts of *motor unit action potentials* which originate in the motor axons firing at high rates (150 to 300 Hz) for a few seconds, and which often start and stop abruptly. The amplitude of the response typically wanes. Discharges may occur spontaneously or be initiated by needle movement, voluntary effort and ischemia or percussion of a nerve. These discharges should be distinguished from *myotonic discharges* and *complex repetitive discharges*.

Neuropathic motor unit potential Use of term is discouraged. It was used to refer to abnormally high-amplitude, long-duration, polyphasic *motor unit action potentials*. The term incorrectly implies a specific diagnostic significance of a motor unit potential configuration. See *motor unit action potential*.

Neuropathic recruitment Use of term is discouraged. It has been used to describe a recruitment pattern with a decreased number of *motor unit action potentials* firing at a rapid rate. See preferred terms *reduced interference pattern, discrete activity, single unit pattern*.

Neurotmesis Partial or complete severence of a nerve, with disruption of the axons, their myelin sheaths, and the supporting connective tissue, resulting in degeneration of the axons distal to the injury site.

Noise Strictly defined, potentials produced by electrodes, cables, amplifier or storage media and unrelated to the potentials of biological origin. The term has been used loosely to refer to one form of *endplate activity*.

Onset frequency The lowest stable frequency of firing for a single *motor unit action potential* that can be voluntarily maintained by a subject.

Order of activation The sequence of appearance of different *motor unit action potentials* with increasing strength of voluntary contraction. See *recruitment*.

Orthodromic Propagation of an impulse in the direction the same as physiologic conduction; e.g., conduction along motor nerve fibers towards the muscle and conduction along sensory nerve fibers towards the spinal cord. Contrast with *antidromic*.

Paired stimuli Two consecutive stimuli. The time interval between the two stimuli and the intensity of each stimulus should be specified. The first stimulus is called the *conditioning stimulus* and the second stimulus is the *test stimulus*. The conditioning stimulus may modify the tissue excitability, which can then be evaluated by the response to the *test stimulus*.

Parasite potential See preferred term *satellite potential*.

Peak latency Interval between the onset of a stimulus and a specified peak of the evoked potential.

Phase That portion of a *wave* between the departure from, and the return to, the *baseline*.

Polarization As used in neurophysiology, the presence of an electrical potential difference across an excitable cell membrane. The potential across the membrane of a cell when it is not excited by an input or spontaneously active is termed the *rest-*

ing potential; it is at a stationary nonequilibrium state with regard to the electrical potential difference across the membrane. *Depolarization* describes a reduction in the magnitude of the polarization toward the zero potential while *hyperpolarization* refers to an increase in the magnitude of the polarization relative to the resting potential. *Repolarization* describes an increase in polarization from the depolarized state toward, but not above, the normal resting potential.

Polyphasic action potential An *action potential* having five or more phases. See *phase*. Contrast with *serrated action potential*.

Positive sharp wave A biphasic, positive-negative *action potential* initiated by needle movement and recurring in a uniform, regular pattern at a rate of 1 to 50 Hz; the discharge frequency may decrease slightly just before cessation of discharge. The initial positive deflection is rapid (<1 msec), its duration is usually less than 5 msec, and the amplitude is up to 1 mV. The negative phase is of low amplitude, with a duration of 10 to 100 msec. A sequence of positive sharp waves is commonly referred to as a *train of positive sharp waves*. Positive sharp waves can be recorded from the damaged area of fibrillating muscle fibers. Its configuration may result from the position of the needle electrode which is felt to be adjacent to the depolarized segment of a muscle fiber injured by the electrode. Note that the positive sharp waveform is not specific for muscle fiber damage. *Motor unit action potentials* and potentials in *myotonic discharges* may have the configuration of positive sharp waves.

Positive wave Loosely defined, the term refers to a positive sharp wave. See *positive sharp wave*.

Postactivation depression A descrip-

tive term indicating a reduction in the amplitude associated with a reduction in the area of the M wave(s) in response to a single *stimulus* or *train of stimuli* which occurs a few minutes after a brief (10 to 30 sec), strong voluntary contraction or a period of *repetitive nerve stimulation* that produces *tetanus*. *Postactivation exhaustion* refers to the cellular mechanisms responsible for the observed phenomenon of *postactivation depression*.

Postactivation exhaustion A reduction in the safety factor (margin) of neuromuscular transmission after sustained activity of the neuromuscular junction. The changes in the configuration of the M wave due to *postactivation exhaustion* are referred to as *postactivation depression*.

Postactivation facilitation See *facilitation*.

Postactivation potentiation Refers to the increase in the force of contraction (mechanical response) after *tetanus* or strong voluntary contraction. Contrast *postactivation facilitation*.

Posterior tibial nerve—short latency SEP (Abbr. PTN-SSEP). *Short latency somatosensory evoked potentials* elicited by electrical stimulation of the posterior tibial nerve at the knee occur within 50 msec of the stimulus in normal subjects. It is recommended that individual response components be designated as follows: (1) nerve trunk (tibial nerve) component in the popliteal fossa: PF potential; (2) spine components: L3 and T12 potentials; (3) scalp components: $P\overline{37}$ and $N\overline{45}$ waves.

Post-tetanic facilitation See *facilitation*.

Post-tetanic potentiation The incrementing mechanical response of muscle during and after *repetitive nerve stimulation* without a change in the amplitude of the action potential. In spinal cord physiology, the term has been used to describe enhancement of excitability or reflex outflow of the central nervous system following a long period of high-frequency stimulation. This phenomenon has been described in the mammalian spinal cord, where it lasts minutes or even hours.

Potential A physical variable created by differences in charges, measurable in volts, that exists between two points. Most biologically produced potentials arise from the difference in charge between two sides of a cell membrane.

Potentiation Physiologically, the enhancement of a response. Some authors use the term *potentiation* to describe the incrementing mechanical response of muscle elicited by *repetitive nerve stimulation*, i.e., *post-tetanic potentiation*, and the term *facilitation* to describe the incrementing electrical response elicited by *repetitive nerve stimulation*, i.e., *postactivation facilitation*.

Prolonged insertion activity See *insertion activity*.

Propagation velocity of a muscle fiber The speed of transmission of a muscle fiber action potential.

Proximal latency See *motor latency* or *sensory latency*.

Pseudofacilitation See *facilitation*.

Pseudomyotonic discharge Use of term is discouraged. It has been used to refer to different phenomena, including (1) *complex repetitive discharges* and (2) *repetitive discharges* that do not wax or wane in both frequency and amplitude, and end abruptly. These latter discharges may be seen in disorders such as polymyositis in addition to disorders with *myotonic discharges*. See preferred term *waning discharge*.

R1, R2 waves See *blink responses*.

Recording electrode Device used to record electrical potential difference. All electrical recordings require two *electrodes*. The electrode close to the source of the activity to be recorded is called the *active* or *exploring electrode*, and the other electrode is called the *reference electrode*. *Active electrode* is synonymous with *input terminal 1, grid 1,* and *G1*, and reference *electrode* with *input terminal 2, grid 2,* and *G2*.

In some recordings, it is not certain which electrode is closer to the source of the biological activity, i.e., recording with a *bifilar (bipolar) needle electrode*. In this situation, it is convenient to refer to one electrode as *input electrode 1* and the other electrode as *input electrode 2*.

By present convention, a potential difference that is negative at the active electrode (*input terminal 2*) relative to the reference electrode (*input terminal 1*) causes an upward deflection on the oscilloscope screen. The term "monopolar recording" is not recommended, because all recording requires two electrodes; however, it is commonly used to describe the use of an intramuscular needle exploring electrode in combination with a surface disc or subcutaneous needle reference electrode. A similar combination of needle electrodes has been used to record nerve activity and also has been referred to as "monopolar recording."

Recruitment The successive activation of the same and additional motor units with increasing strength of voluntary muscle contraction. See *motor unit potential*.

Recruitment frequency Firing rate of a *motor unit action potential (MUAP)* when a different MUAP first appears with gradually increasing strength of voluntary muscle contraction. This parameter is essential to assessment of *recruitment pattern.*

Recruitment interval The *interdischarge interval* between two consecutive discharges of a *motor unit action potential (MUAP)* when a different MUAP first appears with gradually increasing strength of voluntary muscle contraction. The reciprocal of the recruitment interval is the *recruitment frequency.*

Recruitment pattern A qualitative and/or quantitative description of the sequence of appearance of *motor unit potentials* with increasing strength of voluntary muscle contraction. The *recruitment frequency* and *recruitment interval* are two quantitative measures commonly used. See *interference pattern* for qualitative terms commonly used.

Reduced insertion activity See *insertion activity.*

Reduced interference pattern See *interference pattern.*

Reference electrode See *recording electrode.*

Reflex A stereotyped *motor response* elicited by a sensory *stimulus.*

Refractory period The *absolute refractory period* is the period following an *action potential* during which no stimulus, however strong, evokes a further response. The *relative refractory period* is the period following an *action potential* during which a stimulus must be abnormally large to evoke a second response. The *functional refractory period* is the period following an *action potential* during which a second *action potential* cannot yet excite the given region.

Relative refractory period See *refractory period.*

Repair of the decrement See *facilitation.*

Repetitive discharge General term for the recurrence of an *action potential* with the same or nearly the same form. The term may refer to recurring potentials recorded in muscle at rest, during voluntary contraction, or in response to single nerve stimulus. See *double discharge, triple discharge, multiple discharge, myokymic discharge, myotonic discharge, complex repetitive discharge.*

Repetitive nerve stimulation The technique of repeated supramaximal stimulations of a nerve while recording M waves from muscles innervated by the nerve. The number of stimuli and the frequency of stimulation should be specified. Activation procedures performed prior to the test should be specified, e.g., sustained voluntary contraction or contraction induced by nerve stimulation. If the test was performed after an activation procedure, the time elapsed after the activation procedure was completed should also be specified. The technique is commonly used to assess the integrity of neuromuscular transmission. For a description of specific patterns of responses, see the terms *incrementing response, decrementing response, facilitation,* and *postactivation depression.*

Repolarization See *polarization.*

Residual latency Refers to the calculated time difference between the measured distal latency of a motor nerve and the expected distal latency, calculated by dividing the distance between the stimulus cathode and the active recording electrode by the maximum conduction velocity measured in a more proximal segment of a nerve. The residual latency is due in part to neuromuscular transmission time and to slowing of conduction in terminal axons due to decreasing diameter and the presence of unmyelinated segments.

Response Used to describe an activity elicited by a *stimulus*.

Resting membrane potential Voltage across the membrane of an excitable cell at rest. See *polarization*.

Rheobase See *strength-duration curve.*

Rise time The interval from the onset of a change of potential to its peak. The method of measurement should be specified.

Satellite potential A small action potential separated from the main MUAP by an isoelectric interval and firing in a time-locked relationship to the main action potential. These potentials usually follow, but may precede, the main action potential. Also called *late component, parasite potential, linked potential,* and *coupled discharge.*

Scanning EMG A technique by which an electromyographic electrode is advanced in defined steps through muscle while a separate SFEMG electrode is used to trigger both the oscilloscope-sweep and the advancement device. This recording technique provides temporal and spatial information about the motor unit. Distinct maxima in the recorded activity are considered to be generated by muscle fibers innervated by a common branch of the axon. These groups of fibers form a *motor unit fraction.*

Sea shell sound (sea shell roar or noise) Use of term is discouraged. See *end-plate activity, monophasic.*

Sensory delay See preferred terms *sensory latency* and *sensory peak latency.*

Sensory latency Interval between the onset of a stimulus and the onset of the *compound sensory nerve action potential.* This term has been loosely used to refer to the *sensory peak latency.* The term may be qualified as *proximal sensory latency* or *distal sensory latency,* depending on the relative position of the stimulus. ‐

Sensory nerve action potential See *compound sensory nerve action potential.*

Sensory nerve conduction velocity See *conduction velocity.*

Sensory peak latency Interval between the onset of a *stimulus* and the peak of the negative phase of the *compound sensory nerve action potential.* Note that the term *latency* refers to the interval between the onset of a stimulus and the onset of a response.

Sensory potential Used to refer to the compound sensory nerve action potential. See *compound sensory nerve action potential.*

Sensory response Used to refer to a sensory evoked potential, e.g., *compound sensory nerve action potential.*

SEP See *somatosensory evoked potential.*

Serrated action potential An action potential waveform with several changes in direction (turns) which do not cross the baseline. This term is preferred to the terms *complex action potential* and *pseudopolyphasic action potential.* See *Turn.*

SFEMG See *single fiber electromyography.*

Shock artifact See *artifact.*

Short latency SEP That portion of the waveforms of a *somatosensory evoked potential* normally occurring within 25 msec after stimulation of a nerve in the upper extremity at the wrist, 40 msec after stimulation of a nerve in the lower extremity at the knee, and 50 msec after stimulation of a nerve in the lower extremity at the ankle.

Silent period A pause in the electrical activity of a muscle such as that seen after rapid unloading of a muscle.

Single fiber electromyography (Abbr. SFEMG). General term referring to the technique and conditions that permit recording of a single *muscle fiber action potential*. See *single fiber needle electrode*.

Single fiber EMG See *single fiber electromyography*.

Single fiber needle electrode A needle *electrode* with a small recording surface (usually 25 μm in diameter) permitting the recording of single muscle fiber action potentials between the active recording surface and the cannula. See *single fiber electromyography*.

Single unit pattern See *interference pattern*.

Somatosensory evoked potential (Abbr. SEP). Electrical waveforms of biological origin elicited by electrical stimulation or physiological activation of peripheral sensory fibers. The normal SEP is a complex waveform with several components which are specified by polarity and average peak latency. The polarity and latency of individual components depends upon (1) subject variables, such as age, sex, (2) stimulus characteristics, such as intensity, rate of stimulation, and (3) recording parameters, such as amplifier time constants, electrode placement, electrode combinations. See *median nerve-SEP, common peroneal nerve-SEP*, and *posterior tibial nerve-SEP*.

Spike (1) In cellular neurophysiology, a short-lived (usually in the range of 1–3 msec), all-or-none change in membrane potential that arises when a graded response passes a threshold. (2) The electrical record of a nerve impulse or similar event in muscle or elsewhere. (3) In clinical EEG recordings, a wave with duration less than 80 msec (usually 15 to 80 msec).

Spinal evoked potential Electrical waveforms of biological origin recorded over the sacral, lumbar, thoracic, or cervical spine in response to electrical stimulation or physiological activation of peripheral sensory fibers. See preferred term *somatosensory evoked potential*.

Spontaneous activity Electrical activity recorded from muscle or nerve at rest after insertion activity has subsided and when there is no voluntary contraction or external stimulus. Compare with *involuntary activity*.

Staircase phenomenon The progressive increase in the force of a muscle contraction observed in response to continued low rates of direct or indirect muscle stimulation.

Stigmatic electrode Term of historic interest; used by Sherrington for *active* or *exploring electrode*.

Stimulating electrode Device used to apply electrical current. All electrical stimulation requires two electrodes; the negative terminal is termed the *cathode* and the positive terminal, the *anode*. By convention, the stimulating electrodes are called *bipolar* if they are encased or attached together. Stimulating electrodes are called *monopolar* if they are not encased or attached together. Electrical stimulation for *nerve conduction studies* generally requires application of the cathode to produce depolarization of the nerve trunk fibers. If the anode is inadvertently placed between the cathode and the recording electrodes, a focal block of nerve conduction (*anodal block*) may occur and cause a technically unsatisfactory study.

Stimulus   Any external agent, state, or change that is capable of influencing the activity of a cell, tissue, or organism. In clinical *nerve conduction studies*, an electrical stimulus is generally applied to a nerve or a muscle. The electrical stimulus may be described in absolute terms or with respect to the evoked potential of the nerve or muscle. In absolute terms, the electrical stimulus is defined by a duration (msec), a waveform (square, exponential, linear, etc.) and a strength or intensity measured in voltage (V) or current (mA). With respect to the evoked potential, the stimulus may be graded as subthreshold, threshold, submaximal, maximal, or supramaximal. A *threshold stimulus* is that stimulus just sufficient to produce a detectable response. Stimuli less than the threshold stimulus are termed *subthreshold*. The *maximal stimulus* is the stimulus intensity after which a further increase in the stimulus intensity causes no increase in the amplitude of the evoked potential. Stimuli of intensity below this level but above threshold are *submaximal*. Stimuli of intensity greater than the maximal stimulus are termed *supramaximal*. Ordinarily, supramaximal stimuli are used for nerve conduction studies. By convention, an electrrical stimulus of approximately 20% greater voltage than required for the maximal stimulus may be used for supramaximal stimulation. The frequency, number, and duration of a series of stimuli should be specified.

Stimulus artifact   See *artifact*.

Strength-duration curve   Graphic presentation of the relationship between the intensity (Y axis) and various durations (X axis) of the threshold electrical stimulus for a muscle with the stimulating cathode positioned over the *motor point*. The *rheobase* is the intensity of an electrical current of infinite duration necessary to produce a minimal visible twitch of a muscle when applied to the motor point. In clinical practice, a duration of 300 msec is used to determine the rheobase. The *chronaxie* is the time required for an electrical current twice the *rheobase* to elicit the first visible muscle twitch.

Submaximal stimulus   See *stimulus*.

Subthreshold stimulus   See *stimulus*.

Supramaximal stimulus   See *stimulus*.

Surface electrode   Conducting device for stimulating or recording placed on a skin surface. The material (metal, fabric), configuration (disc, ring), size, and separation should be specified. See *electrode* (*ground, recording, stimulating*).

Synchronized fibrillation   See *complex repetitive discharge*.

T wave   A compound action potential evoked from a muscle by rapid stretch of its tendon, as part of the muscle stretch reflex.

Temporal dispersion   Relative desynchronization of components of a compound action potential due to different rates of conduction of each synchronously evoked component from the stimulation point to the recording electrode.

Terminal latency   Synonymous with preferred term *distal latency*. See *motor latency* and *sensory latency*.

Test stimulus   See *paired stimuli*.

Tetanic contraction The contraction produced in a muscle through repetitive maximal direct or indirect stimulation at a sufficiently high frequency to produce a smooth summation of successive maximum twitches. The term may also be applied to maximum voluntary contractions in which the firing frequencies of most or all of the component motor units are sufficiently high that successive twitches of individual motor units fuse smoothly. Their tensions all combine to produce a steady, smooth maximum contraction of the whole muscle.

Tetanus The continuous contraction of muscle caused by repetitive stimulation or discharge of nerve or muscle. Contrast *tetany*.

Tetany A clinical syndrome manifested by muscle twitching, cramps, and carpal and pedal spasm. These clinical signs are manifestations of peripheral and central nervous system nerve irritability from several causes. In these conditions, *repetitive discharges (double discharge, triple discharge, multiple discharge)* occur frequently with voluntary activation of *motor unit action potentials* or may appear as *spontaneous activity* and are enhanced by systemic alkalosis or local ischemia.

Tetraphasic action potential *Action potential* with four phases.

Threshold The level at which a clear and abrupt transition occurs from one state to another. The term is generally used to refer to the voltage level at which an *action potential* is initiated in a single axon or a group of axons. It is also operationally defined as the intensity that produced a response in about 50 percent of equivalent trials.

Threshold stimulus See *stimulus*.

Train of stimuli A group of stimuli. The duration of the group or the number of stimuli and the frequency of the stimuli should be specified.

Trains of positive sharp waves See *positive sharp waves*.

Triphasic action potential *Action potential* with three phases.

Triple discharge Three *motor unit action potentials* of the same form and nearly the same amplitude, occurring consistently in the same relationship to one another and generated by this same axon or muscle fiber. The interval between the second and the third action potential often exceeds that between the first two, and both are usually in the range of 2 to 20 msec.

Triplet See *triple discharge*.

Turn Point of change in direction in the waveform and the magnitude of the voltage change following the turning point. It is not necessary that the voltage change passes through the baseline. The minimal excursion required to constitute a change should be specified.

Unipolar needle electrode See synonym *monopolar needle electrode*.

Utilization time See *latency of activation*.

Visual evoked potential (Abbr. VEP). Electrical waveforms of biological origin are recorded over the cerebrum and elicited by light stimuli. VEPs are classified by stimulus rate as transient or steady state VEPs, and can be further divided by presentation mode. The normal transient VEP to checkerboard pattern reversal or shift has a major positive occipital peak at about 100 msec ($P\overline{100}$), often preceded by a negative peak ($N\overline{75}$). The precise range of normal values for the latency and amplitude of $P\overline{100}$ depends on several factors: (1) subject variables such as age, sex, and visual acuity; (2) stimulus characteristics such as type of stimulator, full-field or half-field stimulation, check size, contrast, and luminescence; and (3) recording parameters such as placement and combination of recording electrodes.

Visual evoked response (Abbr. VER). See *visual evoked potential*.

Volitional activity See *voluntary activity*.

Voltage Potential difference between two recording sites.

Volume conduction Spread of current from a potential source through a conducting medium, such as the body tissues.

Voluntary activity In electromyography, the electrical activity recorded from a muscle with consciously controlled muscle contraction. The effort made to contract the muscle should be specified relative to that of a corresponding normal muscle, e.g., minimal, moderate, or maximal. If the recording remains isoelectric during the attempted contraction of the muscle and artifacts have been excluded, it can be concluded that there is no voluntary activity.

Waning discharge General term referring to a *repetitive discharge* that gradually decreases in frequency or amplitude before cessation. Contrast with *myotonic discharge*.

Wave An undulating line constituting a graphic representation of a change, e.g., a changing electrical potential difference.

Waveform The shape of a *wave*. The term is often used synonymously with *wave*.

Index

Page numbers followed by *f* represent figures; those followed by *t* represent tables.